So—You've Survived Cancer. Now What?

Theresa Kilpatrick
Alexis Hilliar-Hine

Riversmeet Publishing, LLC

So—You've Survived Cancer.
Now What?

Riversmeet Publishing, LLC
Published by Riversmeet Publishing, LLC
P.O. Box 346, Mason, MI 48854

First Riversmeet Publishing, LLC Edition
Published in 2011 by Riversmeet Publishing, LLC

ISBN: 978-1-4507-7072-9
Library of Congress Control Number: 2007012345

Quote from American Greetings Card #4289880
Reproduced by Permission
American Greetings Corporation, ©AGC, LLC

Disclaimers

The information contained in this book is only intended to provide the reader with general information, and is not intended in any way to take the place of advice or counseling given to you by licensed, competent (or, if you so choose, incompetent) health care professionals or health care providers. Should symptoms arise that you question, immediately contact a physician who might be able to help you or who can refer you to another physician who can. The information in this book is basically summary in nature, in large part done in our own quest for knowledge, and should be used as a springboard for your own questions and concerns to professional, licensed, competent health care providers. This book does not provide knowledge of all topics related to cancer, nor does it cover all cancer diseases, symptoms or treatments. While we, in certain cases, did our own brand of "self management," we in no way encourage you to do the same. We were incredibly lucky in our recoveries, and the strategies we used may not work for you. While we do express opinions about various topics, based on our own experiences, this does not mean you should blindly follow our advice. You need to do your own information searches, listen to the people who are helping you and then make appropriate decisions about your health care and procedures.

The information in this book has been gathered from many sources, but the authors of this book do not guarantee the accuracy of the sources. Neither the authors nor the sources listed in this book should be held liable for any of the information you choose to follow. Despite our best intentions and efforts, the accuracy, completeness, reliability, timeliness or usefulness of the information may be out of date by the time this book goes to publication. As the reader, you are encouraged to do your own research, talk to your own health care providers and professionals, and use the information contained herein as a basis to begin your own search for answers.

The authors of this book assume no liability for downloading the websites and cannot guarantee they will be free of any type of virus, infection or code that contains contamination or destructive properties. If you choose to access these websites, or follow the strategies the authors of this book used in their own health care, you do so at your own risk. We will accept no responsibility for your choices and decision-making.

We further state that we are not recommending legal advice. If assistance is needed in that area you should secure the services of a competent, licensed attorney.

We have endeavored to make this book as complete and accurate as possible, but there may be mistakes in content or typographical errors. Again, use this book as a general resource, conduct your own research and listen to your health care provider and/or spiritual adviser.

We also want to state unequivocally that the many people we quote or cite within the book may not at all agree with the positions we have taken, or how we have interpreted what they said.

Now, after all the disclaimers (we do live in a litigious age and with any luck have left nothing out), we hope you will enjoy the book.

Dedication

From Alexis

This is dedicated to all the people who have loved ones who have cancer. This is for every support person who has endured, loved, cried, laughed, worried, prayed and dropped an "F bomb" in the name of cancer support. These people are so very important to every aspect of care. They are instrumental in getting help when we need it, food when we need it (but don't really want it!), the reminder to keep hydrated, and giving a smile, hug or goofy look whenever it is absolutely necessary.

To my "support goddess," my partner, my Andrea: you were and are my rock. You drove me to every appointment, every chemo appointment, and had every neighbor in a two-mile radius on alert with strict instructions of who to call should I need help when you were away. You shaved my head shortly after my first chemo treatment, and in your haste, nicked my ear, which made it even more interesting. You were the first one to see my scars post-surgery. You were the brave one who kept a smile on your face and told me it was O.K., reassuring me while you were terrified inside. You held it and me together when everything could have emotionally careened out of control. There are no words to express my admiration and the deep wealth of thanks I feel for you. Without your strength, my prognosis would have been completely different. You will always have my love, devotion and admiration for being my personal hero, my friend, my soul mate, my soft place to land. Thank you.

To my daughter, Calen: Thank you for taking such good care of me. You have endured so much for such a little person. You are a constant blessing to me. I love you, Pea.

To Dr. Lindsey and all of his amazing staff members: your sincerity, professionalism, honesty and the great care you provided me made me feel like less of a number, and more like an individual being treated by family.

To Red Cedar Oncology, for your laughter, voice of reason, care, concern and support, I thank you.

To Hayes Green Beach Hospital and staff. For every person who had a hand in my case, my care and support, I thank you for an amazing healing experience.

To my "Mims"—thank you for being my Mom and doing it selflessly. I love you.

To my Aunt Terryat: For every phone call and each time you talked me off the proverbial ledge, each hug and smile, for every laugh and cooking lesson (which are one and the same!), for every time you reassured me that "I'm not crazy," I thank you. God sent us on this journey together. He knew exactly what we would need . . . each other! I have learned so much from this blessing . . . this cancer. The comfort and support you gave me are immeasurable and for this we are forever stamped upon each other's hearts. I love you.

From Terry

To Dr. Mark Mills, my physician for 24 years, who thought the "shadow" on the X-ray might be lymphoma before all the test results came back, I thank you. Your abilities and the abilities of your staff at Ingham Internal Medicine to "work the system" in record speed literally saved my life.

To Red Cedar Oncology, Dr. Carol Rapson and all of her amazing, wonderful staff, for their laughter, compassionate care, patience, dedication, knowledge and professionalism, I thank you. You each have added to my life in ways that are immeasurable.

To the staff at Karmanos Cancer Center who gave me new hope for life, I thank you. From the doctors, the nurses, the physician assistants, nurse practitioners, apheresis staff, phlebotomists, and pharmacists, to the food service staff, receptionists, and other behind-the-scenes support staff—all of your continual kindness, compassion, knowledge and concern helped speed me to a complete recovery.

To the anonymous and numerous researchers and scientists discovering medicines, treatments for cancer and blazing new trails in stem cell research, your dedication, commitment and perseverance are more appreciated than any of you could ever imagine. You, the risk takers, the knowledge seekers, have persevered through the darkest hours of stem cell research, opposing political ideologies and lack of funding. I wish I could meet you in person to thank you. James Allen, philosopher, said in his treatise, *As A Man Thinketh*, "The dreamers are the saviors of the world. As the visible world is sustained by the invisible, so men . . . are nourished by the beautiful visions of their solitary dreamers. Humanity cannot forget its dreamers. It cannot let their ideals fade and die. It lives in them. It knows them. It knows them in the *realities* which it shall one day see and know." You are our dreamers, our visionaries, and our saviors.

To friends and colleagues at the Lansing School District (Bev, Brenda, Carol, Cathy, Debbie, Eve, Kristy, Lori, Jim, Rose and Sharon), the Michigan Department of Education (named in the body of the book) and the Van Buren Intermediate School District (especially Pedro and Bonnie) for their generous assistance, listening ears and unfailing understanding when I simply couldn't work or meet you for lunch or had some other crisis that you simply handled, always with grace and alacrity, I thank you.

To other cancer survivors and their families who continue to fight the good fight—and win, I thank you for showing me how to face things with courage, strength, humor, compassion and dignity.

To the still-mourning families and friends of people who did not survive cancer, I honor and thank each of you. Please know that we survivors owe our lives to their sacrifices and the knowledge that was gained during their battles. We owe our very lives to them.

And to my dearly loved family, and friends, who have provided continual love, support, laughter and their own brand of courage as I went through this, I love, bless and thank each of you. When you have cancer, all the other people who are in your life also have it. You don't survive cancer—and thrive—without this kind of love and support.

Finally, to my beloved husband, Tom—my love, my enigma, my companion in this journey through life, my valiant partner in developing patience, tolerance and compassion, my antagonist—always challenging me to be better than I am, my antithetic polar-opposite ally—struggling to be the man of both of our visions, my friend—united with me as comrades-in-arms in this battle against an enemy we can neither see, nor anticipate, my fellow combatant—continually inspiring me as we endure each new challenge and grasp onto every new hope, and my champion—the one who knows me and loves me anyway. We have gone together to God and asked Him to illuminate the darkness that invades our space, so we may transcend our conditions and soar back through these dark shadows, until we once again become the vital and thriving life forms with which we once had been blessed to be. Throughout our lives together, I have learned so many things, but none so absolute or so poignant as the fact that . . . *having cancer yourself is far, far easier than being the caregiver for someone you love who has cancer,* much less your lifetime travel mate. But just as our flames flicker, falter and appear as though they will be extin-guished, the aura and luminosity of life begins to flourish anew, and we continue on our wondrous journey together. Tom . . . I thank you, I commend you, I honor and bless you, and I love you. Today and always, I hold you close in prayer.

Contents

Introduction

We decided to write this book because of our own experiences. We have each had cancer. Alexis (age 33 at the time) was diagnosed with breast cancer and had a double mastectomy after her original doctor, Dr. "X," refused to give her a mammogram because she was "too young". Terry (who had just celebrated her 21st annual 39th birthday) was diagnosed with Nodular Sclerosis Hodgkin's Lymphoma. We have both gone through chemotherapy and Terry through radiation. After Terry's lymphoma metastasized, she had an additional two different kinds of chemotherapy and a stem cell transplant.

We have survived, and survived quite well, thank you, but not without going through some interesting times, both during treatment for cancer and afterward. We both learned early that we would have to become advocates for our own health; we had a responsibility to ourselves, and by extension, to our family and friends, to learn as much as possible about our diagnoses and how best to follow what needed to be done. We also learned a most important lesson: we could choose our attitudes. To fight this disease, we could either play "Poor Me," wallow in it (as Meg Ryan said in *French Kiss*, "until your fingers get all pruney"), or we could choose to be upbeat and optimistic. We chose to be "kick-ass," "we're gonna lick this," and to find all the positives possible in the whole process. And for the well-intentioned people who wanted to make us victims—we graciously, but firmly and ruthlessly, exited them from our lives.

In Alexis's case, breast cancer runs in her family, so she knew what she had to watch for. In Terry's case, there is no genetic history of cancer. When Terry asked her oncologist (Dr. Jason Beckrow at the time) why this happened, he simply said that a gene had gone "wacko." That's probably as good a reason as any.

Terry also knew 34 other people who had been diagnosed with cancer and was talking to them about their experiences AC—"After Cancer." These diagnoses included prostate cancer, lung cancer that had metastasized into the brain, CML leukemia, throat cancer, bladder cancer, liver cancer, spleen cancer, cervical cancer, multiple myeloma, pancreatic cancer, brain cancer, basal cell carcinoma of the lower eyelid, thyroid cancer, and additional cases of lymphoma and breast cancer. (Perhaps the problem is in knowing Terry and people should get a new friend!)

Our life styles actually preclude any predilection to cancer: neither of us has ever smoked, we don't drink excessively, we try to eat properly (although we do have our binges), and we exercise (Alexis jogs and bikes, Terry walks up to four miles a day depending on the weather and her schedule that day). We also both have positive attitudes in life; we look for the good in things that happen to us, and do not dwell on things (for very long!) that can eat at the body and soul.

If one of the things that might cause cancer is stress, we both did have great stress early on in our lives. For Alexis, about three years before she was diagnosed with breast cancer, she had "come out" to her entire family. That statement in itself, "I'm gay," had caused major problems in the relationships within her immediate family. She, of course, was fine with it. As Alexis says, "It was a relief to finally stop all the charades and just be . . . me." Her family, on the other hand, didn't roll with it all that well. Her mother, with whom she had shared everything (well, almost!), had a very difficult time. They were, at best, speaking about once every six months, and then it was only when something really needed to be conveyed.

In Terry's case, she grew up with parents who were both two- and three-pack-per-day smokers, with one parent who was a drug addict (prescriptions), including alcohol (let's stop this nonsense about "drugs and alcohol;" alcohol is a drug). Her father died when she was 16 of a long illness and then it took five years to settle his estate. She worked three jobs at one time to put herself through college so she wouldn't have any debt when she got out. Once she started teaching (and going back to school nights and weekends to get her Master's degree), there were literally years that she only got three hours' sleep at night, if that.

Both of us were full-time students, worked full-time at the same time we went to school, tried to be involved as much as possible with our respective families, and also to have as much of a social life as possible. We often thought there should be more hours in the day, but then we realized if there were, we would simply pack additional activities into those extra hours.

Since we are aunt and niece, we had the opportunity to compare notes. "Is this . . . happening to you?" "Yes." "Is that . . . happening to you?" "Yes." Then we laughed, and asked each other what we were doing about it. Most of the time, we knew little we could do. Whenever we talked, at the end of each discussion, we would say, "Now what," or "What next?" Thus, the unintended seeds for this book had been planted.

As we searched libraries and bookstores for any information about "AC" (after cancer), we discovered there are tons of books for being diagnosed and for going through cancer treatment, but very little for what happens to you after cancer. A cursory cruise through the Internet revealed some information about cancer survivorship, some of which is included in various parts of this book. Hopefully we have given credit where credit is due. If not, we will try and make those corrections at a future date. We apologize, in advance, for any such omissions by our AC brains.

One of the things we couldn't wait for was to be "normal" again. After surviving cancer, we discovered there is no such thing as "normal," and we will never again have a "normal" life. But this is true of life in general. Each experience you have in life, each person with whom you come in contact, touches you in some way. You can never go back to being the same person again. This is true whether you are a toddler taking your first steps, a teenager learning how to drive, graduating from high school or college, surviving the trauma of losing your (first but not last) "true" love, giving birth the first time, becoming a grandparent for the first time, experiencing the death of a friend or family member . . . and having cancer or other diagnosis of an illness. There's no going back to what was.

You want desperately to be "normal" again, but there are all these strange things that are happening to you because of the cancer treatments you have received. Your body and emotions were one way BC (Before Cancer). They changed while going through treatment for cancer. And now AC, everything is changed again.

Please don't misunderstand—we are immensely grateful for being alive! Immensely, humongously, gi-normously grateful for being alive!!! Those of us who survive cancer, or any other life-threatening diseases or events, are perhaps much more fully aware of how precious our lives are, how precious every breath is that we take, and how much we have to appreciate. We also come to know how every minute of every day is to be cherished.

We are thankful for: the last chemo treatment, the peach fuzz we optimistically call hair the minute we find it...anywhere! We are thankful for no more steroids and anti-nausea medicines (although a blessing during treatment, it is really a relief not to have to take them anymore). We are thankful for every touch, hug, laugh, sunrise, smile, and breath. However, we are also human, and will have bad days. PLEASE, PLEASE, PLEASE!!! Do not remind us, "At least you have hair." If we feel we are having a bad hair day, we are allowed, just as you are. Or Alexis's favorite, "You should just be thankful to be alive!" *No one realizes this fact more than a cancer survivor.* We're sure a few well-meaning, ill-timed people have gotten their frames climbed for iterating that sentence. Cancer makes you sensitive, perhaps overly sensitive, which can be both good and bad.

Things seem to become magnified. Our symptoms "AC" are depression, weight gain, short temper, rage over the simplest of things, impatience –with everything, need for control -when there is no need, and as Alexis says, you develop a low "bullshit" meter. These are just a few of the symptoms people experience after cancer. More will be covered later in the book.

Cancer tweaks your tolerances. For example, Alexis has no tolerance for tape. Any kind of adhesive she finds intrusive, and refuses to have it stuck to her. We both have a low level of tolerance for rudeness (directed at anyone) and ignorance, which we know cannot be helped, yet at times feel compelled to voice our opinions, which may not be productive either!

In 2010, cancer became the number one disease in America as the leading cause of death, taking over the position held by heart disease for many years. The good news is that although cancer holds the highest death rate, as time passes, there will also be greater and greater numbers of cancer survivors, as researchers continue to learn and find out more about cancer, and develop more effective ways to treat it.

We both recognize we have been incredibly lucky, so very, very lucky, and now it's time to give back, to "pay it forward," if you will. If this book can help anyone, either a cancer survivor, or the caregiver for a cancer survivor, a physician who is taking care of a survivor, or someone who has lost a loved one to cancer, someone who has been recently diagnosed or who has had their cancer metastasize with a "notso-hotso" prognosis, we will feel we have been truly blessed all over again. Our prayers now focus upon making our experience have some purpose that benefits others. Once you have read our story, we hope it leaves you with feelings of hope, of optimism and of empowerment, along with some pertinent scientific medical information and resource referrals, practical solutions to survivor conditions and a look into a variety of philosophic and spiritual thoughts, but perhaps, most importantly, we hope you find peace in the knowledge that you are not alone.

So please, sit back, relax, and walk through this unimaginable journey with us. Experience the highs and lows we have encountered, laugh with us as we find the humor all along the way, and cry with us as we lose some of our direction and focus toward the ultimate goal—living. Just as these journeys have been for all other cancer survivors, the stories are incredible!

So—You've Survived Cancer

Miranda's Story

Miranda Kreiser was diagnosed with Acute Lymphocytic Leukemia (ALL) when she was *20 months old*. For the next two years of her life, she had chemotherapy. At such a tender young age, she was poked with needles every time she went to the doctor or hospital. When she was diagnosed, she was given very little chance of surviving the chemo. However, the doctors told her parents that even as short a time-span as nine years earlier, there would have been nothing they could have done to cure her. Today, fortunately, between 70–90% of young children diagnosed with ALL respond favorably to treatment.

At a time when young kids are learning to socialize with other children, Miranda was isolated from them because her immune system would not tolerate exposure to childhood diseases. She and her parents watched as other children, many of them friends, died from cancer. She was only 10 years old when her father, Mike, died of colon cancer. Her father wrote an essay about his experience with cancer, and also wrote individual letters to his wife, each of his children, his brother and to his parents. Miranda Kreiser graduated from Grand Ledge (MI) High School with all As. She was also the Captain of the Pomming for a Cure Relay Team. She is currently attending Grand Valley State College with a major in nursing. Miranda's grandmother, Rose (also mentioned in this book), had throat cancer. (Thanks to Miranda's Mom, Sherry Kreiser-Crouch, for the synopsis above and for her permission to include Miranda's background. Sherry attributes Miranda's survival to research, which has come farther for ALL than it has with colon cancer.)

What follows is Miranda's story, taken from the essay required as a part of her application to college. She has graciously allowed us to share it with you:

So vividly I remember walking into his dark hospice room, anticipation and deep hopelessness conjoined with an atmosphere too peaceful for words. Leaving my ten-year-old innocence at the enormous oak door, I quietly approach his bedside, and look down to a stranger's weak, frail body. Sitting down to gaze into his jaundiced eyes, I get a glimpse of the strong, healthy soul I have known my entire life. Grasping his large, bony hand, I am holding onto "the smartest," the "strongest," "the best driver in the whole world," but I am not holding onto a victim of cancer. I am looking into the face of the bravest man I have ever met, my hero, my Father.

Moving on after the tragedy of losing a parent to cancer is difficult; moving on after the tragedy of losing a parent to cancer as a cancer survivor is devastating. Most grieving children have to deal with the question of "Why did God take Daddy?" or "Why did Daddy die of cancer?" My thoughts, however, were much more complex. "Why didn't Daddy survive the cancer like I did?" "Why did God let me stay?" "What makes me so special?" For what seemed like an eternity, these guilty thoughts consumed my mind as I tried to find the reasons behind life's twisted ways of exposing such vulnerabilities. After countless days of anger, tears, and confusion, I came to as close an understanding as possible to God's "unfair ruling." Whatever the reason, whatever the justification, He must think I have some pretty amazing things left to do in this second chance at life. As the daughter of the late Michael Kreiser, who bravely overcame cancer's sufferings with dignity and pride, I decided to see to it that these amazing things get done.

For years I have diligently worked to achieve success, not only in the name of my survivorship, but also for the thousands whose legacies will end at the hands of cancer. My perseverance toward academics and leadership has not only accomplished an all "A" honor roll, but a continuation of my Father's beliefs in a strong education. This dedication toward pursuing excellence in everyday life because of my Leukemia is a reflection of the strength, among many other gifts, my diagnosis instilled in me. My survivorship fuels this passionate outlook to help other children through their journey of cancer with the same tenacity, courage and willpower my journey has given me. My dream of making a positive impact on this world is obtainable with a promising tomorrow, a tomorrow that starts with a chance at higher education. A degree in nursing will not only fulfill these dreams of making a difference in fellow cancer patients' lives, it will exemplify to the world that there is hope, a light at the end of a traumatic but monumental experience. I thank God every day for my cancer, for it has not only left a scar upon my chest, but the zest in my heart to change lives. I have no doubt that with a higher education, these aspirations will be achieved, for I am strong; I am driven; *I am a survivor.*

Alexis's Story
Our Journey

This is the story of our journey. It is a part of our life that needs a bit of a forward, a history if you will, to explain. Let me tell you a bit about my family. At the time this all occurred, I was 33 years old. My partner, Andrea, and I had been together 4 years and we shared a daughter from my prior marriage.

Just before Thanksgiving, 2007, I was running on the treadmill. Nothing unusual for me to do; I distinctly remember because I was wearing a black string bikini top. I wasn't in the greatest shape, but I figured what the heck, I am at home, who cares? I finished my three miles and went to take a shower. During the shower, I noticed that my left breast hurt. It wasn't a sharp pain; it was just sore. I felt it . . . nothing unusual. Honestly, it felt like I had torn some breast tissue. The area where it was sore had a little indentation in it, which I didn't find weird at all. I kept reminding myself that these boobs had been through a lot. They had swelled to gigantic proportions when I was pregnant, and then they had had "the air let out of them" when I subsequently lost 100 pounds. They were dense, fibrous, floppy and affectionately called "Fruit Roll-Up boobs" by my best friend and partner, Andrea. Her theory behind it was, "I think you can just roll them up and tuck them neatly in your bra!"

I remember thinking I had covered all the bases. My gynnie lady, Dr. X, had said for the past two years that even though my boobs were all the before-mentioned things (I had not discussed Andrea's nickname for them with her!), she thought I could begin having mammograms at the age of 35. She assured me there was no reason to begin testing me at 32 or 33, even with the history of breast cancer in my family. I had been running hard and wore a less than supportive bikini top. I told Andrea that night before bed and we agreed to get it checked. Thanksgiving was coming, so I made an appointment to see my primary care physician, Dr. Dorothy Mondejar, the following week. Silly, but at that point, it was only for peace of mind for me. I knew that Dr. Mondejar would come in, mash around on my 33-year-old floppy boob and say, "Don't worry, they are lumpy!" I was convinced that would make me feel better. So I waited for the appointment, and my boob continued to ache.

Keep in mind that during this time, Andrea was, to say the least, angry. She had already been through breast cancer with a former partner, and under no circumstances, was "going to go through it again." When I brought the lump to her attention, she freaked. According to her, I was overreacting and had no idea what I was talking about. I knew she was reacting out of utter terror and would be just fine, once she calmed down. She didn't go to my first appointment with me. She refused.

So on Wednesday, November 28, 2007, I kept my appointment with my primary care physician. I knew it would take her two seconds to mash around on my breast and give me the reassurance that everything was fine. She told me, "Probably fibro adenoma, benign, but still need to send you for a mammogram. I just need to make sure." I remember thinking, this was okay. She was doing her job and I trusted her. She was taking action to make sure it was nothing, which I still believed. The office receptionist told me that she had made the mammogram appointment for December 8th, which seemed a long time away. Later, as I thought about it, my impatience and concern finally got the best of me. I called the mammogram center at Hayes Green Beach Hospital in Charlotte, Michigan, and filled a cancellation spot they had for the following Tuesday, December 4th.

On December 4th, I had my mammogram. It was not as bad as "people" had said it would be. It *was* a little unnerving to see a sea of little pink breast cancer ribbons everywhere I looked. I reminded myself that was their job; they needed to increase awareness. I just kept repeating over and over in my head, "I do breast exams all the time. I do breast exams all the time!" The mammogram tech was nice and could tell this was not very easy for me emotionally. She asked if I had heard horror stories about mammograms and my response came flying out of my mouth. I guess what shocked me was not my honesty, but how quick I said it. "I think that everyone has heard a horror story or two in their day, but honestly my partner had a mammogram a few months ago, and she said she liked it and that it felt good!" The only thing this girl could say was "Okay!" which was shortly followed by, "Let's get started!" I left the radiology center feeling proactive and a little lost. My impatience was going to be a problem. "No results will be available for a few days," was not what I wanted to hear. So we waited . . . and life went on.

During this time, I had just begun nursing school at Kellogg Community College in Kalamazoo, MI. My first clinical rotation was at Evergreen Manor, which is a nursing home. On Thursday, dressed in my "blueberry" uniform, cell phone on my hip, I went to my clinical at Evergreen Manor. This was all transpiring at the end of my first semester of the nursing program. Around 9:30, my phone rang. Dr. Mondejar's office had received the results of the mammogram. The nurse said it showed a "NODULE" in my left breast. I felt like they had just spent two days to find a medical word to describe the lump I felt in my boob. I wanted to scream, "NO, REALLY!", but I didn't. The nurse on the other end of the phone was very nice and understanding. They were sending me for an ultrasound, which was "procedure" in this case.

I had done a little, and I mean little, research on breast stuff, simply because I didn't want to freak myself out with too much information. I asked why they weren't sending me for an MRI. The nurse said the ultrasound would be the definitive tool they needed to help them know what was going on in my breast. Needless to say, I was upset and needed to suck it up. My clinical instructor, Logan, and I had gotten close in the past semester and I felt she needed to know. I explained the situation and she quickly became the voice of reason. She helped me get through that day, because she genuinely cared about me, and about what was happening to me. (Sign of a really great nurse.)

The nurse called me back and told me my ultrasound was scheduled for Monday, December 10th. I called Andrea and told her everything I knew at this point; the waiting was getting to her, too. We were at the mercy of the system with no answers and no quick passes to the front of the line. Andrea said she and Pea (our nickname for our daughter—it is short for "Peanut") would go with me for the ultrasound. I wanted Monday to be here and the results to be back and everything to be alright. What I wanted and what would happen did not turn out to be the same thing. With each new step, my mental anxiety was building and my impatience growing, and Andrea could tell.

We both had questions and neither one of us had any of the answers. Together, we would get through it, with lots of talking, crying, "what if"-ing, praying and an alcoholic beverage here and there.

On Monday, December 10, Andrea, Pea and I all piled into the car and went for the ultrasound. It was pretty uneventful, with the ever-popular conversation at the end. "We'll have the radiologist read this and call you with the results in a few days." It was hard to not try to read the expressions on the faces of the people doing the exams. They had practiced not reacting, just as I did when I went to work. It wasn't their job to give me results, nor would it be fair to either one of us.

Wednesday, December 12, Dr. Mondejar's office called with the ultrasound report. The radiologist's report had deemed my "nodule" to be "suspicious" and they were going to send me to a surgeon. I remember thinking, "This is not happening! This means I could really have breast cancer. NO . . . this is NOT happening."

I think my state of shock began with that phone call. I remember feeling dazed, and my mind began to run. That night Andrea and I sat in the hot tub and chatted. We were both on the same page. We knew I had to have a biopsy, and we needed a plan of attack for afterward. I told her how I felt and she almost seemed relieved. I did not want to mess around with saving any part of these boobs if they had cancer in them. We decided then and there that if the biopsy came back positive for cancer, I would have a mastectomy. Andrea was so strong and sweet, she told me she didn't care if I had boobs or not, hair or not, or arms or not, as long as I was here, we would be just fine. She was already beginning to be my rock and helping me to exhale. I love her for that.

It was around this time that Andrea and I decided to start telling a few people. Andrea's Aunt Terry, who from here on out will be Ter-ryat, was very close to us. Both she and her husband had been dealing with their own forms of cancer, and Andrea knew she would not only be a great support, but a wonderful resource to us. We both spoke to her that week, and we could hear the positive in her voice. She reminded us she was just at the end of a phone anytime we needed her.

On Tuesday, December 18 Andrea and I met with Dr. Hugh Lindsey. He is a very nice man of very few words. He did not blow sunshine up our asses. He had a plan of attack before we walked in the door, which was nice. He came in and introduced himself and did a breast exam. He asked me who found the lump, me or my primary care physician. I told him, me. I was thinking to myself, there is no way any doctor would find a lump on my body before I did!! Come on!! He was very calm, and very serious. He sat with both of us and said plainly, "We are, of course, going to be doing a biopsy of the lump you found. There is also a secondary area of concern that showed up on your mammogram. We don't know if that is a separate site or if it is attached to the first site, but that will have to be biopsied as well."

When he got to "secondary area of concern" I stopped listening. He showed us both of the areas and told me there is no way I would have felt the second one, and that it was good the mammogram had detected it. By this time, I was reeling and Andrea knew it. I asked Dr. Lindsey if they could biopsy them both at the same time; he said no. This was only because it would do too much damage to the breast, and they needed to keep the swelling and risk of infection down to a minimum.

Andrea spoke up and said, "So we are going to do the first biopsy tomorrow, right?" Dr. Lindsey smiled and said no. He told us that what was there had probably been there for a while, and that waiting until after the holidays would not change the outcome of any biopsy. He wanted to do the first biopsy on January 4th. We did at some point during this conversation tell him that if it did come back positive, we had already discussed having a mastectomy. He listened and said we could make that decision after the results came back. I was close to losing it and Andrea could see it. I said "thank you" out of sheer politeness, and I heard Andrea do the same. Dr. Lindsey said if we had any questions, we could call the office at any time.

Again, "secondary area of concern" was all I heard. I was beginning to cry when Andrea stood up and grabbed my arms, looked me straight in the eyes and said, "Let's get out of here." She ushered me to the car and I proceeded to fall completely apart. She was just as upset, but holding it together much better than I was. She drove directly to Players, a local pub in Charlotte, which just happens to be around the corner from the hospital and the doctors' offices, and parked outside. She kept saying, "It'll be fine." I could hear her talking to her dad, asking him to come over in a little while. She walked me in and sat me down at "our" table. Trish, the waitress, could see something was wrong and just asked what we wanted. I cried my way through two coolers and Andrea through a large beer. I felt like our world was spinning out of control, and neither one of us could stop it. We both decided to put it on the back burner until after the holidays, not only for us, but also for Pea. We needed to breathe . . . and wait.

The holidays went well and things seemed to go at a normal pace. We talked about the biopsy as if it were years away. Most of our friends and immediate family were up to speed on my "status" and were in "prayers and good thought" mode. As the 4th drew closer, Andrea, Monica (Andrea's sister) and I began to make some plans. They were both going to go to the biopsy with me. Support, whether it is physical, emotional or spiritual, is wonderful.

Noon came quickly on Friday, January 4. Pea was still out of school on Christmas break, so Penny (Andrea's Mom) came to stay with her. Monica arrived and offered to drive to the office. Dr. Lindsey and Cheryl (a nurse from the operating room at HGB hospital) were in during my procedure. Cheryl was very nice, and altogether it went well. It was uncomfortable, but Dr. Lindsey never lied to me. If it was going to sting, it did or if it was going to be noisy, it was. It took all of 45 minutes and I got a huge ace bandage/sports bra when I was done. I was sore, but nothing horrible. Dr. Lindsey said that because of the holidays, the labs and offices were very busy trying to play "catch up" from all the time staff had been away from the office. He said they would call with the results as soon as they arrived, and that we should not expect them on Monday.

Monica drove us home, and what we had waited so long for was over. I actually felt better, as if I had done everything I could and now the waiting was not on my shoulders. I felt proactive, which made the mental gymnastics I had been doing a bit better over the weekend. I wasn't planning on hearing from the Doctor's office on Monday, so when the call didn't come, I was okay with it. I suppose in a small way, it was me clinging to the normalness of the day . . . the day when I still did not have cancer.

On Tuesday, we found our house phone had gone out on Saturday. I do have to admit the quiet was nice. We called the phone company and they said it would be fixed by Thursday at six P.M. I kept my cell phone by my side all day, and called Dr. Lindsey's office and told them our dilemma. My cell phone rang a little before five P.M. Andrea had said that if they were going to give us any bad news, they would just call us into the office. When I heard Dr. Lindsey's voice, I wasn't worried. Then he said it, the words I wasn't expecting to hear over the phone, the words I had dreaded ever to hear.—"I am sorry to have to tell you this, but your biopsy came back positive. *Y o u   h a v e   c a n c e r.*"

I know he kept talking, but I didn't hear a word he said. Andrea saw the look on my face, and I began to cry. I couldn't move or think clearly. Andrea told me to put it on speakerphone, which was a difficult task to perform. She caught the tail-end of him saying we needed to write down any questions we had, and that he would answer them all on Friday, our next scheduled appointment for my biopsy follow-up. He said he knew we had a ton of questions swimming around in our heads, and that if we needed anything, to call the office. He said because of my age, he was going to schedule some other tests, and that one of the nurses from the office would be calling to set those up with us. I don't remember the conversation very clearly, but in trying to listen and understand everything he said, it didn't seem to last that long.

I was reeling when I hung up, trying to regurgitate what he had said before I put it on speakerphone. I sat on the couch and began to cry. Andrea held me in her arms and just said, "Oh, my God", over and over. Next thing I knew, she was on the phone. "We need to get Pea out of here. She can't know, not right now. She can't see us like this." I agreed with her; it was not the time for Pea to see us crying and upset. Andrea called her Dad (Tim), who said he was on his way. Then she called Monica, who changed her plans with a moment's notice and said she was on her way, and that she would be there soon. Carol (Andrea's step-mom) was actually the closest to us and was at the house in about 10 minutes. Andrea told Pea she was going to get to spend the night at Grandma's and Grandpa's and to get her stuff gathered. She did it without question. I stayed upstairs and yelled my good-bye to her and told her that I loved her. I wanted to hug her so tightly, but I was sure she would know something was wrong. Before she left, she asked Andrea if something was wrong with her eyes. Pea is such an intuitive child; she seems to see right through people and knows if someone is upset. Andrea simply told her she had been rubbing her eyes. Then she gave her a hug and told her to have fun. I heard Andrea give Carol a hug and then they left.

Shortly after they left, Monica arrived. She walked in, determined to let us know everything would be all right. She gave us both hugs and the first thing she said was, "This is going to be okay, we are going to beat this!" The second thing she said was, ". . . and if you get bigger boobs than me when you get your reconstruction, we are really going to have problems." She had a huge smile on her face. It meant so much to me to have her with us, bringing humor even at a time like this. Tim arrived shortly after Monica and immediately swept Andrea into a big hug. I think at this point, we were all crying. Everyone wanted to know what the doctor had said and what was going to happen next.

Next, I thought, what's next? I wanted to jump out of my skin, I was so anxious. I kept thinking, No really, this wasn't happening. I have breast cancer? This day, and the week following, would prove to be what I called my "face on the floor" time. I was deflated, and all sorts of things were flying through my head. Things I couldn't justify with any rational answers. Nothing felt concrete to me anymore.

There were a few things that were real for me. I loved my life and I loved my family and I didn't want to lose that. Andrea spent the rest of the night sort of leading me around. I was in a fog . . . she was my rock. She was my reality, and even though we were both in shock, I remember her strength and her voice telling me over and over, this is going to be all right. We sat in the hot tub that night. It was good therapy, to force our bodies to relax. It seemed to take the sting out of the day. It seems silly now but the only thing I could think of, in between crying, was "Stupid Boobs." As we sat in the hot tub, there they were, just floating. It was hard to look at them and think of what was going on inside of them. I felt as if they had betrayed me. Stupid boobs, I would think, and then we'd cry some more. Neither of us slept well that night. I suppose I should have expected that. I went to bed thinking something I don't think I ever had before. "What will happen tomorrow?" That question crossed my mind, and so did fear—a big shuddering moment of fear, as I thought it.

Sometime early Wednesday afternoon the cell phone rang again. It was Barb, from Dr. Lindsey's office. I told her to hold on so I could put her on speakerphone so Andrea could hear everything too. Barb told us there was no indication the nodule I felt in my breast was anything other than the primary site. However, due to my age, the doctor wanted to send me for some other tests. He wanted me to have CT scans, called "CAT," of my chest, abdomen and pelvis. A CT scan is a radiology machine that looks like a big doughnut. The bed they put you on zooms you through the middle and it takes slices of pictures of your body. The CT scans were to detect any other masses or "areas of interest" in the rest of my body. All right, I thought to myself; CT scans are no big deal—I can fly through those.

Barb then went on to say that Dr. Lindsey wanted me to have bilateral breast MRIs and that the only places in Lower Michigan that did them were Michigan State University and an imaging place in Flint. (An MRI, or "Magnetic Resonating Image," uses magnetic imaging and can pick up what a CT scan cannot.) I had to have bilateral (two-sided) breast MRIs, as well as the before-mentioned CT scans of my abdomen and pelvis. The MRIs of my breasts were looking for the extent of the existing tumors, and a look at the right breast, just in case anything small was noticed that the other scans hadn't found. I wanted them done now, so I asked her to put me with whoever could get me in first. Both Andrea and I agreed; we were ready to go. She further explained we could get it all done at the same time in Flint, and the benefit of going there was that if they found anything they had the capability to biopsy it that afternoon. That sounded great, I told her. Sign us up. She said that we could go to Flint on the 15th, but in my head I was thinking, why can't we go tomorrow? I told her that seemed a very long time away, and questioned why we had to wait for so long. The nurse said they could make an appointment relatively fast and could have the results of the tests before my surgery date. That way we, too, would know the results before I had surgery.

She did say she wanted to block off some surgical time for me. At this point, Andrea and I knew what we wanted to do. There was not a doubt in our minds. I told Barb I wanted "it" or "them" off. Sign me up. Let's get this show on the road! This was said with a bit more confidence than I had felt at the beginning of the conversation. Barb said she was blocking off time for the surgery on the 23rd of January. More waiting. I could hardly believe it. Why so long, why not tomorrow? Barb said they needed time to get all the results back. I told her to block off the time, and then I asked her if they had a surgical "will call" list: just in case someone cancelled, we could be ready. She laughed a little, but said no. She was very calming, and did her best to reassure us these tests were all necessary in order to make sure I didn't have cancer anywhere else.

In the back of my mind, I know I had heard what she said. PRECAUTIONARY, I knew what that meant, and had been on the other side of this before . . . trying to reassure patients that we needed to do a certain procedure, just to make sure. The only thing I could think of was the possibility it was somewhere else. My mind went crazy again. Andrea reeled me in well, and told me she was happy they were being so very careful with me. Barb said we could call if we had any questions, and that we could ask all of them on Friday at our appointment with Dr. Lindsey. Then she said goodbye.

I think this was the day we initiated the "phone tree." We had to make what seemed like a thousand phone calls. Now was the time to get everyone on board and up to speed. Between the two of us, we called all our friends and family and let them know what was happening. It was hard to rehash the timeline over and over again. Everyone was very supportive, and willing to drop things at a moment's notice if we needed anything.

Unfortunately, the phone calls didn't get any easier. Telling people that someone they love has cancer is not easy. It is hard because you know you are going to shock them with your news. It broke my heart to hear one of our friends crying on the other end of the phone. They, just like us, needed time to recover. Terryat was a great sounding board through all of this. She offered to do some research for us on breast cancer. I couldn't look at anything negative; I think it would have shoved me over the edge. Over the course of the next ten days or so, we spent a lot of time on the phone, updating people. I think it goes without saying that anytime anything new happened, or any news at all became available, we called everyone. This took its toll on Andrea. It was a hard job, so we tackled it together.

The next few days seemed to go by at a snail's pace. We spoke with everyone we knew and updated them on what was happening. It was hard; everyone had all sorts of questions we just didn't have answers to yet. If we weren't calling someone, someone was calling us. The phone never seemed to stop ringing. It was around this time Andrea began asking me to call my Mom. Right after we had found out, I was just too angry, confused and frightened, and felt somewhat out of control. I hadn't spoken, I mean really spoken, to my Mom in a long time and I didn't want to unleash on her just to let her know. Even though I said no, or sometimes, not yet, Andrea didn't let it go. She didn't pester me; she just kept reminding me that it was the right thing to do, and that I knew she had to be told.

On Friday, January 11, we met with Dr. Lindsey. I was up early and eager to go, but why, I have no idea. I felt like he could give me some kind of closure, I suppose. He came into the room and reiterated what he had said on the phone. I had breast cancer. He called it *infil-trating ductal adenocarcinoma*. What a mouthful. We asked about staging (the stage of cancer I was in; stage 1 is basically everything would be fine; stage 4—kiss your ass goodbye), and he said he wouldn't be able to do that until we knew exactly what was happening with my lymph nodes. Shortly after, he began "informing" us about our options. The only thing I could think was: Tell me when you are going to take my boob off! He started with the lumpectomy speech, which I know he was just doing his job by regurgitating it to us. The next was the mastectomy, which could go one or two ways: I could either have one or both taken. As of right now, he said that taking the right breast would be completely precautionary. I thought to myself, I like precautionary, so I said, "Let's go for it."

I knew Andrea was thinking the same thing. He said his course of action for me was definitely to do a left-sided mastectomy and possibly, a right-sided one as well. In his opinion, taking my age and my hormones into consideration, I would most likely have to have the other breast removed within the next five years. That, of course, was based on the assumption I would not get a lump in the right breast in the meantime. All of a sudden, this all seemed so crazy to me. I just wanted to scream, "Take them both off!!! Now!!! Tomorrow!!!" but somehow, I didn't. I tried to take a deep breath and to regain my composure, so I could listen to what he was saying to us. It took just a moment.

Andrea and I looked at each other; neither one of us wanted any room for error. Dr. Lindsey went on to tell us about our appointment in Flint, and that he would get the results back to us as soon as he could. Andrea wanted statistics, facts, chances, survival rates—something! Dr. Lindsey responded that only two percent of all the women who have breast cancer are my age. My hormones were going to play a huge part in my treatment and in my outcome. He wasn't giving us anything to go on, and it wasn't making Andrea feel any better. He was essentially saying, ". . . we are going to make all these plans, but we can't give you an outcome, because we just plain don't know."

After he finished talking, we sat for a minute, trying to absorb it all. I wanted him to say, "Alright, you have cancer and we are going to take it out tomorrow, and you will have a good chance at recovery." Well, that didn't happen, not even close. We told him we didn't want to take any chances, and didn't care if the breast MRI came back clear on the right, we wanted them both gone. Why have a time bomb lashed to my chest? That just seemed silly. I had a plan, and I actually felt better. Andrea on the other hand, seemed to be going in the other direction.

This is the point where I need to take a break from this little journey and explain a little more about "us." Andrea and I fit very well together. She is a loud speaker, her voice projects, where I am soft-spoken. Andrea used to remind me all the time that she had to turn up the volume on all the phones because she could never hear me. If you add anxiety and stress, it seems to increase those things, no matter who you are. She would get louder and faster, and I would get softer and slower. That is just us. It is how we function and why we function so well at times. I am the soft and squishy mom and she is the "black and white" mom. My point in telling all of this is to say we never have our "face on the floor" moments at the same time. That is a blessing we have come to embrace. This was one of those times, and I knew it. I was holding onto hope, and she felt like the wind had been taken out of her sails.

We told the Doctor what we wanted and he agreed. He told us if we changed our minds, we could tell him not to take the right breast, even as late as on the day of surgery. I knew in my heart there was no chance that would happen.

This period, from the time I found the lump until the day of surgery, was when I was truly shown the strength of family, the power of prayer, and the depth of love. Keep in mind that up until this point, I had yet to mention anything to anyone on my side of the family. All of my support, prayers, and love were coming from Andrea and her "kin," if you will. She had asked me once or twice if I wanted to call my Mom and I had told her no. I was angry and still wasn't in the right place in my mind to call her. A few days later I woke up after having spent the night dreaming about my Mom. When Andrea woke, I told her, "I want to call my Mom today." She smiled. I loved her for that. She never pushed, never judged; she just suggested and waited. I know that girl knows me—in and out, up and down, back and forth— she really knows me.

I called my Mom the day before we were scheduled to go to Flint. I remember it clearly, which is kind of odd. I asked her if my step-dad was home and she said no; he was at the office. I just didn't want her to be alone when I told her. Nevertheless, I told her. The words came out slowly, and I know it shocked her. But amazingly, her shock turned into strength in a matter of minutes. She wanted to know everything, so I told her. First, I told her the surgery was scheduled and when, and then I told her we had made the decision to have both breasts removed, no matter what was found by the doctors in Flint during the tests.

The phone call was about a half-hour long, and Andrea listened to the whole thing. She wanted some kind of insight into my Mom. I couldn't blame her. I do remember telling my Mom things were going to be hard during the next few weeks and would be even more so given this tension within our family. I told her I was not trying to push anything down her throat, but that I would like, before this whole thing gets started, for her to just meet Andrea. She, without any hesitation, said, "Alexis, that is a non-issue. I am sure we will." I could hardly believe it.

We ended the conversation shortly after that and I promised to call her with the results of the scans in Flint. She told me she loved me and that she would be talking to me soon. It was a very emotional day.

Calen (aka "Pea;" when Calen was born, I called her my "*calen*dar girl") spent the night with Carol and Tim so she could get on the bus, and we could be on our way to Flint on Monday. Sunday night, when we said our goodnights to Pea, she gave me a big hug and told me to be a big girl and that it would all be okay. She then asked her Mom Jo (Andrea) to take good care of me, which Andrea promised to do. It was hard not to cry. Pea is very intuitive, she feels everything, and we are very blessed to have her.

Bright and early Monday morning, January 15, we left for Flint and, lucky us, there was a huge storm early that morning, leaving the road conditions (for lack of a better word) crappy. Andrea drove nervously the entire way to Flint. . . . Nothing like a little stress to add to our big stress. Yikes! We arrived on time and began to fill out paperwork. This nice woman came over and asked me if I had finished drinking my contrast for my CT scans. Darn! I had no idea I was supposed to be drinking contrast. She came back shortly with two bottles of grape juice. She told me when to drink one and then the next, and that they would be calling me for my MRI in a few minutes.

We sat for a bit and they called my name. I told Andrea I would be back in a few minutes and left with the tech. I changed into a gown and was escorted into a room with a table and a big machine. I am truly thankful I have had many years of experience with "procedures" and "scans" with my job. It completely took the anxiety out of the big looming machine through which my body was going to be taken. I was told I had to have an IV for the MRI, and that it would take from about 35 to 45 minutes. Oops! Sorry, honey! I know how Andrea hates waiting and not knowing anything.

They started my IV and told me I would be lying flat on my stomach, with both of my boobs hanging down through the machine. (Ha, I knew eventually the floppy things would come in handy!). They told me it would be very noisy and gave me a pair of earplugs. Great, this I wasn't expecting. No worries, still calm. I lay down on the table and they positioned me the way they needed me to be. I put my earplugs in, and they gave a little squeeze ball to me. The tech told me if I needed anything, to squeeze the ball and she would come to see what I needed.

After about five minutes through the first part of the procedure, I began to feel horrible. The grape juice/contrast was running right through me, and my stomach was starting to cramp. I broke out in a sweat and tried to breathe through it. It was not working, so in a panic, I squeezed the ball. Then I waited, squeezed again, and waited. Pretty soon the tech was at my head asking what was wrong. I told her I needed to get up and go to the bathroom. I was sure I was absolutely going to explode. She told me I only had four minutes left, and that if they stopped they would have to wait three hours to do it again. I held my breath and began to count off four minutes. When the other techs came to get me and my boobs out of the machine, I pulled my earplugs out and said, "BATHROOM!" I think she knew that I wasn't kidding. She scooted me out across the hall and into the nearest bathroom. Mental note: grape juice equals diarrhea.

Once that was all taken care of, I returned to the room and finished my MRI. Next came the discussion about keeping my IV in. I had to have it in for the CT scans, and told them I would like to keep it. Long story short, I forgot I was in Flint, and the risk for using my IV access for drugs was viewed as greater here. There is less trust in the inner city of Flint than there is in Lansing, as far as drugs are concerned. The health care professionals choose to completely eliminate the liability of drug users using IV sites by not allowing them off the premises. I laughed and told them that if the risk was that great, they could take it out because we were going to get breakfast. I think I shocked the techs because they tried to reassure me the only reason they had to take it out was because they were worried the IV would clot-off. Hmmmm.!?!

Needles to say (pun intended), we had the IV taken out and went across the street to Bob Evans for breakfast. About an hour or so passed and we returned to the imaging center for the CT Scans. This time they brought Andrea back to another waiting room where she would not be so far from me. They poked me again for the second IV, no big deal and away we went. It took about 30 minutes from start to finish. When I was done, they told me to wait in the room across the hall. I asked them to get Andrea. She came in and sat with me, and we waited. The head imaging tech person, I can't remember his name, came in and promptly spilled the beans. "The radiologist who will do your procedure today will be in shortly."

WHAT PROCEDURE? We were spinning again. Did that mean they had found something new, or they were going to biopsy something old, or what? Next, two radiologists came into the room. Both women were fairly attractive. We began firing our questions: "What did you find?" and, "Why are we just now finding out about a procedure?" They explained nothing else had been found in the breast MRIs, which was good. They had not had time to read the CT scans yet, so that was still pending. They were under the impression we knew I would be having a sentinel lymph node biopsy in their office. Sentinel nodes are the lymph nodes that will first be infected if the cancer has spread outside the breast. That, I told them, we did not know. They said it would help to stage the cancer, and help Dr. Lindsey know better what he was going to encounter when operating.

I had done the other biopsy in my doctor's office; how bad could this be? Boy, was I wrong. Radiologists and surgeons are two completely different kinds of doctors. But then again, breast lump biopsy and lymph node biopsy are, too. They set me up, the same as the last time, only this time Andrea got to sit in the room with me, thank God. They used ultrasound to find The Lymph Node they wanted to "suck stuff out of" and got me in the correct position.

Until now, I had experienced only minimal pain. I remember her saying they were going to extract part of the lymph node and heard the machine start. I can't even begin to tell you how much it hurt. I began to cry and Andrea was up and out of her chair, with her hands on my legs, keeping me on the gurney. I was shaking, it hurt so badly. I told them once was enough, and they would have to stop right then. I told her where the pain was coming from, and she said she was nowhere near there. I don't know if she crossed the last incision site and the biopsy site or what, but I was done. Andrea came up to my head and smiled, and then said the most precious thing: "You are being such a sissy." I smiled. She was, and is, exactly what I needed.

The doctor finished what she was doing and they put pressure and ice packs on the site in my arm pit. I was scared and Andrea knew it; she never left my side, although she did say she would not sit through one of those again, and they would need to knock me out if they were going to do it again. I wholeheartedly agreed. On the way home, we called a few friends and family and told them about the day. When we got home, we rested and waited.

Between January 15 and February 19, we had to make some big decisions. How were we going to handle this topic with Pea? My Mom was offering help anywhere it was needed, so we took her up on it. She volunteered to take Pea while I had surgery and recuperated a day or two at home, and she would be down to pick her up. We sat Pea down and had a family meeting. We told her my boobs were sick and the doctor was going to remove them. We told her I would have to stay in the hospital for a few days and that she was going to stay with my Mom, who she calls "Jamma." At best, Pea was scared and unsure, but who wasn't at this point? She agreed to go with Jamma, and then we spent the next few days reassuring her that I was going to be fine, that everyone was going to take great care of me, and that we would all be back home together very soon.

Over the next few days and in the past few weeks, Andrea had talked to my Mom on the phone, but they had yet to meet. Although I couldn't see it at the time, cancer was a blessing. It was the impetus that would finally put things in perspective, and bring us together.

My Mom was coming to get Pea and take us out to dinner. Andrea was a ball of nerves, and so was I. Despite the tension in the air, because my surgery was growing closer and closer, my Mom swooped in like a paratrooper—in the Army of HOPE! She, in the most definite terms, said, "We are going to do whatever we have to. We will get through this!" I think I will remember that hug from my Mom forever. Dinner went well. After we hugged and kissed Pea goodbye, we told her to have fun, and that we would call her every day so she could talk to me.

January 23, the longest day in history. We had to be at the hospital early because I had tests that needed to be done before the morning of surgery. Neither one of us slept that night, which I suppose is natural. I got up before the alarm and took a shower. I remember being in the shower thinking, "Stupid boobs." I got dressed in comfy clothes and got Andrea out of bed. Neither one of us knew what to say. Anxious, scared, weak, and nauseated are all great words to describe how I was feeling that morning. I just kept thinking, "You just have to get through surgery, just get through surgery!"

We arrived at the hospital with a gigantic exhale and got escorted to a bed in pre-op. I did the usual, confirming my name, date of birth, allergies, meds, and got into a fashionable gown. I got an I.V. and they began filling me with fluid. Shortly after we arrived, I had to go to Radiology for "the tests". Since I was having both breasts removed, they were concerned with lymph node involvement. They had to inject both breasts with dye that would help them find my sentinel nodes. These are the nodes that will show positive first for cancer, if the cancer has spread beyond the breast. Not necessarily fun having some radiology tech trying to hold your floppy "fruit roll up" boob in one place while a radiologist injects your breast in five spots around your nipple. Stupid, stupid boobs!! The right breast hurt, duh. The left breast, since it had been biopsied twice, was damned near unbearable. I couldn't help but cry, which got to the radiologist. He was a very nice man who kept reassuring me he was almost finished. Once that was complete, I was wheeled back to the holding area where Andrea was waiting. She asked if I was all right and I told her what happened. She gave me a hug and tried to make me feel better.

Slowly family and friends began showing up to wait with Andrea. They all came in for a minute to say hello, and give me a hug. There were a few people that just completely lost it and had to leave the room. Sometimes, despite people's best intentions, it becomes too overwhelming for them. That is when you must do the best you can to reassure them, even though you are rather overwhelmed and frightened yourself.

The anesthesiologist came to get me with both of the nurses that would be in on my case. I started to cry; I didn't want to leave the safety of my holding area and Andrea. I was bawling pretty hard when they wheeled me into the O.R. (operating room). Just as I was thinking, "Someone, give me something to make this terror go away," they did. The next thing I remember is quite cliché. I was moving, feet first, down a hallway with lights whizzing by. I remember Andrea being there and a voice telling me that I was going to be moving. I was in surgery for nine hours, during which time, I found out later, they had called a "Code Blue" on the med/surg floor. When you have a loved one in the operating room and they are yelling over the speakers "Code Blue" and Surg, you tend to flip out. Andrea had a lot of people to sit with her and calm her fears, which helped when she thought they were talking about me. I don't remember much of the first few hours after surgery. I had the anesthesia spins really bad when I woke up. The nurses were great about trying to get me some pain meds. All I wanted was something to keep me from puking. I fought to sit up so I could help myself not to throw up. I faded in and out over the next few hours. I know I saw my family and friends during that time, which was so nice. They needed to see that I was "all right", which is code for breathing, and also wanted me to know they cared. I got back to my room around five P.M. By the time everyone was gone, it was nine or ten. Andrea was by my side the entire time, and I knew she had to be exhausted. She watched as the tech and the nurse checked my blood pressure and pulse every hour to make sure I was recovering well and medicated enough so I wasn't in pain. This went on for the next six hours or so. Around five in the morning, I woke up. Yep, I woke up, and I was ready to go. The hospital staff had brought in bedding and a pillow for Andrea to sleep in my room. The girl had not yet been to bed, watching every breath and every exhale I had made. She had been asleep for about ten minutes, when I called to her. "Honey. . . ." She was up and standing next to me in a second. What was wrong, what did I need? I told her my ass was numb. She was not impressed. She told me to just relax and wait for a while. I repeated my problem ". . . . honey, my ass is numb." She told me she had just gone to sleep and the new shift would be coming on soon. I knew she was tired, but I also knew the rules. If I got up and walked around, I could have the catheter taken out of my bladder. I also knew I would be one step closer to going home. I pleaded my case, and not too subtly, ". . . so I'm just supposed to sit here while my ass is numb?" That got her up and moving. She hit the call light and the nurse came into my room. I was up walking around, and had the catheter out in the next half hour. Today was a good day.

I slept most of the next day, and had quite a few visitors. Andrea snuck out and got me a grilled chicken wrap from our favorite bar,

Players. The next day, Dr. Lindsey came in to do a dressing change. I couldn't look, and Andrea knew it. She put on the best "calm" face she possibly could, and told me everything would be all right. I started crying part of the way through. This was scary—me, with my arms over my head, not watching, as a doctor was pulling bandages off my chest, a chest I could hardly feel. The nurse got emotional and excused herself. Dr. Lindsey started talking to me, telling me how everything looked great and that he was almost done. Andrea never waivered; she smiled and told me again everything was fine. A little while later, I was being discharged. I was sitting on the side of the bed waiting for the nurse to come in. When I stood up, I was shocked. I had a huge dent in my hip. I told Andrea, "Look at the size of my ass!" Remember all that fluid they started in the pre-op area? Well it hadn't stopped. I had successfully gained a ton of extra water weight and it had settled where I had settled . . . my ass. The nurse just laughed, and told me it would take a few days for my body to process all the extra fluid.

On the way home, Andrea tried not to run over any sticks or rocks or bumps. She was so careful—it was adorable. We finally got home, and I set myself up in the bonus room of the house. The last place I wanted to be was in bed. I had been there for two days and was trying to do everything I could to not act or look like I had just had major surgery. Shortly after we got home, friends and family started arriving. We finally gave up locking the front door, and just put a note on it that said, "Come on in . . . we're upstairs!"

Calen came home a few days later. She was hesitant and nervous and needed to know I was all right. I had talked to her on the phone while I was in the hospital, and told her I was fine. But, she needed to see me. Once she saw me and hugged me, she was better. A few days later, we showed her my dressings and my drains and how they operated, which made her feel even better. She was a trooper from then on. She helped me empty my drains and watched for infection every day. She was amazing!

On February 18, I realized life was speeding along as I recuperated. I got a phone call from one of my close friends from class. She was in tears, trying to explain something horrible. Dana, the girl I had been seated next to during my first semester of nursing school, the one I borrowed highlighters from, ate lunch with, joked about other students with and shared my breast cancer story with, was found dead in her home. She had hung herself. Her death was very, very hard for me to deal with; it just did not seem possible, and I could not begin to understand why she might have done this thing. Life certainly can hit you from many directions, at any time, and in ways that totally change your perspectives.

On February 19, we woke up bright and early, which must have been adrenaline, because it wasn't excitement. We had to be at HGB by 6 A.M. to have the infusaport inserted. After we got to the hospital, everything seemed peaceful. Everyone in pre-op knows us, which made things easier. I got a little Versed (a tranquilizer) to calm me down prior to leaving Andrea, which also seemed to make things easier.

The next thing I knew I was back with Andrea. Wow, piece of cake. No nausea, nothing. We were home by 10:30 and I took a nap. Andrea tried, but couldn't. I was feeling pretty good by now; chemo starts tomorrow. Chemo will be administered at Red Cedar Oncology, with Dr. Carol Rapson. Her office is in Charlotte, where we live, but because of the dangers of administering chemo, we were going to her Lansing office, which was at that time across the street from Sparrow Hospital, just in case . . .

On February 20, I woke up and took off all of my steri-strips. Steri-strips are pieces of tape that will stick to skin, and were placed by doctors directly across my fresh incision from the infusaport. The tape was bad again; I guess I just wanted it gone. By this time, my loathing of tape had grown to gigantic proportions. Kevin was my nurse, and he is wonderful. He carefully explained everything and acknowledged my concerns. Accessing my port hurt a bit, but nothing too bad. Terryat and Tom popped in for a few minutes and then left (Tom had had his treatment that day, also). When all was said and done, it took about four hours. I left feeling tired, drained and wanting to go home. I was so glad Andrea was here with me. She took such good care of me; I didn't have to worry about a thing. In all the hurry to get home, I misread the anti-nausea medicine schedule and missed the first dose. Oh, did I pay for that! Around 10:30, I was in tears in Andrea's lap. I felt sick, I looked sick and I thought I smelled sick. I got the nausea under control later that night, and spent the next three days sleeping.

Three days later, I felt better and obviously needed to get up and do something. Once I got over the nausea and off the Compazine, I felt like doing more. There was a lot going on at home and then, there was Dana's funeral. Andrea told me I shouldn't go, and I knew she was right. I shouldn't expose myself to any more germs than necessary. I guess that was solved, so we didn't go to the funeral. I took some Tylenol to curb the headache I had had brewing for hours, and went to bed.

The next day I was sitting next to Andrea while she played Zelda (one of my favorite pastimes); I was playing with my hair and when I brought my hand down, I had somehow pulled a ton of hair right out of my head. Nervous habit, I suppose. Andrea looked up at me and said, "Honey, nice bald spot!" It was coming out *everywhere*. Tomorrow I was scheduled to have more chemo, and after tomorrow—two down and two to go.

Andrea and I were watching a movie sometime around the first of March. After the movie had finished, she asked me when I had washed my hair last. I knew this was a trick question. I lied and said a few days ago. She had that look in her eyes. She told me she had noticed my hair was coming out and that it was covering the back of my robe. Nope! No! This was not happening! Then she said it, the words that I knew I would hear, but didn't want to hear. "Honey, I think it's time to shave your head." I immediately began to cry. No! No! No! Due to the fact I was going to need some huge convincing, we went where we always go to fix the day's problems, the hot tub. An hour later, a few coolers and ten pruney fingers and toes later, we were in the bathroom with the scissors. We tried the Demi Moore- G.I. Jane method, which didn't work; we just got the shaver stuck in my hair. We switched methods and she put my hair in a ponytail and cut that off. I started drinking again. Andrea then just started cutting, as close as she could to my head. All I could hear was the snip- snip- snip- . . . as I tried not to watch the hair falling to the floor. Andrea was on a roll and got a little excited; somehow, she managed to snip my ear. Blood began running down my ear and neck. I was crying, and as Andrea was apologizing, we pressed onward. Once she was finished, she immediately put me in the shower, so she could get all the hair off the floor quickly, just to make sure I wouldn't see it at all. We got some of the hats Andrea had ordered in preparation for this day, one we both had known was coming, and got me into my pjs (pajamas). We took some pictures a little later that night. Crocodile tears in my eyes, hat on, smile on my face, we had made it through another day with cancer.

A few days later, on March 10, I went to take a shower and as I was lathering, a large amount of pubic hair fell out. I called Andrea just because I wanted her to see!! It just kept coming out! Yikes! I am so glad she/we decided to shave my head last week. I really don't think I could have handled a huge clump of the hair on my head coming out in my hand like this had. Andrea got teary eyes. She said it was just kind of sad. I think it was emotionally harder for her than it was for me.

My next chemo day, March 14, was much better than the first. I knew what to expect. Kevin was there, which was nice for me. Wow, little things are really starting to bother me. That Huber needle hurts. I let out a quiet, "SHIT," while he was accessing my port. I just kept repeating to myself, "This means I am half done." I was tired when we left and spent the rest of the day lying on the couch, sleeping off and on. The next day felt like my fifth day of the first treatment. I even went to the store with Penny. Wal-Mart was a hoot. One of the cashiers "helped" me through a "you scan it" line. She was lifting my groceries and scanning things. She was concerned and asked me if I was gonna puke. I must have looked like crap. I told her no, but thanks, and then the questions began. Is it breast cancer? Then it came, the statement I can never let go. "I'm sure your husband loves you whether you have hair or not." Without hesitation I answered her. "Yes, my partner is very supportive. She has been wonderful through this entire thing." The woman turned to me and whispered, "You're a lesbian?" I answered, "Yes." She got a big smile on her face and said, "You go, girl!" She then launched into some story I half listened to about a friend or a cousin who was also a lesbian. It took forever to get out of Wal-Mart. I was thankful for her willingness to help and her honesty, but, Andrea, please understand this is why it takes me so long at the store!

The third day of chemo I was a wreck—tired, pale, weak, short of breath. Andrea went to work; watching me sleep had become a necessary pastime of hers, and not a fun or welcomed one. I knew she was a phone call away. B.J., a friend, was going to be stopping by the house, and Carol was home if we needed anything.

By the time B.J. and her sister got around to coming by, Andrea was already on her way home early. She thought it was best, and she was right. She met B.J. and her sister, Shelly, in the driveway. Shelly is a nurse and needed to come in and assess me for herself. She sat down next to me and took my pulse. First, Andrea went and got my stethoscope. Shelly listened to my lungs, which sounded all right. They all gave me hugs, and then I got sent straight to bed. I don't think I moved until the next morning.

I went back to school on Monday morning. Sitting in class was a piece of cake both days but I was wiped out by the time I got home. I took my first quiz and exam—100% and 92%, respectively!!! Thank God the chemo brain was only affecting my short-term memory. Wednesday was my first clinical day. It took all I had to stay moving and awake. Wow, was I dehydrated, hardly seeing at all. This was one of those days when my everyday angel was doing her daily stuff and I found a surprise angel in my path. Her name was Mary H. She was teaching a pre-natal class at the hospital. My clinical instructor thought it would be a good idea to go to neo class, because labor and delivery was so slow. She "recognized" me immediately. She is a ten-year cancer survivor that has an amazing gift of "calm." She gave me a hug and during her parental relaxation segment, told the other girls and me to practice as well. She talked everyone in the room through a meditation session and gave me a back rub while she talked us through it, so I just closed my eyes and breathed. The most amazing part of my first clinical was Mary, my unexpected angel.

Which brings me to support people. Everyone needs them and has them in their lives. You cannot have cancer and not have it affect the people who love you. I can't emphasize that enough. You may be the one with the disease, but your support people are the ones who have the tougher job. After all, they are the ones we look to, to make everything all right.

April 24th was my final chemo treatment. Yippee! This was the only treatment I was truly dreading, because I knew it would be the worst. A few days before this, I received a call from Barb, in Dr. Lindsey's office. She was the person who had called and set up all the tests in Flint just after I had been diagnosed. She told me she was on the board for the Susan G. Komen Foundation and the three-day walk was coming up soon. They wanted to interview me, videotape it and play it during the walk. I was stunned. I told her I would love to, however my last treatment was coming up and I knew it was going to be bad. She told me to wait and see—if I was up for it; if so, then I could come out and do the taping.

Unfortunately I spent quite a bit of time in bed after that last treatment. Wow, did that knock the wind out of my sails. During the next few weeks, I spent time finishing up classes and building my strength back. It was all downhill from there. Piece of cake, I told myself. I began feeling better and decided it was time to write the letter to Dr. "X", as we shall call her. If you recall, she was my initial physician, the doctor who insisted I was too young to have a mammogram. The letter I wrote and sent to her is in the back of this book in Appendix A. I never went back to see her. I didn't think seeing her was worth the $15 co-pay.

I have to say I did have a few defining moments during this time. I was in nursing school, doing chemo, had no hair, was having problems concentrating and was attempting to take tests along with everyone else. I remember sitting in class taking a labor and delivery exam. Keep in mind that most everyone in class was well aware of my illness, and that my bad days were truly bad days. That being said, if I coughed, sneezed or tried to get up to go to the bathroom, everyone was aware of it and ready to help if I needed it. Well, I was taking this test and sneezed. This was no little sneeze either; it was huge! I opened my eyes, and looked down at my exam and realized I had sneezed OUT ALL of my eyelashes! Now, you have two choices at this point. You can either completely lose it and cry, or you can accept it and move past it. So I chose the latter; without moving my head, I took a big breath in, and blew the eyelashes off my paper. The few people who were watching this unfold burst into laughter. I finished my exam and felt like I had given cancer a big black eye that day.

Once I understood how my body was going to react to chemo, I realized I didn't have to stay in bed the whole time. It took about a week for me to get through the bad days after each chemo session. So the other two weeks I had before the next treatment, I spent getting back to basics. I began walking on my treadmill. Once week one was over and I was feeling better, I increased my pace. Once that went all right, I began to run. The day before the next treatment, I was running just like I had before. Then it was time for me to get chemo the next day, and I would start the cycle all over again.

Once summer arrived, I started biking. My sister-in-law, Monica, and I were going to participate in the DALMAC. The DALMAC is a bicycle ride that begins at the campus of Michigan State University and goes to the Mackinaw Bridge. We take four days to travel and camp at scheduled stops. The first day is ninety-one miles and you bike from Michigan State University to Central Michigan University's campus. That being said, I needed to train. I spent the summer riding my bike and going to class. I had a goal: I wanted to complete this ride. I was nervous, not so much about the ride, but about everything else. It's hard to hide the fact I didn't have any breasts. I was going to be out in public in tight clothes, without Andrea. Would people be staring at me? Would anyone ask me what happened? Monica swooped in and took all my anxiety away. She told me she would be with me every day, and would hold up a towel for privacy in the community shower, if I needed it. There was no way I would ever be hurt or made fun of with Monica around. She is another one of my angels! I completed the DALMAC and she got me on video climbing "the Wall". It was amazing—another black eye for breast cancer.

Many times I have pondered getting implants. I do want to get them, and feel it is yet another step toward closure for me. One of the reasons I want to get them is simply because my clothes just don't fit the way I want. I have prosthetic breasts, and wear them occasionally, but I only wear them for short periods of time and never to work. It took one time of doing CPR (Cardiopulmonary Resuscitation) and having them slap against my chest for me to realize I couldn't be knocking the wind out of myself doing my job just to look nice. I suppose it's just not for me. I am me and fine with how I am now. Will I get implants? Yes. Will I get them because I am ashamed of my flat chest and how I look? Absolutely not!

Terry's Story
Travels with Tom

All life is an experiment. The more experiments you make, the better.

—*Ralph Waldo Emerson*

I didn't meet Tom, my husband, until I was 41 (or, as I refer to it—my 3rd annual 39th birthday). As it turned out, for years he had only been one mile from where I worked. He was (and still is) in the wholesale produce business, started by his father over 40 years previously. As a child, I had always seen myself with three kids, two boys and a girl. And, lucky me, that's what I had once I married Tom. (However, their names were not what I had picked.) By that time, my nieces were all grown up with lives and families of their own, but we remained close. Each of them is one of the most precious components of my life. Tom's family, his kids, grandkids, brothers, sisters-in-law, his twelve nieces and nephews, their spouses and *their* kids, have also become integral parts of my family. My life is infinitely richer than I could ever have imagined it would be for having all of them in it.

It has been a truly interesting marriage, primarily because we are absolute opposites in most all things. Tom is so far to the political right, he sometimes makes former Senator Jesse Helms look like the 'middle.' (Of course, to Tom, I'm so far to the left, I make Reverend Jesse Jackson look like the 'middle.') He loathes change, and I thrive on it. He is impulsive when it comes to spending money, but needs years to think something through if it will involve change. I am a planner and organizer and do everythingjustasquicklyaspossible, and I am good at making snap decisions, especially when it comes to chocolate. He paces incessantly when he's bored, but falls asleep immediately when I get out my "honey-do" list, and is particularly adept at pacing when I'm trying to work. We have about 3,800 square feet of house space, but he feels compelled to alternately pace and hover in the 125 square feet of space in the "library" where my laptop is set up to work, where the laundry gets done, books are available for reading and where I store some of my craft materials. Those traits we both share unquestionably are our commitment, love and devotion to each other, and to our family and friends, which are most likely the characteristics that carry us through the rough patches every marriage goes through from time to time.

Tom (who is Tom III) and I went to England and Ireland about three weeks after we were married and took his parents, Tom Jr. and Marion. Tom's Dad was *VERY* Irish, and was really upset at the thought of going to England, but toward the end of the trip admitted that England was prettier. We were there for 20 or so days, at the end of which, Tom and I knew we wanted to go back again and again. On our next trip in 1991, we met Tony and Jean Coburn, who had "hire cars" in London, and the four of us became friends. One of their activities into which they graciously folded us was the London to Brighton Antique Car Run, held the first Sunday in November every year; in order to participate, all the cars have to be dated from 1904 *or older*. It is quite an event, but I will have to save the descriptions of our adventures for another time.

Tom and I went to England, Ireland, Scotland, Wales, Spain, France, Portugal, Guernsey, Jersey, Alderney, Sark, and we even gambled in Monte Carlo (big spenders that we are—$20 each). We travelled to Europe more than 20 times in about 15 years. Life was amazing. Grandchildren started to be born, as did the great-nieces and –nephews. The St. Patrick's Day parties continued (a family event that raises money to buy clothing for needy children; usually between 900 to 1300 people attend and we did all the cooking for the event). Birthday parties were given, weddings were celebrated, graduations and baptisms were attended, yearly family reunions took place, as did all the other ordinary, every-day life events we take for granted.

And then, the unthinkable happened.

At the end of August in 2005, Tom, in his usual matter-of-fact fashion, came home and said, "I don't know if I have one day left or ten years." After playing "20 Questions" to try and figure out what he was talking about, he finally told me his PSA (Prostate Serum Antigen) test done near the end of May was 192.8 (the normal range is 0–4, or depending on the type of lab procedure that is run, can be 0–6). This simply had to be a mistake. How can "normal" be 0–4, and his be 192.8? Mistake, mistake, mistake! No way! Impossible!!!

It was at this point that Tom told me he had taken himself off Proscar about 3 years ago. (Proscar is a drug that is given to men when their PSA is rising; it may help delay the onset of prostate cancer.) Please do not ask why it took him all this time to breathe a word about this to me. I have absolutely no idea, and have searched for possible reasons so many times. As everyone knows, early treatment is key to cancer survival! Was he avoiding the reality of it for himself? Was he thinking if left alone, it would go away? Was he trying to shield me from this? What on earth could he have been thinking for three years? I suppose I shall never really know, but this day was the beginning of a new reality for us.

He was retested in September by his primary care physician, internist Dr. Craig Wheeler, at Ingham Internal Medicine. When you first meet Dr. Wheeler, he immediately puts you at ease and you can tell this man knows his business. What's more important, as time went on, he could put all the tests in perspective and in a way that was easier to understand. This time Tom's PSA was 461.9. Between May and September, a little over four months, it had gone up 269 points—for you mathematicians, a 240% increase. Dr. Wheeler said the odds were

Tom had a virulent form of prostate cancer, but he would refer Tom to various doctors and have him undergo a bunch of tests to make sure. What we discovered in this part of our journey was that there had to be a lead doctor, and since Dr. Wheeler was Tom's primary care physician, it would be him. However, as time went on, it became increasingly difficult to get copies of the test results back to him (and us) no matter how many times his name (or ours and the other doctors) was put on the list.

It's hard to describe the gamut of emotions you go through when faced with something like this. When you hear the word "cancer," anything after that is simply not heard. Any other words seem to be muted, slurred, and on slow motion. "Cancer" rolls around in your head, reverberating, drumming, screaming out at you all hours of the day and night. Shock, numbness and feeling off-balance become your new way of life. Cancer is always something that happens to someone ELSE. And this is one club no one is in a hurry to join. The initiation rites can be frightening and the yearly (or monthly) dues are far too high.

One of the emotions that came to the forefront early was *ANGER*. . . . Anger at Tom . . . Anger when I found that he had been self-medicating, Anger that he believed every quack alternative medicine magazine or booklet that came through the mail rather than his doctors, Anger that he had taken himself off medicines the doctor had prescribed because he thought he didn't need them and those quack magazines said were dangerous, Anger that he might not live long enough to celebrate our 50th wedding anniversary, Anger that he might not live long enough to see the grandchildren grow up and have children of their own. This gut-wrenching, paralyzing anger lasted for several months. Regardless of all my efforts, I simply couldn't get past the anger.

What finally stopped the anger was the realization that this horrible prostate cancer had happened, we had to deal with it (not that we weren't anyhow), that the anger was totally destroying my inner peace, not to mention our relationship, and it wasn't helping anything in the situation. I hardly recognized myself anymore. I had to stop fighting and accept that what had happened, had happened. There was nothing I could do about it. I could either choose to be angry all the time, letting the anger eat me alive like a gangrenous injury, or I could choose to find the positives in this situation. Had I not always believed in the positives of every circumstance? Was I not a proponent of "life is what you make it?" I could choose to be angry, or choose to move on with life, to enjoy whatever time we would have, to live in the "now" of the moment, rather than festering, fussing and fuming all the time. There is still the frustration of his fervent belief in those quack magazines and self-medicating (all of which have proved to be harmful, but does he listen? Nooooooooo . . .), but since he stopped using credit cards, I don't have to worry so much about a strange package arriving in the mail once a week. Whether he wanted to or not, Tom had joined the "cancer club," and I was an associate member of the club no one really wants to join.

Around the same time, Rose (Miranda's grandmother), a high school classmate of Tom's, had also been undergoing a battle with throat cancer. She would go through several struggles while battling this type of cancer, including a laryngectomy (removal of the larynx or voice box and restructuring the neck area to separate the airway from the nose, mouth and esophagus), then infections, then more surgery to repair the opening in her throat where the prosthesis was to go, as well as procedures every three months to stretch her esophagus. Another high school classmate had bladder cancer. Another high school class-mate was also diagnosed with prostate cancer. The daughter of another high school classmate was diagnosed with breast cancer. The big "C" just seemed to be popping-up everywhere, surrounding Tom.

Tom was referred to a urologist, Dr. Rafid Yousif. Dr. Yousif radiates calm, confidence, compassion and competence and over time was always about a year ahead of the curve in terms of what would happen next. Dr. Yousif performed a biopsy. About six little snips were taken off the prostate. This was to determine Tom's Gleason Score. The Gleason Score is a convoluted mess, but it's very effective and a good predictor of prostate cancer and chances for survival. It looks at the patterns of cancer cells, which are then broken down into two differ-ent scales. Each pattern is rated from 1–5 and each scale gets one of those numbers. Generally speaking, if your *total* score is 5–6, it is clas-sified as a low-grade tumor. A score of 7 is classified as intermediate, and 8–10 is a high score. The score of 8–10 has an unfavorable out-look, with a strong correlation between the Gleason Score and death rate. The PSA number and the Gleason score are used in combination to determine a likely outcome of prostate cancer. Tom's Gleason Score was 4 on the first scale and 3 on the second, for a total score of 7 out of 10, which put him in the intermediate range. That, in combination with his PSA of 461.9, did not bode well for his prognosis. The cancer had metastasized into his bones and his lymph nodes. Tom was diagnosed as having Stage 4 metastatic prostate cancer (see the section on staging later in the book).

Where do you begin to even treat something like that? Because of Tom's prognosis, all treatments would be palliative in nature. His cancer was too far advanced for any type of radical treatment—radiation, implants, prostate removal or (shudder, shudder) castration. As it turns out, this type of cancer feeds on testosterone, so all the testosterone in his body had to be killed. Tom was put on female hormones to try and combat this, as well as monthly intra-venous Zometa for the bone cancer. He was also put on Casodex, Eligarde and Uroxatral. A few months later he was put on DES, Cytoxan, Prednisone and Warfarin (generic Coumadin). Because of the drugs he was taking, his cholesterol and triglycerides went up, so to combat that, he was given Simvastatin. Some of the drugs raised his glucose level, putting him at risk for diabetes. At some point, it was determined the Eligarde wasn't working, so he was changed to monthly injections of Lupron. It became a monthly balancing act to keep up with his physiological changes because of the treatment medications, and the additional medications needed to counteract the side effects of the primary medications he was taking.

My best friend, Linda Kent, was the first person I told (before Tom told me he didn't want anyone to know). Really, Linda deserves her own book about what a friend is; she has brought great joy to my life! If you look in any dictionary under "friend," I know it has to say, "See Linda Kent." We have known each other for 38 years. We have been through happy times and sad times, through good and bad times, through special magical times, through difficult life-changing times, through fun times (Linda and I taking turns praying to the "porcelain goddess" one night when we had too much fun) and professionally stressful times at work (after one particularly grueling day we left work, and made an all-nighter of it, ending up at some bar in Bitely. Those were the best nachos I have ever had and I don't even really like nachos.) She makes this incredible cheesecake. When I do something particularly stupid, she is the first one to point it out, but in such an unobtrusive and inoffensive, yet firm way, you know that particular behavior has to stop if you want to stay sane, a decent human being and live a long life. She is always one you can count on for good advice, unwavering loyalty, intuitive insights, genuine compassion and the greatest sense of humor you could ever imagine. With us, the laughter never ends.

So there was no one better to turn to than Linda, nor was there anyone other than Linda I wanted be with, when I got the news about Tom. I had to go to the pharmacy to pick up the first of what would prove to be several regular, mostly weekly, rounds of medicines for Tom. When I came out, much to my surprise and in answer to my silent prayers, Linda was there, waiting for me, with tears in her eyes as she gave me the best hug of my life.

We had to tell his family. Tom didn't want anyone to know, but the doctor ruled that out by saying at least Tom's kids and immediate family had the right to know. (And believe me when I tell you Tom is also not the least bit thrilled with this section of the book, but if "two have become one," my story is nothing without his story. Tom hasn't exactly given his blessing but he has grudgingly accepted that his story is necessary to be included in this book and has even gone so far as to suggest changes and more accuracy.) (Whew!) Tom refused to go to talk with his kids, so I went and met them at our usual restaurant in Battle Creek—Don Pablo's, a halfway point for all of us. His kids, Lori, Tom IV and Matt and our daughter-in-law, Michelle were told on what would have been my late Dad's 108th birthday. I took that as a good omen; my Dad was watching out for us, and things wouldn't be as bleak as they felt right then. As I spoke, I vividly remember Lori's hand shaking uncontrollably while she tried to take notes and sort through all the information we had to talk about. The faces of Tom, Matt and Michelle were in total shock and ghostly white as we went through how this all came about. Aside from Tom, their next biggest concern was: Did they tell their own kids? At that time, the grandkids ranged in age from 3 to 13. If so, what did they tell them? I didn't know what recommendations to offer, and apologized for having zero ideas. In reality, I hadn't even gotten that far in my thinking (but later in the book, we have provided some suggestions on how to talk with kids in age-appropriate language on such sensitive topics).

We had to tell his Mother, who at the time was 85. No parent wants to hear that his or her child might possibly pre-decease him or her. After the initial shock began to wear off, she took the news with her usual courage, grace, dignity, inner strength and common sense, and asked how she could help. She wanted and got my word that I would always—ALWAYS—tell her the complete truth about whatever was going on with her son, and would NOT sugar-coat any of it! I have, <u>bar none</u>, the WORLD'S BEST MOTHER-IN-LAW. Tom's three brothers and two sisters-in-law, Jack, Colleen, Dan, Gail and Tim, also had to be told. And then they told their children (much to Tom's cha-grin), all of whom were adults, many with their own children.

Tom really didn't want anyone to know, so to try to honor his wishes, I didn't tell my nieces for a long time. It was only after about a year, when I had "dropped off the map" that they asked me what was happening with me. The line they were walking was trying to respect my (our) privacy and yet manage their own concern for both Tom and me, still showing how much they cared and wanted to be there for both of us. Before I had told them, they had thought I was sick and withholding the information from them.

Even repeating the same information over and over brought no comfort, nor did the telling ever become any easier. Tom comes from a large and close family, so gradually the word spread, to cousins, aunts and uncles and their friends, much to his displeasure. (In fairness, the family and friends of a person with cancer also need their own support group as this disease runs its course.) I would run into Tom's family members in the grocery store, at a gas station or in a department store, and have to go through the same story again and again. It hurt even to breathe after awhile.

After the initial anger went away, emotions went for me from shock and numbness, to a different kind of anger, this time not blam-ing Tom (well, maybe a little), but the situation. <u>*NO!*</u> This was not how it was supposed to be. We were supposed to celebrate our 50th wedding anniversary, be in pretty good health, still have all of our mental faculties (good luck with that), surrounded by our many great-great grandchildren, not to mention the great-great-great-nieces and –nephews. Research became my focus to try and cope with this. My life-links also became family and friends, who helped with their senses of humor, their compassion, their understanding and their listening abilities. A good friend, Marc (another person that Linda, Ricardo, Pat and I "grew up together with" in the Lansing School District), had also been diagnosed with prostate cancer and became a wonderful sounding board.

Tom was referred to oncologist Dr. Carol Rapson, but she was out of the office when the appointment was scheduled, so we met Dr. Jason Beckrow. The first thing that went through my mind was: He's so young! Is he even through medical school yet?!? Yes, he was. He was up front about everything, including Tom's life span, estimated at being between three to five years, but could be as short as six months. However, he added, with medical advances, Tom's life span could be much longer. What we had to be careful of in all of these treatments was that Tom didn't become "hormone refractory"—his body didn't develop immunities to any of the drugs. If that happened, then there would have to be a search conducted to look for something else that might work to try and prolong his life. Dr. Beckrow had only been in practice about a week at that time, so Tom might have been his second patient ever.

It was important to me to also know the human being inside the doctor. Right away, we discovered we were both voracious readers and were going through similar quests in terms of spirituality (he was raised Catholic, and I grew up a kind of holy roller-Evangelical-Pentecostal-Baptist). Over time, we began swapping books to read and having incredible discussions about philosophical and spiritual issues. Kevin, one of the many exceptional nurses in the office, was also very well-read, so between the three of us, we never lacked for interesting topics about which to read and talk. When you're waiting for someone who is hooked up to an IV for hours on end, and you can't go anywhere, stimulating discussions are a must, if you are not getting caught up on your sleeping.

We asked how high a PSA score could go. All doctors are cagey about answering this. They mumble something, evade the topic, say "Ummmmm" a lot, then change the subject or rush off to see another patient. Tom happened to run into a man at the pharmacy who also had prostate cancer. They exchanged scores. (The typical man exchange—"My (whatever] is larger than your [whatever].") That man's PSA was over 1,000. He died about six months after the exchange of information. So if you were wondering how high a PSA score could go, it's at least 1,000, and I've heard rumors it can be 12,000. Tom's 461.9 seemed right then a blessing. It gave us hope for the future. In fairness, it's important to remember that with all medical tests and scores, each patient is an individual and one man's PSA of 12 might be significantly worse than Tom's 461.9. As the doctors and nurses say, "It's just a number." But it's an important number, and frightening, downright terrifying, to a layperson.

We sought a second opinion and after doing research on the Internet, discovered that, at that time, Memorial Sloan-Kettering (MSK) in New York City was ranked #1 in the nation. Our appointment was held on Tom's late Dad's birthday, so we considered that a good omen, too. There is no way (father) Tom would abandon his son. Tom had immediately started treatment upon the diagnosis of his cancer, and MSK was the only cancer treatment center that would look at a patient who had already started treatment. We drove the twelve hours to New York, taking all the X-rays, biopsy slides, doctors' reports and other histories. After consultation and reviewing everything, the oncologists ranked Tom's Gleason score as 9 out of 10, which was significantly worse than we were originally told; in one breath we went from "intermediate" to "high grade," with the least favorable outlook. We really didn't want to hear that. However, they did confirm the protocols Tom was undergoing to be the best possible treatment. There were no trials being conducted for which Tom qualified. They also recommended that if things took a nose-dive at some point, Dr. Kenneth Pienta at the University of Michigan was an excellent prostate cancer doctor and researcher, and was much closer to home than New York. When Tom and I left, we each had different viewpoints about the consultation. I had gone there to know more about the disease, and whether or not the protocols were the best available. Tom had gone there thinking he would be cured by the end of the day, or maybe the end of the week, and if not, there was surely a trial taking place that would cure him shortly. That is certainly understandable.

Treatment started, and one of the first things that happened was a "discussion" between two of the doctors about who would administer the medications. The primary reason for the debate (even though it was never stated) was that there would be money in the pockets of whichever doctor gave the medications. We weren't too concerned about who administered the drugs, but I made it clear Tom was NOT going to be caught in the crossfire of this skirmish, and that neither Tom nor I worshipped at the doctor altar. The drug administration issue was settled pretty quickly. After that, things went along pretty well. Tom tolerated the drugs, had absolutely no pain from the bone cancer, and was able to carry on his normal life. The only exception was that he couldn't lift more than 60 pounds because of the bone cancer. This restriction would make it difficult for him in his business; a great deal of the produce comes in boxes or bags that weigh 100 or more pounds. Tom was clearly going to need to rely on others at work.

We visited the oncologist once a month, the internal medicine doctor once every six months, and the urologist once a year like clockwork. Tom would get his treatments or medical updates, and then off we'd go until it was time for the next round of appointments.

In 2006, I started to cough. I attributed it to the "Michigan cough" and ignored it. It was a dry cough, not painful, and eventually it would go away. It always had. I was fatigued all the time, just a wee bit stressed out, and was also undergoing thyroid treatment so I ignored everything. I had been working hard to lose weight, so wasn't too concerned when the scales showed I had lost 81 pounds. In fact, I was delighted; I had never been in a size 4 in my life. Regardless of the cough and weight loss, I ignored it. I knew Tom had to be my primary focus. We were geared up for battle. This was not intended to be the act of a martyr, just a part of the sorting-out process for determining what priorities had to be sustained. A cough and weight loss were simply way at the bottom of the list.

In September 2006, a very close friend, Pat (a member of the group we all "grew up with" in the Lansing School District mentioned earlier), was diagnosed with CML Leukemia (Pat is the epitome of "unconditional love"). She was diagnosed on her grandson's first birthday. Another person had become a member of the cancer club. Pat is a couple of years younger than I. I had held her newborn first daughter, Alita (who was fascinated with my long red hair), and later her second daughter, Lilia, just after both of their births. The numbness within me continued to grow as Pat began her journey through cancer. Like Tom and me, Pat had never smoked, always ate good food, was not a drinker, was active (you should see her dance) and there was no history of cancer in her family (Unlike Pat, Tom's Mother had uterine cancer about 40 years ago, from which she has become a long-term survivor, and Tom's Dad, a multiple decade smoker, died from lung cancer).

A day before Thanksgiving, I was carrying down boxes of ornaments to decorate the Christmas tree, which I always start the day after Thanksgiving. There are 15 stairs in our house going from top to bottom. I tripped and fell down the entire flight of stairs, trying desperately not to break the fragile ornaments in the boxes. (You will be happy to know that effort was successful.) As I got up, I realized my ribs on the left side hurt a bit, but I didn't think anything about it. Maybe a little strain, maybe a bruise, maybe a fracture, but Christmas was coming. The house had to be cleaned from top to bottom and decorated; presents had to be bought and wrapped; candy had to be made (batches upon batches each of Irish Crème fudge, English Toffee and chocolate-covered cherries); kolaches and pies had to be made and frozen; cookies had to be baked; the silver had to be polished; kitchen cabinets had to be cleaned; there were parties to be attended; the house needed to be prepared for overnight guests, and all the normal festivities had to be scheduled.

Now, if you can believe this, in mid-December, Tom fell down the other stairs just six days before our 60-person Christmas party (we have two sets of stairs in the house). As a result, he had to have surgery on his ankle two days before our little party. (*Note to Self: Next house NO stairs!) He was completely homebound, in a wheelchair to get around, and had to sleep downstairs. The sofa bed had to be made up every night and taken apart every morning. A (male) friend came over and suggested that Tom should have a little bell to ring to summon me whenever he needed something. (The body has since been buried in the backyard.) Tom wisely thought twice about that little suggestion, and decided not to do it.

Our Christmas is always celebrated the Sunday before Christmas. We have Santa and Mrs. Claus come to the house for all the grandkids and great-nieces and –nephews. I make silk ribbon stockings for each of them that they use until they're 16, the last year they can sit on Santa's lap. The kids do their stockings first so they don't see Santa drive up in his white Oldsmobile. My cough was worse, my ribs still hurt, but it was nothing debilitating. That year we had 30 kids under the age of 16 to sit on Santa's lap. During this time, even the adults get to briefly feel like they are five years old and can once again, fall under Santa's magic spell. The kids all know the *real* Santa Claus comes to our house, and the ones in the stores are his helpers.

A couple of days after Christmas, when most of the house was cleaned, the shopping for next year's Christmas was started (love those 50% off sales), and all the decorations were put away, I went to the doctor because the ache in my side was still present, and so was the cough. My doctor of 24 years, internist Dr. Mark Mills, examined me; then he had an X-ray taken. Dr. Mills is an incredible doctor. He is kind, gentle, considerate, knowledgeable, a great listener and makes you feel like you are his only patient. Every question you ask he treats with respect and takes the time to explain things. The appointment was at 8:30 A.M. By 10:00, he was on the phone saying that the X-ray showed a "shadow" of a tumor that was quite large. He thought it might be lymphoma, but wanted to send me to several doctors and to get a variety of tests run. Oh, a tumor, which everyone knows means "a growth." That's o.k. Just a tumor . . . Everyone knows a growth can be removed, no worries. Everything's fine . . . Cough, ouch! Cough, ouch! Cough, ouch! At least there are no broken ribs, no pneumonia, no lung cancer, nothing dire—just a tumor. Simple, problem solved . . . It'll probably even be outpatient surgery.

In January, after several more X-rays to rule things out, it became apparent this was more than just a tumor. Dr. Mills asked me if I had a preference of oncologists, one I would specifically like to go to in order to find out what was really going on in my body. Of course, it had to be Dr. Rapson's office, with all of her great staff. Before the referral was made, we happened to have had an appointment with Dr. Beckrow for Tom. There was shocked disbelief on his face, and those of the staff, when they were told I might also have cancer.

Dr. Beckrow referred me to a pulmonologist, Dr. Gauresh Kashyup. He put me through this horrible lung test that involved being in this tiny enclosed chamber, then inhaling and exhaling all the air in and out of my lungs. Finally, you have to inhale and hold it for eons; your face turns purple and red and blue with the effort.

Now the rounds of tests started in earnest: one was a PET (Positron Emission Tomography) scan done at Michigan State University (incidentally, MSU has some of the most cutting-edge research being done in cancer). I asked why a PET scan and not an MRI (magnetic resonance imaging) or CT/CAT (computerized axial tomography) scan. The answer was that each test gave a different picture. A CT/CAT scan is basically a detailed X-ray of your organs or tissues in a three-dimensional cross section. An MRI is similar in that it also creates a three-dimensional cross-sectioned image of your tissues and organs. A PET scan looks at abnormal increases in sugar consumption by your body (cancer feeds on sugar and high fructose corn syrup), which can then be correlated to a CT scan, if necessary. An injection of a radioactive glucose would be given. Cancer cells grow rapidly, which means they need a lot of sugar so they gobble up the radioactive glucose. A PET scan can help diagnose whether you have a benign or a malignant tumor, as well as watch for recurring cancer and monitor how you have responded to the chemotherapy and/or radiation treatment(s). In my case, Dr. Beckrow needed to know the extent of the tumor and whether it was malignant or benign.

Ultimately, I was referred to a surgeon's office; his name was Dr. Divyakant Gandhi. He showed us one of the X-rays. The tumor went from my collarbone down to my diaphragm, and wrapped around my heart. "Media Stinum" (what I heard; it's really "mediastinum") was a new terminology, which had absolutely no meaning to me. **_CANCER_**!!! screamed my brain! Dr. Ghandi explained the mediastinum is the area between the lungs and includes the heart, the veins and arteries leading to the heart, the trachea, esophagus, the lymph nodes, and bronchi (the "tubes" that go from the trachea and deliver air to and from the lungs). Dr. Gandhi performed an outpatient surgical biopsy, which was just a little slit at the base of my throat, because the "growth" was so high up in my neck. The diagnosis came a few days later: *Nodular Sclerosis Hodgkin's Lymphoma.*

Dr. Beckrow then ordered a MUGA—**Mu**lti-**G**ated **A**cquisition— test to make sure my heart could tolerate chemo. I remember a large machine and several tests from different angles being conducted. I think I had to drink something so my heart would show up better, and then wait a couple of hours before the actual test was conducted. By now, with all the tests and procedures, either for Tom or for me, everything became a blur, one thing seamlessly morphing into another, one day after another with a medical something-or-other scheduled on the calendar. (Long after things slowed down a bit, I looked it up: a MUGA looks at how the heart is functioning; it is a moving film of how the heart beats. Radioactive Technetium 99 is injected into the bloodstream and becomes attached to red blood cells in the heart. A gamma camera then detects the Technetium 99 in the blood cells in the heart. The MUGA measures and monitors how well the heart is ejecting blood with each heart beat, especially in the left ventricular chamber. Since chemo can be hard on your body, the doctors need to make sure your heart is strong enough to tolerate it and also need a means to determine if or when chemo or other medications need to be stopped. This test is much more accurate than an echocardiogram and has the added benefit of being non-invasive.)

The next thing that had to happen was a bone marrow aspiration, which in contrast to the MUGA, was a vivid memory, forever etched in my brain. Will this hurt? I asked Dr Beckrow. No, I was assured. So, in I went to Dr. Ronald Horowitz at Sparrow Hospital in Lansing, who gave me a local anesthetic. Will this hurt? I asked. No, he kindly, gently, soothingly and confidently assured me. They all lied. It hurts!!! When Pat had one, she left fingernail scratches on Ricardo's arms. If any of you ever have to have one, remember, _none_ of the doctors involved have _ever_ had one, so regardless of what they say, GET KNOCKED OUT!!! (And you can feel free to tell them Doc Terryat said so.) For the other two bone marrow aspirations I had to have, being totally anesthetized is the only way to go. (This will be repeated later in case you didn't focus this time.) If you want, I can even give you the names of some of the amazing anesthetics they have available today. One of them left me grinning for over an hour when I came out of surgery, although the double vision took some getting used to for the first hour. It was a real disappointment to find out there was only one chocolate bar, not two.

As the word started to be spread that I had cancer (unlike Tom, I can't keep my mouth shut, and I realized and accepted I was going to need a tremendous support system), the love and compassion of family and friends was incredible. If you have cancer, you cannot get through it alone! You need the love, support, laughter, tears, anger, insights and opinions of everyone who is in your life or who comes into your life. It's not just you who has the cancer. All the people who are in your life, whether for 5 minutes or for 40 or 60 years, also have it. Their lives have been deeply impacted, too, and somehow, with everything you will encounter as a cancer patient, you must not ever let that fact get lost in your mind. You most likely will not be able to help those you love, except perhaps through the acknowledgement of what they must be going through with you. Let them know you understand.

It was at this time, one of my close friends said something that has stayed with me, and probably always will. Truthfully I can't remember if it was Pat or Rose. The expression that got carved into my brain and my heart was: "**_I have cancer, but cancer doesn't have me_**." That also helped me realize if I was going to get through this, I would have to ruthlessly weed out of my life those people who were "downers." This doesn't mean that peoples' initial shock and disbelief couldn't get talked about. We all needed to do that. What it did mean was that anyone with a negative or depressing outlook on life _as a lifestyle_ had to go. NOTHING of a negative aura or energy could come into my space. To fight this disease meant having people around me who would look at the positives and offer unconditional support, being a part of a cheerleading squad, so to speak, and NOT walk around saying "Oh, poor you." Wallowing in self-pity was not going to help. It was NOT "poor me"—this was going to end up being a gift, a blessing, in some way or another. And people have to be able to crack jokes about cancer so it does not feel so overwhelming. (For example, "Just think of all the money you will save not having to have haircuts or getting your hair colored!") Oops, you may need to be sensitive about your timing with some of the jokes I have heard, but for me, laughter has always been good for any of the dark days that tend to come along periodically.

On January 21, 2007, I got an e-mail from Jean in London, our travel friend. Her daughter, Nicky, 21 years old, was diagnosed with a rare form of ovarian cancer called *dysgerminoma*. Nicky had discovered the lump on Christmas Day while taking a shower. She underwent surgery to remove a large tumor and her right ovary. The surgery had gone well, and she was now scheduled to undergo massive doses of chemotherapy. ". . . cancer does NOT have her."

I had to have another outpatient surgery to install an infusaport so the chemo could be administered. Dr. Gandhi again did the honors. An infusaport is a little metal and plastic gadget that gets inserted into the upper left portion of your chest. It has a long tube that goes directly into your heart. Over time, that became important because you didn't have to have IVs in your arms during the administration of chemo. There is more mobility, which you need—with all the fluids going into your body, you do have to frequently go to the bathroom. (Why, in books and movies, except for *The Goonies*, do the characters never have to go to the bathroom?) Even with me having TB (Teacher's Bladder—the ability to go all day without having to go the bathroom), I still had to go a couple of times during the treatments. An IV would constitute the risk of getting dislodged, and then have to be repeatedly reinserted. (As an aside, what was amazing was how my body coped with that foreign contraption. Additional veins formed to carry the blood in and out of my heart. They would be unsightly if you are wearing a bathing suit, but definitely a lifesaver. Good thing my two-piece bathing suit days are long gone.) What I didn't know at the time was that there could be adverse side effects with an infusaport—but mine gave me absolutely no problems. Another friend had problems from day one. I subsequently learned that each doctor has his or her own opinion about the advisability of using an infusaport.

The infusaport was installed (again, outpatient surgery) on Monday, February 13. Tuesday, February 14, Valentine's Day, was my first chemo session. I was to have five hours of chemo every two weeks for six months, from February through July. Lynette, another of the compassionate and competent nurses in Dr. Rapson's office, did the honors and walked me through what was going to happen. Tom and I had joint infusions that day—Tom, his Zometa and other drugs; I had chemotherapy. Dr. Beckrow stood well over six feet tall, was on the cutely chubby side, and had a puckish grin on his face all the time; I thought he should dress up as a cherub, carry around a little bow and arrow and wear a diaper. I was sure I could find some wings. He turned bright red and said he wanted nothing to do with it! We all joked about bringing in candles and violins to enhance the ambience of our "togetherness" in cancer. They put us in a private room and drew the curtains just in case we got to feeling frisky, but they said definitely no loud kissing, moaning and/or slurping was to occur. They needn't have worried. They gave me great drugs to combat the nausea, but the chemo was exhausting. And, like Alexis, I had to learn the hard way to take the anti-nausea pills *as prescribed* once I got home.

At the time of diagnosis, I had naturally curly, long "strawberry blonde" hair that came down almost to my waist. At some point I could lose all my hair because of the chemo, so I decided it would be less traumatic to pull out wads of short hair rather than long. I had it cut to just below my ears and decided to donate the rest of it to Locks of Love. I kept it initially, because if my hair grew back in a different color, which was possible, I wanted to be able to take it to the hairdresser to match the color. (Vanity, thy name is woman.) And besides, maybe, just maybe, my hair wouldn't fall out at all, but even if it didn't, short hair would be easier to take care of while going through chemo.

The kind of chemo I had was called ABVD, which stands for Adryamycin, Bleomycin, Viablastine and Dacarbazine (aren't you glad you asked?). The great anti-nausea drugs were Emend, Aloxi (given through IV), Kytril and Compazine. A steroid, called Decadron, was also given. The day after each chemo session I got two injections: Neulasta, because of the low white cell count, and Aranesp, for the low hemoglobin. Because the chemo drugs can cause constipation, I took Senokot under Dr. Beckrow's care (you do have to be careful how much you take). All vitamin supplements I had been taking to keep myself healthy (including Vitamin C) were discontinued, because they conflicted with the chemo. The only ones allowed were calcium tablets with Vitamin D. Later on, magnesium oxide and potassium gluconate were added, because chemo depleted these nutrients from my system. Warfarin (generic Coumadin) was prescribed to keep my blood thin and slippery to prevent clots with the infusaport. I had to be careful not to cut myself and not to get bruises. A bloody nose could be dangerous. My eyelashes and eyebrows fell out, as did the hairs on my body. The good thing with all the hairs on my body falling out was I didn't need to shave my legs or underarms. (Or is that TMI—"Too Much Information"?) But the hair on my head stayed right there; just could not believe it.

For the first week after each chemo session, I could hardly get out of bed the next morning. This usually lasted a week or so, and by the second week, my energy would start to come back. All the bedrooms in our house are on the second floor. One time during the week of chemo, I was so exhausted I couldn't make it upstairs into the bedroom, and I fell asleep on the hall floor. I could drive in for treatment and back home (probably shouldn't have done that), but was then totally exhausted. Some days I'd try to go into work. I'd no sooner get there, than I'd have to turn around and go right back home. Work, and having things to do, was important for me. There was no time to really dwell on what was happening. I could stay focused and positive.

Eating was another challenge. By nature I'm an "opportunistic grazer." I was once kicked out of an all-you-can-eat place. As long as food didn't have anchovies, oysters, scallops or clams on it or in it, any food was fair game (remind me sometime to tell you about *barbacoa*, a Mexican dish that is wonderful; it's a cow's head on the center of the table. . . . Never mind, I just did.) I had to learn to eat smaller portions and several times a day. Sometimes the food would just "stick" in my throat, and I'd have to wait a bit before having another bite.

Sleep was now always interrupted. When or if there was any real sleep, it was for short periods of time. There were nights when I'd get up around 2:30 A.M., craving a baked potato with a pound of real butter and a ton of sour cream. Thank goodness microwaves had been invented; I could never have waited for a potato to bake in a conventional oven.

And then, what we had dreaded happened. Tom became hormone refractory. A referral was made to Dr. Kenneth Pienta, Professor of Internal Medicine and Urology, Associate Dean for Clinical and Translational Research at the Comprehensive Cancer Center at the University of Michigan. He was the one who came highly recommended by Memorial Sloan-Kettering. We met with him and nurse practitioner, Nancy Egerer, and Tom was taken off some meds and put on new ones. Both Dr. Pienta and Nancy were fighters and would stop at nothing to help Tom. In time, I would also discover that no matter how much research I did, Dr. Pienta always was familiar with not only the research but most likely knew the researcher who was involved.

Finally, after about five months of chemo, in June, my hair started to fall out in handfuls. In total, it took about three weeks for it all to come out and leave me bald. But with that loss came the good news: the PET scan done in June showed the tumor was almost completely gone. Radiation was the next step to once and for all completely kill this cancer. I was sent to a radiation oncologist, Dr. David Debiose. This was another interesting experience.

We first met Vicky, the cheerful receptionist who efficiently took care of things. Next, we met Melissa, the radiation oncology nurse (she would eventually be diagnosed with breast cancer). She was funny, and eased our concerns right away, all the while taking care of business. Dr. Debiose spent about an hour with us going through what the current PET scan showed and what the radiation procedures would be. We had ample time to ask questions and were not rushed. (*Note to All: Always, always, always have questions written down before going into any doctor for any reason; leave ample space to write down the answers to your questions.*) He explained that first of all, a form would be made that would cradle my head so it wouldn't move while the radiation was being administered. I would have to have "tattoos" put on my body so that every time I had radiation, the radiation beams could be lined up to go to the proper places. My body had to be positioned exactly right each time, and both the form and the tattoos would help with this. I would have 18 consecutive days of radiation except for the weekends. Because the radiation would be aimed from close to my throat down to my diaphragm, Tom was concerned whether my salivary glands would be affected. The answer was "probably not." There was the likelihood I would develop radiation burns and have difficulty swallowing, but there were medications to help with that.

Next, I met Ken, one of the radiation techs. Ken is a friendly, put-you-at-ease kind of guy. As it turns out, we both love to cook, so over time, we were able to exchange recipes. The form that would cradle my head had to be mixed up from a powder. I laid my head on the table and the form . . . um . . . formed around my head. The form was warm to the touch, and if it hadn't been over 90 degrees outside that day, it would have been quite pleasant. Air conditioning is truly a blessing.

The tattoos came next. Ken had to make little nicks in my skin and then fill them in with black ink. The size of the nicks was about the diameter of a sharp pencil point. I had one by my throat, and 2 on each side by my ribs. To do this, I had to be fully uncovered from the waist up and have my arms spread out on that hard, narrow table. (Trust me, boobs this old should never be in that position.) Ken got up on the table and, aiming down, used a digital camera to take pictures of my front. Ken tried to be nonchalant about it, with an 'I've-done-this-a-million-times-before-no-worries' kind of attitude, but it was still a bit disconcerting. After the 3rd or 4th picture, I told him that if these pictures somehow ended up on the Internet for sale, I wanted 50% of the proceeds.

While the tattooing wasn't really painful, if I had ever considered having some of those glorious tattoos put on my body, my appetite for that has been completely eliminated. There is no way I would ever put myself through any more needle pricks than absolutely necessary, except for future medical procedures. I kept wondering how people got their whole bodies tattooed or even a shoulder or with something as small as a flower. Please forgive me, but deep down inside, I think anyone who would put him- or herself through this voluntarily, must surely be masochistic, or drunk.

The day finally came to start radiation. We had just come back from our annual week-long trip with four of the grandsons. I showed up promptly at 7:00 A.M. in order to be the first appointment of the day every day so I wouldn't be waiting and waiting and waiting for my turn. Ken, once again, did the honors. There was radiation aimed at my front in six different sections and one radiation burst through my back. One burst lasted as long as 13 seconds (by my count—one chim-pan-zee, two chim-pan-zee . . .); another burst was only about 3 seconds. Ken told me not to move while the radiation was being administered. Dear God, please don't let me sneeze or have to scratch any place (but that wasn't nearly as bad as the PET scan which takes 25 minutes and you also can't move a muscle).

I did develop radiation burns on my front and back, but while it was a little unsightly, it wasn't hideous or really very painful. The medicine that was administered, Xclair, for the burns worked wonders. I also developed the inability to swallow for a few days, but again, a medicine, #675 Lidocaine (I wonder why not #674 or #676?), helped me swallow and I only lost about five pounds. The burns cleared up quickly and when my swallowing returned, so did my appetite.

In September I had another PET scan. The tumors were really shrinking, and were almost totally gone. Was this going to mean I am a cancer survivor?

It was during this period of time I began to realize how much cancer had been a gift for me. Eventually, I would identify or become aware of 9 reasons for this, and I'm still looking. The nine reasons I have found are described near the end of this book.

By November, I was feeling great. My energy level was returning (although an afternoon nap was still a requirement on most days; thanks to Rose, I was prepared for this). I was able to work some 16-hour days on occasion and not be totally whacked the next day. I could take grandkids, two great-nieces and one great–nephew on adventures. In short, the world was a beautiful place. All my blood work started coming back in great shape. There was only the PET scan left to do in November confirming how well things were going, and all of us—doctors, nurses (Lynette, Amanda, Kevin, Julie, Gretchen, Michelle, Katrinka), Sue the amazing, incredible, comforting and friendly scheduler, Helen and Margie the billing clerks, Shirley the receptionist, Linda the phlebotomist, friends and family—thought we had this thing licked!

Along with the "ups" in early November, 2007, in the on-going cancer saga, there was also a big "down". A friend and another Lansing School District colleague, Rod Doig, in his 40s, died from cancer after a heroic battle, one that had included several remissions.

Shortly after Rod's death, I walked into the MSU PET scan department ready to take on the world. I knew there was no way the cancer had returned; I felt too good. It was time to get on with my life.

So, it was with a sense of confidence in mid-November that I returned to Dr. Beckrow to get the good news of my recent PET scan. My hair was finally starting to come back in—but it was brown! *BROWN*! It had taken me my whole life to make peace with being a redhead, and now it comes back in <u>*BROWN*</u>?!? The good news was that my hair was still naturally curly and thick, so that was o.k. Hello, hair dye (except I found out I couldn't dye my hair right away with any type of coloring because of the potentially cancer-causing chemicals.) It was a couple of weeks before my birthday, a milestone birthday, the si . . . six . . . the s-word birthday. Dr. Beckrow was unexpectedly solemn when we came into the examining room. Not a good sign . . . .

The cancer had metastasized, he gently explained. It was now below my diaphragm, with additional tumors by my right lung, kidney, liver, and back again underneath my heart. It was unknown whether it was the same cancer or a different cancer. It had metastasized way too quickly, especially with all the chemo and radiation that had been administered. We discussed options. Dr. Beckrow said we could wait until after another biopsy and an official diagnosis was made of the type of cancer and even wait another two or three months after that to decide what I wanted to do. If it was lymphoma again, he also suggested another option be a part of treatment, a stem cell transplant, after additional chemo. The decision was almost instantaneous . . . definitely chemo <u>AND</u> the stem cell transplant. Let's get this show on the road—the sooner the better. After all, I have a lot of life yet to live!

So another bone marrow aspiration was done, and I was out like a light—no local anesthetic this time. The only good news from the bone marrow aspiration was that the cancer hadn't metastasized into my bones. Another biopsy was ordered to take place. This time I could not receive an anesthetic. I had to be wide awake, because during the type of ultrasound I had to have in order to do the biopsy, and to help them find where they had to insert the needle, I had to be fully conscious and able to follow directions *(something I don't do well even under ordinary circumstances)* about my breathing—to breathe different ways and to hold my breath upon command.

Before going in for the newest procedure, I learned about Alexis and the possibility she might have breast cancer. For a moment, my heart nearly stopped beating, and I had trouble getting a breath. Regrettably, because of where I was in terms of re-diagnosis and treat-

ment, I would not be able to be as much of a support to either of them
as they had been for me, except emotionally, of course, and to be one
of their cheerleaders. The good news was that Alexis and Andrea had
each other and their daughter, and my other niece, Monica, would also
step in to help. I knew, without a doubt, she would fight along side
them, just as hard as Andrea and Alexis would be doing.

Dr. "Mitch" Mitcherson performed my biopsy. He is a highly
skilled surgeon and was very funny. And so young! When I looked at
Dr. Mitcherson and reflected on Dr. Beckrow and all the other doctors
I had had, they were all so young! They looked like twelve-year-olds.
*Why is it when I was growing up, all doctors looked as if they were
older than dirt, as they should, but now, they look young enough to
literally be my sons?* Something is surely wrong with this picture. I
know it can't be me!

I was horribly nervous before the procedure and asked again if I
couldn't be totally "out" for this. The first bone marrow aspiration
done with a local anesthetic was still fresh in my memory, and for the
other biopsy I was "out." Really, "out" is the only way to travel. Both
Dr. Mitcherson and the nurse said that with all the drugs they were
going to give me, I truly wouldn't care about anything. They were
right. I could get used to living my life like that. Wa-hooooooo! Talk
about taking a trip and never leaving the farm! They were *incredible*
drugs! At that point, I clearly understood Dow Chemical's old adver-
tisement: "Better Living through Chemistry."

Dr. Mitcherson had great difficulty in getting a large enough sample for the biopsy because of the locations of the tumors, but he persevered. The needle had to be placed just so, I had to hold my breath just
so ("not so deep a breath" or "deeper breath" or "exhale completely
and hold it" or "I said a *shallow* breath, dammit!"). He had a pleasant, gentle voice and when he said," Holditholditholditholditholdit" I
didn't mind too much. But talk about waiting to exhale!!!

Just after Thanksgiving and my s-word birthday, we met with Dr.
Beckrow. The biopsy confirmed it was lymphoma again, but this time
a whole different chemotherapy regimen had to be implemented. I
would have to be in the hospital for this next round of chemo so it
could be administered 24 hours a day for five days, once in January,
2008, and then, again in February. It would be a much more aggressive
treatment this time. I told Dr. Beckrow that I simply couldn't be in the
hospital for five days, and that I would stay for three. And was it o.k.

for me to take my laptop, not only to be able to get some of my work completed, but also to be able to have e-mail so I would not feel so isolated? (Yes.)

In early December, I had to go to the Karmanos Cancer Center in Detroit to meet with their doctors to see about a stem cell transplant. It was my last and only hope. If the stem cell transplant wasn't successful, or if I was not deemed eligible to receive one, my life would be considerably shorter. With the original diagnosis of lymphoma, my odds of survival were about 90%. With the metastasis, those odds were cut by one third, to a high of about 60%, or to as low as 35%. That was certainly a wide range of difference; I really could not understand why the odds were so disparate. Actually, I liked the 90% odds much better. But, if the stem cell transplant was successful, there were hopes for TOTAL REMISSION! Now that was something I could live with!

The doctor I saw in December was internationally renowned, Dr. Voravit Ratanatharathorn, the clinical director of the Karmanos Cancer Institute stem cell transplant program, and leader of its bone marrow transplant (BMT) team. Everyone calls him Dr. Voravit. Dr. Voravit was responsible for developing the BMT program at Karmanos in 1980, as well as the one at the University of Michigan. The Stem Cell Coordinator was Anne Marie Campbell. She became a tremendous ally and a great source of information and comfort. At the first meeting, Dr. Voravit was questioning whether I actually had lymphoma, because people "my age" usually do not get lymphoma. He was also concerned about whether I could tolerate a stem cell transplant at "my age." At that point in time, stem cell transplants weren't normally done on people "my age"—over the age of 55. I told him I wasn't 55—I had just celebrated my 22nd annual 39th birthday so there should be no worries. He was not amused.

We also met Simon, the oncological pharmacist. He originally came from England, so we spent the first hour talking about places we all had loved. After an hour, they finally came to find him to counsel other patients and we still had to go through the drug list and what would happen while I was, as Simon says, "in hospital" for the stem cell transplant. He too, is a voracious reader, so we exchanged names of books that we each had enjoyed.

Another battery of tests was given. Finally, Dr. Voravit was convinced I did indeed have lymphoma, and could "probably" tolerate a stem cell transplant quite well, even at "my age." He said that my general health condition did not reflect someone of "my age," and that I appeared younger. I decided not to remind him about my many 39th birthdays.

We also discussed my wearing contact lenses. Dr. Voravit was adamant they not be worn during the stem cell transplant because of the extreme risk of infection should the lenses not be cleaned properly. This would be a problem for me. I'm legally blind without them, and would not be able to do my work for the Michigan Department of Education (MDE). We finagled around about this for some time, and then Dr. Voravit decided since I was no longer an irresponsible youth, that if I promised to completely sterilize my hands before applying the cleaning solution, someone "my age" would probably make sure the lenses were cleaned properly. He also concluded if the drops for the dry eyes from the chemo could be in individual packets so the risk of infection from using the same bottle was eliminated, it would probably be all right for me to put in my lenses. Back I went to Dr. Ken Marton, my absolutely wonderful eye doctor for about 30 years, who had the perfect solution for the dry eyes. Problem solved. While I may seem to be making light of this process, it was—no fooling—a real concern. Dr. Voravit was simply doing his usual magnificent job of assuring complete success of the stem cell transplant. As an aside, had I had to have a donor for the stem cell transplant, the odds are I wouldn't have been able to wear my contacts. The restrictions would have been much more stringent.

We went to Karmanos on the Saturday before New Years. I had to learn to give myself Neupogen shots. As a result of this process, I learned I could never become a drug addict. *(Do you see all the positives that are coming out of this? If ever I had wondered about becoming a drug addict, now I know my response.)* Tom and I went down to Karmanos for the 7:30 A.M. appointment so I could learn to give myself shots. I'm not a crier by any stretch of the imagination, but this truly frightened me. I cried when Anita, the kind, gentle, understanding, soothing, incredibly patient nurse, put the needle in my hand. I cried when I learned how to "prep" the needle. I cried when I had to take the needle and place it over my thigh (the other option was my abdomen, but that really freaked me out, even though she said it would hurt less). My hand shook while I tried to steady it. I knew I had to be successful the first time (although I had primed several friends at home to be on hand if I couldn't do it). Finally, I took a deep breath, *closed my eyes* and plunged the needle into my own thigh.

It didn't hurt! It did NOT hurt! It was like a little mosquito bite. Anita was right! It didn't hurt! But even so, I hated doing it and would be glad when I wouldn't have to do it again. I felt deep empathy for people, especially children, who were diabetics and had to do this all the time. This became an incentive for me to keep my weight down and my exercise up. The Neupogen shots, 960 mcg, had to be given every twelve hours on the dot for three days. I had to get my blood tested every day (another poke of a needle) for those three days to make sure the shot was increasing my white blood cell count and priming the stem cells to be available. (As an aside, each of these shots costs $6,000.00. Blue Cross/Blue Shield wouldn't pay for it *because it was self-administered.* Would they rather pay for hospital staff to administer the shots, which would significantly increase the costs? And we wonder why our health care system is in such a mess? And for heaven's sake, please don't suggest the federal government run health care—they can't even balance the budget, let alone live within a budget like the rest of us mere mortals have to do. Fortunately, the staff at Karmanos was able to find a way to fund the shots. They were magnificent. In fairness, I should also say that BC/BS did pay the entire amount for the stem cell transplant—about $150,000, for which I am extremely grateful. What I keep questioning though, is their reasoning ability and common sense. Wait until we get to the part about the dental work and the kiddie vacs.)

All I could say was, "I was glad this old year was almost over; it was definitely NOT one for the record books." And I was absolutely sure the New Year would be better.

On January 2, I went to Karmanos to have the stem cells withdrawn. Fortunately for the stem cell transplant, I was able to be an "autologous" donor—I could donate my own cells. In this I was lucky. A huge percentage of people have to find a donor, which most frequently means long waits to find a match, high rates of rejection and life-threatening infection. (*PLEASE– IF YOU OR YOUR FRIENDS AND FAMILY ARE BETWEEN THE AGES OF 18–60, PLEASE-PLEASE-PLEASE-PLEASE-PLEASE BECOME DONORS. THERE ARE SO, SO MANY PEOPLE IN NEED AND WAITING—YOU TRULY CAN SAVE LIVES! IT'S A SIMPLE, PAINLESS PROCEDURE—A Q-TIP TO SWAB THE INSIDE OF YOUR MOUTH. THAT'S IT. MORE ON THIS LATER.*)

We went to the 10th floor at Karmanos where they have the "apheresis" unit. There were eight beds, all to be filled that day with people who either needed a stem cell transplant, or were going to be donors. My nurses were Monique and Erica, both of whom lived in Windsor, Ontario, Canada (really not that far—just across the bridge, but it sounded a long way away; it's another country, for Pete's sake), and commuted every day to/from work. During lunch, Steve took over monitoring the machine. I hope the description below doesn't gross you out, but it was a fascinating procedure. Having so much going on at once took away the fear of the unknown and instead, became a great learning experience. (As Marc always says, ". . . how the problem gets defined dictates the solution.")

We got started at 8:00 A.M. A harpoon (or so it looked) to withdraw the blood was inserted into the vein in the crook of my right arm. Another needle was inserted into the vein in my left arm to return the blood. Fortunately I have large veins—as one nurse said, she could stand in the doorway and still hit my veins (poor Tom—he has such tiny veins that also roll; it usually takes three or four or even seven jabs when he has to have blood work done; one time it took 45 minutes to find a vein). The machine that separates your stem cells from your regular blood isn't all that big, but it is a complicated machine. And it's a very finicky machine that has to be monitored constantly. Once the blood is withdrawn, it goes through tubes, around a coil, through another part of the machine that actually does the withdrawing of the stem cells, and then the rest of the blood goes back into your left arm. You have to keep your right arm absolutely, completely, entirely, totally, and unequivocally, you-betcha, uh huh, STILL, or it throws the machine into a conniption fit. The stem cells actually are on the top of the tube and have to be siphoned off and placed into a little plastic bag. They are salmon- or light-peach- colored.

Lunch was one sandwich with a see-through sliver of turkey and no condiments. I didn't know anyone could slice meat that thin—I held it up and you really could see through it. But, I suppose beggars shouldn't be choosers. At least the sandwich was already cut in half, so I didn't have to negotiate trying to cut it.

About 3:00, the "bag" lady (the one who collects the stem cells and takes care of them while they are frozen, waiting to be used) came in to collect the three bags that had been filled. Then, she had to run tests to make sure there were enough stem cells available to do the transplant. Because the machine had been acting-up all day, there was some concern there weren't enough stem cells. We talked about whether to be disconnected from the apheresis machine and come back the next day, or to just keep going. I asked if it was possible to just keep going, even though by then I was exhausted. The thought of going back home and then coming back the next day after another 1-1/2 hour drive one way, and being harpooned all over again was NOT appealing. They said they would keep going until 7:00 or 8:00 that evening just to see what would happen (some people have needed 16 bags of stem cells to have an adequate amount, because stem cells most usually exist in very small numbers in the blood). If there still weren't enough stem cells, there would be no other choice but to come back the next day. And I'd have to give myself another set of those Neupogen shots. I can't tell you how excited I was after hearing that.

At 4:00, the bag lady came rushing back to the room. At this point, about a half of bag #4 had been filled. She said, "Stop! Stop! We have more than enough stem cells." Upon hearing her, I envisioned myself with a huge bag of fireworks to set off in celebration! Instead, I just let out a huge sigh of relief! Because my arm had been in one position for more than eight hours, it took several minutes before I could actually bend it. I was so tired, and was ready to go home.

Now, keep in mind, my husband is a good man, but there are times he simply doesn't seem to use a lot of common sense. When we got out to the car, he had decided he wanted to go sightseeing in Detroit (he is famous for going on these "wild goose chases" at the most inappropriate times). He wanted to look at all the neat buildings (Detroit does have some incredible architecture). Needless to say, after a few choice words, he decided that he could sightsee another time.

A week later, I was at Sparrow Hospital in Lansing for more chemo. This type of chemo was called ICE—Ifosfamide, Carboplatin, and Etoposide plus Mesna (I'm so glad they thought to include Mesna, whatever that is). The same anti-nausea shots and pills were also administered, along with drugs to combat potential fever, a real risk with this type of chemo. The great thing about being in Sparrow Hospital for the around-the-clock chemo (apart from the nursing staff, who were absolutely wonderful to me) was their food—it was amazing. They have a menu you can pick and choose from, so even when you don't feel like eating, you have something that might appeal to you. And, as a side cost-containment benefit, there was less waste because you were eating something you really wanted or at least could tolerate. Rumor has it the chef at Sparrow had come from a really good restaurant. My system tolerated the drugs very well, no nausea, no other side effects, so the tempo of administering them could be increased. What had to be watched was my temperature, to make sure it did not spike. Since my immune system was now practically non-existent, I understood this was a real danger. And I stayed in the hospital three days, not the five days the doctor said it would take.

Everything was going well. I was quite tired, but still able to do things. And then my temperature spiked two days later, which meant another couple of days in the hospital to get it under control. *(Note to All: Have someone contact your doctor to call ahead to reserve the room in emergency—you get right in.)*

From January 31 to February 10, additional Neupogen shots were administered every day to raise the white blood cell count. This time they were administered by one of the nurses at Dr. Rapson's office, or during the weekend, a Sparrow Hospital lab technician gave the injections.

My hair fell out much more quickly this time. By the third week in January, I was completely bald. When I woke up in the morning, my pillow would be covered in hair. Since it was wintertime, flannel sheets were on the bed; you can imagine what a mess that made! I had to be careful washing my hair so it wouldn't go down the drain and plug it up. People asked me why I didn't simply shave it off and be done with it. I think it was just because I was curious what it would be like this time. How long would it take? Would it come out in splotches, or evenly? Would any remain? Near the end, I was left with a little patch of three or four wisps in the front-center of my forehead. I had not realized what an incredible amount of hair there is on our heads. Even losing it as quickly as I was, it still took about a week to become completely bald.

By February, when it came time to have the second round of chemo, I asked Dr. Beckrow if he could speed up the insertion of the drugs so I could go home sooner. He started out trying a little at first, with the normal wait times between sessions. Then, toward the end, it was one right after the other, rather than having to do all of the waiting between units. There weren't any additional side effects, so once again, my system had tolerated it quite well. (That's not to say it would be the same experience for someone else.) I was still in the hospital just a couple of hours shy of three days. And this time, my temperature did not spike.

Then suddenly, in mid-February, about two weeks before entering Karmanos, Tom developed a blood clot in his right leg that went from his ankle to his groin. This was caused, in part, from the medications he had to take. Dr. Pienta had told us the previous August at our first appointment with him that blood clots were a possibility, and that it was going to be absolutely necessary for Tom to exercise. Not being fond of exercise and not feeling particularly well, Tom became somewhat of a couch potato between August and February, which, of course, helped lead to the formation of the blood clot. Because of all the drugs I was on, as well as all the chemo I had had, my immune system was really compromised. I had to be careful not to catch a cold, and not to be exposed to any germs or diseases. This meant I shouldn't have gone with Tom to the hospital, because of—ironically—the exposure to germs that large numbers of people can carry. Once again, Tom would find himself housebound for a couple of weeks, and he had to keep his leg elevated. And once again, wisely, he decided not to get a little bell in case he needed something.

With my immune system compromised, I could not take any of my grandkids or great-nieces and –nephews on adventures, or attend their birthday parties. It also meant I couldn't go with Alexis to any of her appointments, if she had wanted me to. Whenever I went out in public (to the grocery store, for example, at 4:00 A.M., when there weren't many people around), I had to wear a mask and sterilize the handle and tops of the shopping carts to prevent any likelihood of transference of germs or disease. When the day came for Alexis's double mastectomy, I had to stay home. The waiting was interminable. When Andrea's phone call finally came, telling me Alexis had done well in surgery, you can't imagine the relief we all felt. Of course, there was no other oncologist for her to go to other than Dr. Rapson.

Are you getting bored yet? O.K., O.K.! I'll speed things up. But just remember—when it comes time for you to write your story, you will also think every event is critical for you to capture all that is so fascinating about what has happened to you. It will never occur to you that everyone will not be standing in line, having waited all their lives, just to hear it. Well, maybe they will be!

On Thursday and Friday, February 28 and 29, I had to go to an oncological dentist, Dr. Lynne Moseley, at Karmanos. She and her staff, Donna and Hanan, are amazing. Dr. Moseley is the first dentist ever in my life with whom I haven't been afraid. The X-rays showed I had at least 20 cavities from the chemo, and had to have three teeth extracted because there were abscesses. (The stem cell transplant would have been delayed if there were any kind of infection.) It was either have the teeth extracted and give the infection time to drain, or wait to have root canals done. I didn't want to postpone the stem cell transplant. Blue Cross/Blue Shield didn't cover the teeth extractions, either, even though Dr. Moseley found something in the BC/BS hand-book for physicians that said they could. But—they did, as I mentioned earlier with gratitude, cover the cost of the stem cell transplant.

On Monday, March 3, the day after our wedding anniversary, and the day before my admission into Karmanos, I had to have a PICC line inserted. (That was also the day BC/BS decided to cancel my insurance; turned out they hadn't posted the check that had been sent to pay the monthly invoice.) "PICC" stands for a "peripherally inserted central catheter." The infusaport was not usable to administer the stem cells— the PICC line had a wider tube. They were going to use Lidocaine to deaden the area to insert the PICC line. The tube went into the periph-eral vein, inside the fleshy part of my upper left arm (that could have been a struggle, let me tell you!) and was fed into a large vessel near my heart. In one of life's many ironies, I was originally going to have a PICC line installed to administer the chemo rather than an infusaport—until it was explained to me that the PICC lines often had to be reinserted about once a month. Hello, infusaport! For the PICC line to be installed, the nursing staff trussed me up in a sheet, with only my head and upper arm exposed. A monitor was placed above the out-patient surgical bed so I could watch the whole thing. It was fascinat-ing to watch the line get inserted, how it was moved to negotiate the veins, and finally to the vessel where it needed to be. The surgical staff wasn't sure I would be able to drive afterward, so Linda had volun-teered to come with me, and took the day off work to do so. As it turned out, I was able to drive home. (And again, with our bodies being the wonderful and amazing machines they are, small blood ves-sels eventually formed around the site where the PICC line was installed to help carry the blood.)

Finally, the day came when I was to be admitted into Karmanos: Tues-day, March 4, 2008. When it came time to get me to Karmanos, Tom still couldn't drive, so long-time friend David Callaghan and his partner drove us to Karmanos. David, a couple of years younger than I, had just had a stroke the month before, and was now walking with a cane. But he seemed more than willing to be of help to us, and for both of us, it was great to have friends along.

The intake nurse was Tania, who has since become a good friend and *"mi hijita"* (my daughter). She gave me the pick of rooms available, and because I needed to use my laptop for the work I was doing for the MDE, I got the only room with a desk. A good omen!

Dr. Voravit said I would be in the hospital for at least four weeks, maybe longer. I said three weeks. (More positive thinking, a goal for which to aim. Goals and milestones became important during this process.) At Karmanos I had to have another six days of around-the-clock chemo called BEAM (snappy acronyms for all three of these types of chemos, aren't they?)—BCNY (Carmustine), Etoposide (VP-16), Ara-C (Cytarabine) and Melpholan (Aekevan). They also administered DMSO (dimethylsulfoxide). The purpose of all this chemo was to really, once and for all, destroy what remained of my immune system. I could not have the stem cells reinserted unless all my blood work numbers were at or hovering near zero. This meant all of my white blood cells, my red blood cells, everything, would be gone. This also meant all the childhood vaccinations ("kiddie vacs") I had gotten would be destroyed and would have to be replaced a year after the transplant. On March 11, there was a day of rest from the chemo. (Six days shalt they labor, then on the seventh day, there was rest.) Because Karmanos was 99 miles from home (one-way) and the weather so bad, very few people could come see me, which made the visit from my Dear Daughter, Deb, and her friend, Sue, all the more enjoyable. They live in the Detroit area.

March 12, 2008, 9:00 A.M. This is my new birthday. This is the day when I was given my life back. The stem cell transplant team came in to insert the 3-1/2 bags of stem cells back into my body. They said I might throw up. No, I said. That's not going to happen. But I did-beautiful, spectacular, projectile vomiting. The stem cells come to you frozen. They have to thaw them just a tiny bit. If they melt too much, they are unusable. There is only a twelve-minute window to get each bag fully administered. The stem cells feel rather cool when they are being inserted, but not uncomfortable.

Now began the wait to see if the transplant had been successful. The next 100 days would be crucial. I had been told the risk of an uncontrollable infection and even possibly death was a very real possibility.

This was a really "down" time for me. Really depressing. My concentration was zero. I can usually go through a 700-page book in about two days (the seventh Harry Potter book was done in slightly over nine hours). I had taken a book to read about John Adams (written by David McCollough) while in the hospital, as well as another five books given to me by friends (there were another fifteen at home waiting to be delivered once these six books were done). Much to my dismay, I couldn't read more than a paragraph, or sometimes even a sentence or two a day. Even magazine articles couldn't be finished in a day. My energy level was non-existent, and the nurses and physician's assistant kept pushing me to walk. Inside myself, I said, "You have one of these procedures and let ME urge *YOU* to walk!" Of course, they were right—the more exercise you get, the quicker you would get better. Simon had said this would happen but I had not believed him, not for a second. I finally hit bottom, and had to struggle to get out of bed to go to the bathroom. All my blood work scores were at zero or very close to it. A chart had been put up on the wall across from my bed so I could see the way things were going.

Compounding my condition, the food went beyond intolerable, all the way into the unimaginable. I knew immediately when the food trolley came off the elevator. The smell was horrific and the door to my room had to be shut. I stopped eating and lived on one can of Ensure (chocolate flavored) for breakfast, lunch and dinner, supplemented by one of those teensy tiny 2-tablespoon cups of chocolate ice cream. The food that is served has to have the living daylights cooked out of it to kill any bacteria to prevent any damage to your system. The other huge concern for the medical staff was that I would lose too much weight, making my body even more vulnerable to an irreversible infection. Each day, I kept remembering that Sparrow Hospital menu you could choose from to eat what you liked (within reason). Why couldn't Karmanos do that? The unrelenting sameness of the food ("If this is Monday, it has to be a dried out sliver of tough turkey breast with school paste gravy") was . . . pardon the pun . . . hard to swallow.

Then, another miracle occurred. Well, not a miracle, since a miracle by definition is unknowable and indefinable. What had occurred was knowable; it was a direct result of the brains and dedication of many heroic researchers who struggled against all odds, including the lack of adequate funding and opposing political ideologies that obstructed life-saving progress. But it felt like a miracle to me, in the sense of it being awe-inspiring, filled with wonder.

After receiving four pints of blood, as well as the countless other drugs administered to bring the blood cell counts up, slowly, millimeter by millimeter (inches were too big an increment), I began to feel better. Concentration was still a thing of the past, but at least I could do one lap around the hall (there were 16 laps to the mile). Every day, I got better and better. Toward the end I could do four laps two or three times a day, but being tethered to the wheel-rattling IV trolley that administered the drugs through the PICC line was a nuisance, and cramped my style. (Taking a shower tethered to that was also an experience. I couldn't get the bandage or line wet because of possible infection; it had to be wrapped in plastic food wrap to protect it, which meant the shower had to be taken with my left arm stuck outside of the shower. You should try it.)

The last week I was there became better in the food department. The hospital food was still horrible (worse than normal hospital food). Fortunately, another nurse, Rita, who has also become a good friend (and is now going through her own battle with breast cancer), took great pity on me when I was craving hummus. After checking with about twenty people to make sure it would be safe, her mother made me fresh, homemade, from-scratch, authentic old-country hummus. You have no idea how good that tasted. My mother-in-law, Marion, sent me homemade macaroni and cheese. I asked Tom to stop at Red Lobster on his way down to pick up an order of Fettuccine Crab Alfredo and some of those garlic-cheese biscuits they make. Tom also left me some money so I could occasionally do take-out when the nurses went out to get something. And the hospital continued to serve "food" three times a day, every day, even though I had made it patently clear I couldn't even stand the smell of it, let alone eat it. (Talk about waste and the high cost of hospitalization. . . .)

I had made up my mind to leave the hospital on March 23, the birthday of nieces Monica and Jennifer. It also happened to be Easter that year, which I thought was appropriate: a new beginning, a resurrection from the (near) dead, a regeneration. (Meaning no disrespect for those of you who might be taking offense.)

It didn't happen. My counts were still too low to be safely released from the hospital. I was in such a hurry to go home, to be in my own place, to lay my head on my own pillow in my own bed, to be any-where other than a hospital; you could never imagine the anxiety and the anticipation. Patience, be mine!

Finally, Tuesday, March 25, three weeks to the day after I had been admitted, I went home. In order to prevent any unpleasantness, I requested of Tom that we go straight home—no tours today, please. Then, if you can believe it, he "got lost" (after having made ten or twelve trips previously to visit me at Karmanos), but when I raised myself up from the back seat, which I was lying across, and said, "I will drive," he somehow managed to find his way back onto the high-way quite quickly. We were really on our way Home!

At home, I couldn't prepare food. Fortunately, we are blessed with many, many friends and family who brought food to the house. Sharon brought two kinds of homemade soup (it was so cold outside still, and I just have not ever seemed to be able to get warm since the transplant, that the soup was like a burst of sunshine all through my body), Made-line brought authentic homemade Italian stuffed shells (her store, Fabi-ano's Candies, makes incredible chocolates; the shells were ALMOST more welcome than the chocolate), Janet brought chicken salad, Nancy brought some "Mug'Ems" recipes and the mugs to make soup in the microwave, Betty sent homemade burritos, Pam brought salads and quiches, Gail brought a vegetarian dish. *(The problem with listing these friends and their dishes, is that inadvertently, some people will be missed; please accept my apologies for any oversight.)*

I had made several dishes before going into the hospital that were in the freezer. But more than almost anything, I was craving fresh fruits and vegetables. The only problem with fresh fruits and vegetables was that none of them could be prepared before bringing them to our house because of all the air-borne pathogens they carry on their exterior. All fresh fruit and veggies had to be prepared right here at the house before serving. Extra care had to be taken to make sure all the dirt was washed and completely removed. Cooked veggies were O.K., after they had been thoroughly washed. As I thought about food after such a pro-longed dearth, I found myself craving Chinese, Thai, Mexican, Middle Eastern and Indian foods (there is no good place in our area for Tan-doori chicken). You name it; I had a taste for it!

Additionally, I could not clean house—oh, gosh, golly, gee, what a shame! *That* prohibition ended all too quickly for me! But just as I have been so blessed by my friends throughout this journey, wouldn't you know another friend had a friend who had a friend who cleans houses for free for women who have cancer. Can you believe that? The main foundation (please send a donation) was "Cleaning for a Reason" (their website is listed in the back). Susan came out and gave me four free house-cleanings. Her cleaning business is "Helpful Hands" in DeWitt, MI, for women in that area who have cancer and need some help. The process, whether you are in Michigan or not, is that your oncologist has to send in verification to Cleaning for a Reason that you do have cancer. They will contact someone in your area who is a member of this organization. Unfortunately, there are not enough people doing this, so men who have cancer are unable to participate. When Rod was dying, I tried to see if it was possible for Cleaning for a Reason to send someone over to help his wife, thinking she would rather spend time with him than clean house. They said it was simply not possible.

I could not get my hands in soil (or even mow, which I enjoy) because of the bacteria. Although my husband is in the wholesale produce business, I had grown container after container in past summers of tomatoes, green peppers, jalapeño peppers, Brussels sprouts, and herbs. (Corn, carrots and green onions don't really do well in containers, but if you have a big enough pot, potatoes do nicely.) On Memorial Day weekend, my mother-in-law bought four tomato plants so I could have fresh tomatoes for the summer.

They said I had to keep the PICC line in for at least a month. I said one week (it would *never* be used again, and besides, it was a real pain to have to sterilize every day, change the bandages every day, figure out how to sleep with it, hope it didn't become dislodged, which it did quite often while I was at Karmanos, and to keep wrapping it to take a shower). They said I couldn't drive for two months. Of course, I said one week; being "incarcerated" for the past couple of months was driving *me* around the bend! I promised I would go grocery shopping at 4:00 or 5:00 A.M., when there were few people out and about, wear a mask (they are hot and uncomfortable and stuffy), and sterilize the handles of the cart. They said I couldn't be around little kids for a few months because of all the germs they can spread around. Now *that* made sense, so I complied, although it meant missing great-nephew Kole's birthday on March 31. They also said I needed to still wear the mask for a couple of months whenever I went outside, which also made sense. I am nothing else, if not rational, so I was most obedient and followed the rules.

Things happened rapidly after that. By mid-April, when the weather started getting nice, I was back to walking two miles a day, and by the end of May, I was doing four miles a day. On one of these walks I forgot my hat so I was walking bareheaded with no hair. About a mile from home I saw a little girl, maybe three or four years old, who eyed me with great curiosity and told me her name was Olivia. She came right up to me and asked, "Are you a boy or a girl?" I immediately thought to myself, wasn't that great?!? The total, pure honesty and innocence of children never ceases to amaze and delight me! I quickly explained I was a girl who had been sick, but was now all better. At this point, a large golden retriever came bounding up, wanting to jump up on me, lick me, hug me, crawl all over me, wanted its tummy rubbed—and I couldn't be around pets at that time, either. (If we had had pets, we would have had to house them somewhere else for a few months.) Olivia kept eyeing me with curiosity, admired my earrings and my socks, and then asked what color my hair would be when it grew back. I told her just about the color of her dog. She liked that. Now, I think of her and her purity of spirit often; it lifts my own.

In April of 2008, Dr. Beckrow left Dr. Rapson's practice and we elected to stay with Dr. Rapson. It was a hard decision to make; we had grown quite fond of Dr. Beckrow, were very appreciative of his care, but Dr. Rapson had years more experience and had been in the same area for many years. She had been the "go-to" person if Dr. Beckrow had any questions, and we would never have been able to find another group of nurses, scheduling, or other staff as wonderful as these people had been to us (you don't even feel the needle prick when Linda, the phlebotomist, draws your blood; the staff members were easily 50% of the reason we decided to stay with Dr. Rapson). My other concern was that Dr. Beckrow would move from practice to practice because he was so young, and at that time, Tom and I needed some consistency in our lives, as far as medical issues were concerned. While I thrive on change, you have to evaluate what is best, and the best choice for both of us was staying with Dr. Rapson.

By the end of April, if none of the grandkids had colds or the sniffles, I would be allowed to attend our grandson Zachary's birthday party—without a mask. Oh freedom, at last, no mask in public anymore. Perhaps, I would no longer scare all the little children, except of course, for dear little Olivia, who showed no hesitation whatsoever. Not all children had been so brave.

As May came, I was feeling all the exhilaration of spring and was anticipating the entire rebirth occurring in nature. But as life tends to do, just as you are least expecting it, the tables were turned over and over. May, beautiful May, became a devastating month. My dearest Linda was diagnosed with lung cancer that had already metastasized into her brain. After recommending that she go to Dr. Rapson also, I was firmly told by staff there were no discounts for multiple referrals! They were kidding, of course, and the levity was briefly helpful. Linda's condition, however, was horrific, far worse than any of us realized at the time. Dr. Rapson took an aggressive approach to treatment for Linda. She also had to undergo chemo and intense bursts of radiation on her skull. Linda had now begun her own long, slow nauseous, painful, exhausted and frightening journey toward becoming a cancer survivor. Whatever happened now, my heart and my prayers were with Linda.

June was a bit of a tense time for me. I had to have another PET scan. The last time there was a three-month gap between scans, my cancer had metastasized, so it was somewhat (NO—quite!) unsettling to have the PET scan done. The good news is that I have had so many PET scans now, these wonderful nurses at MSU, Jane, Michele and Tracy, know me by sight. That's also the bad news, I suppose. After a few days, the results of the PET scan were ready. Hold your breath—drum roll please—"NO EVIDENCE OF RECURRENCE OF DISEASE."

What could I say, I was thrilled and overwhelmed; I felt as though I would scream, but ever-so-quickly, my mind jumped to the day of the next PET scan. What was the future going to hold for me? I knew deep down in my heart the results were going to be just the same—I was on my way to becoming a cancer survivor.

In July, Tom and I were able to take our annual week-long vacation with seven of the nine grandkids. In previous years, we had taken four of the grandsons to Kentucky, Tennessee, Pennsylvania, and Virginia, but this year, we were taking three 7-year-olds for the first time (including a set of twins) so we stayed in Boyne, Michigan, just in case any of the new ones got homesick. They are all boys and like most boys, have some trouble picking up after themselves and getting their dishes into the sink (they must think the Good Housekeeping Fairy is around). I was exhausted when we got home. Every other day, there were four to six loads of laundry, and I tried as much as possible to have home-cooked (but often store-bought frozen) food. They loved the homemade burritos (thanks to Betty's recipe, which were made and frozen before the trip). I took 84 burritos with us to Boyne; I brought home 4; they even wanted them for breakfast. They also liked my homemade nachos. We made plastic-bag omelets for one of the breakfasts (even today when they stay for overnights, this is one of their big requests; I'm going to have to rethink this because of the BPA issue; see #10 in the section titled "Steps to Take to Reduce Your Risk of Cancer or to Reduce Your Risk of Metastasis "). My hair was only a little peach fuzz at that point, but they took it all in stride.

The summer of 2008 had passed, and September, with all of its awesome coloratura had arrived. It also brought with it another benchmark date, the six-month post-transplant appointment at Karmanos. Once again, the results of the PET scan showed *"No evidence of recurrence of disease."* I did not have as immense a reaction as I had to the first clear scan, but I was no less grateful or overwhelmed with my good fortune. And my hair had started growing back; this time it was more reddish, like it is supposed to be, and had hardly any grey. It grew back just enough for me to drive to Maryland so I could celebrate my last remaining aunt's 90th birthday (she has Alzheimer's) with her, and I did not have to wear a hat.

In December, my ability to multi-task started to come back. I had been mega-dosing on blueberries after reading an article about them (it appears blueberries stimulate the production of new neurons in the brain). One day, it all of a sudden dawned on me I was folding laundry while waiting for pages to download from the Internet, answering the phone, finding information for our trip with the grandkids to Boston in 2009, getting my schedule organized for work the next day, monitoring the pots of Irish Crème fudge and the English Toffee on the stove all at once—and keeping track of all of it. That was a good day. However, Sharon later informed me we really needed to learn to "uni-task," and I think she's right (Sharon has recently been diagnosed with MS). I'm still very easily distracted, though and need a quiet environment to do the work for MDE. If I get off track, I have to start whatever I was doing all over again. I'm not used to that. It's maddening, annoying and frustrating! Sure, I know it's getting better, but not fast enough for me. In remembering that AC, we all want our lives to go back to "normal," it is difficult to accept that this may be my new "normal." Aha, a new challenge to overcome!

In March of 2009, the one-year post-stem cell-transplant appointment was held at Karmanos. All my blood work was back to normal. The PET scan showed "No evidence of recurrence of disease." That was good news. It doesn't mean the cancer is gone. It will always be there, but it isn't progressing and the tumors are all gone. Originally they had said I would need to return every six months to Karmanos, but as long as Dr. Rapson was seeing me every six months, and since I was doing so well, they felt there was no need to see me more than once a year. *IF MY CANCER HAS NOT RECURRED BY 2013, I WILL BE CONSIDERED "IN REMISSION."* At that point then, I will officially be a cancer survivor.

March 12, 2009, was also my first birthday of the stem cell transplant. Pam, a friend of 40 years and colleague I work with at the Michigan Department of Education, the one who brought quiches and salads when I got home from Karmanos, brought in a cake with a big number "1" on top. We also had other goodies to celebrate, including Suresh's surprise of bringing Indian food. Another one of the great blessings in my life has been to find work with this amazing, tremendously talented, bright, funny, capable group of people (Ricardo, Rachael, another Linda, another Pam, Evelyn, Rob, Suresh, Kim and Bill).

In April of 2009, Acyclovir was removed from my medication regimen; it was being prescribed to prevent me from contracting shingles (as we age, we run a greater risk of getting this; if you had chicken pox as a child, you will always carry the virus, so I was quite vulnerable). I also had to have all my "kiddie vacs" (childhood vaccinations) readministered. Once again, Blue Cross/Blue Shield refused to cover the costs because I was "over age" to have them, even though their own coverage and benefits manual states that this is, under certain circumstances, a covered medical service. My situation met all of their stipulations for a covered circumstance. Finally, after several letters, even more phone calls and months of waiting, they finally agreed to pay most of the $700 cost. What—would they have preferred for me to have contracted a childhood disease, and then have to pay the hospitalization? (In May 2010, I had to have the second round of kiddie vacs administered. And, guess what? Blue Cross/Blue Shield again refused to pay. I thought, oh NO! I'm going to have to fight another battle! But this time, however, when I called, I discovered the insurance would only pay for the vacs within 24 months of a stem cell transplant. The second round of kiddie vacs I had taken had been administered at 26 months. So for those of you who are going through this process, check with your health insurance company for the fine print on kiddie vacs for adults; then check with your doctor to see if you can get the second round at 9 months after the first round, and not wait the full 12 months between the two.)

I also can't take the shingles vaccination because it is a live virus. It would *give* me shingles, rather than protect me from getting it. I can't sit next to anyone who either has an active case of shingles, or has been recently exposed to them (currently, nephew Chris has them, so I can't go into the warehouse if he's there and has an active rash). I also began to get my teeth fixed—all 25 cavities were filled and one tooth was extracted that had split down the middle all the way to the root.

As I write this, November 2010, life couldn't be better. Even winning the lottery would not add anything to my life, considering how tremendously well I am feeling and how well my friends are doing. There is nothing I can't do. During the summers of 2009, 2010 and 2011, I had eight containers filled with different tomato plants, several pots of herbs and could once again mow the lawn. I haven't felt this good in so many years, I feel as though I could fly and look down at this earth with a new perspective because of all the wondrous blessings that have been bestowed upon me. If you didn't have to get leukemia or lymphoma first, I'd heartily recommend getting a stem cell transplant! Last year I managed to shave off a few seconds in my walking. I do a mile now in about 14.5 minutes. Not bad, considering all this old body has been through. (And, maybe because of the stem cell transplant, my hair hasn't needed "coloring." There's much less grey in it now than before I ever got sick.) Family and friends have become more important, the sunsets have become more intense, the laughter of children is merrier, and meeting new people provides opportunities to learn new things and to embrace new friendships, which take on deeper and richer meanings. Doing the research for this book has brought me in contact with people all over the world, whose support, encouragement and knowledge has been immeasurable and deeply appreciated. Life is GREAT!

The pace of cancer research continues to accelerate (although it seems excruciatingly slow when you're going through it), which is exciting. The February 2009, issue of *Scientific American* includes an article entitled "Nanomedicine Targets Cancer" by James R. Heath, Mark E. Davis and Leroy Hood. Nanomedicine not only targets cancer, but also other diseases such as diabetes. As the article points out, prostate cancer usually grows so slowly (up to 30 years to become fully manifested), it usually doesn't really have much impact on men. In fact, most, if not all, men will develop prostate cancer as they get into their 70s and 80s. Most men will die *with* prostate cancer, not *from* it. The danger arises if and when the cancer metastasizes. Researchers are in the process of identifying the networks in prostate cancer cells to distinguish between "regular" prostate cancer and prostate cancer that has the ability to metastasize. The goal is to make earlier and more accurate identification possible to preclude unnecessary surgery, radiation or chemotherapy, as well as the pain, incontinence and impotence that can accompany these types of treatments. Nanotechnology can also drastically reduce the dosages of medication required to treat different types of cancers.

And while we are on the subject of prostate cancer, the July 23, 2009, issue of the Johns Hopkins Health Alert mentions that Vitamin D might constitute a "ray of hope." Taking sufficient, not excessive, doses of Vitamin D may reduce the risk of the onset of prostate cancer. It may also help to halt the growth and spread of prostate cancer if a man already has it. (Probably because Tom's prostate cancer is so far along, the Vitamin D hasn't helped very much.)

In the March 2009, issue of *Scientific American* an article appeared, entitled "The World's Smallest Radio," by Ed Regis. According to the article, chemotherapy not only kills cancer cells, it also damages the healthy cells. Radio-controlled drug delivery systems in packages, patented by a company called Zettl, are close to being used to molecularly target cancer cells. The claim is that the radio signals will release drugs only into tumor cells.

Medical advances that used to take centuries to discover and test are now happening in accelerated time periods. People used to say, "Just think—100 years ago it was discovered that washing your hands before surgery would reduce the risk of infection." Then it was "Fifty years ago, we discovered that combining different kinds of chemotherapy could lead to increased survival rates." When I reflect back on my journey through cancer, even in just these brief three years, much has happened. When I got my cancer, stem cell transplants weren't routinely done for people of "my age." While they still aren't common-place now, more and more people even older than "my age" are successfully receiving them (one lady at Karmanos was 73). When I started the stem cell transplant process, if my cancer had metastasized for a second time (third time to have cancer), I would not have been able to be my own donor again. Just in the last year, that has become a possibility. However, the chances of success are only about 35%, but that's far better than zero. I have now reached the age when they would not use my own stem cells, because it is felt they would be "weaker" and less effective than if acquired from a younger donor. And if I had to have another stem cell transplant, my risks would be substantially increased, in terms of the speed of recovery. I could not get away with most everything I did in using my own stem cells the first time. Should I need a second stem cell transplant, if they were to say "No driving for a month," I might be lucky it were only one month, and I probably would have to spend the full five weeks in the hospital the doctor expected.

It won't be too much longer when people will be able to say how "barbaric" treatment for cancer was only 25 or 10 or even, 5 years ago. But for those of us who received that "barbaric" treatment, which was state-of-the-art in our time, we are immensely grateful for it. Please, continue the "barbarity" until something better comes along. Please, all you bright researchers, doctors, nurses—continue your excellent work. You are our lifeline to the future, just as we who have gone through this process are lifelines for those yet to be diagnosed.

This is about the seventh re-write of this section, begun in May 2009, and it is now November 2010. Throughout the eight-month period, until November 2009, Tom had been doing magnificently. Even though his PSA had been creeping up, there was really nothing about which to be overly alarmed. We knew in November he was becoming hormone refractory again, but the questions were: do we start Taxotere? Do we change the dosages of the medications that were currently being administered? Or, do we wait and see if the PSA will stabilize? Then in January, he was hospitalized for a urinary tract infection and damage to his right kidney and one wall of the bladder. Three of the medications Tom had been taking—Cytoxan, DES and Zometa—can all damage the kidneys over time. At the same time, his creatinine levels (measure kidney function) continued to rise, going from 1.31 when he entered the hospital, to 1.51 in four days, and by two months later, it was at 1.9. The three medications were removed from Tom's regimen to see if his kidneys would resume normal function. They did not. His PSA at the time of release from the hospital was 10.2; one week later, his PSA had jumped to 17.9. Furthermore, we were also dealing with his rising triglycerides, which were over 1100, and his cholesterol level, which was almost 300.

At our early March appointment with Dr. Pienta, he wanted to wait one more month before making any decisions about starting Taxotere or doing some other form of medication. Dr. Rapson concurred. Given Tom's response (the dropping of the PSA to 15.9 and his creatinine level decreasing slightly to 1.7), it was decided to wait one more month before making a decision. Both of the oncologists were reluctant to start Tom on Taxotere too soon, because Tom remains pretty much asymptomatic for cancer, and the side effects of the Taxotere might be worse than all he's going through now. His only real symptom is excessive fatigue, caused in part by the medications, but also because the cancer may be regrouping and getting ready to make more trouble. In the meantime, Tom was to continue the Cytoxan, and they would monitor all levels closely.

Also in March, Dr. Yousif, the urologist, ordered more tests to either confirm or assuage his belief that the prostate cancer cells were migrating to the kidneys and bladder. If his cancer was migrating to the kidneys, radiation would be the only option. Tom was scheduled for a scope near the end of March and an ultrasound on his kidneys for the end of April. In the interim, Tom was hospitalized with dehydration along with a flare-up of the urinary tract infection. The admitting doctor, Dr. K., kept Tom in the hospital for three days, with the last day supposedly for running more tests. On Tom's second day in the hospital, Dr. K. said to cancel Tom's scope, because he said he needed to run more tests on the third day, when the scope was scheduled. We had asked if there was any way possible for him to run the tests the second day so Tom could have the 9:30 A.M. scope done as scheduled, but Dr. K. said no; he was going to be running his tests on Wednesday morning. When Dr. K. came into the room at 7:15 A.M. on the third day for his morning rounds, I asked what tests he was going to run that morning—Wednesday morning. He said he wasn't and would be discharging Tom. He knew full well Tom had been scheduled for a scope that morning at 9:30; we were trying to find out whether or not Tom's cancer was migrating, but for some unknown reason, he delayed discharging Tom until Wednesday, making it impossible for us to make that appointment. I suppose we had not properly or sufficiently worshipped at the doctor altar, to pay the expected obeisance.

At the April 5 appointment at the U of M with Nancy, the nurse practitioner, Tom had another PSA done; it was 22.5. Taxotere was to be delayed for one more month because the antibiotic Tom had been on in the hospital could have artificially raised the PSA (same scenario we had in February). What we faced, should Taxotere be the next decision, was: The Taxotere would reduce the numbers on the PSA test, but at the expense of increased fatigue and other side effects such as nausea, increased bone/muscle/joint aches and hair loss. Median survival once Taxotere is administered is 18 months; that means that while 50% of the people live less than that, it also (positive attitude) means 50% of the people live longer than that. There were supposed to be some new drugs to treat prostate cancer coming out in the summer of 2009; the FDA (Food and Drug Administration) did not give its approval. The rumor mill said two of the board members who had to give approval denied it because they were associated with a competing pharmaceutical company. Another trial involving 500 men was ordered, before approval could be considered. It is now November 2010; Tom's PSA is on the rise again, nearly tripling since July. And adding to our concern, his recent bone scan showed a new spot of cancer on his sacrum, the upper part of the tailbone.

In October, we visited four of Tom's doctors in one week. Only one of the four reported much that was very hopeful. Dr. Yousif thought the prostate cancer might be migrating into both the kidneys and the bladder. On the other hand, Dr. Rapson thought the prostate cancer might be migrating into the sphincter muscle in the bladder. Dr. Wheeler found none of the recent tests encouraging. And, last but not least, Dr. Pienta told us of a new Phase 2 trial that might help Tom. In order to participate, you have to have any kind of cancer that has metastasized into your bones. This process, called MLN 1202, involves antibodies and is not chemotherapy. There are forty test sites around the nation, with only twenty treatments at each site. Three IV infusions will be administered to qualified subjects, two weeks apart. There are no guarantees it will do anything. There are also no guarantees any more of the treatment will be made (the drug costs $2 million for each treatment). There are no guarantees, even if more were made, that Tom would qualify to participate in the trial. Dr. Pienta was very clear; this is not a cure. This trial could buy him time and might do some good. Ultimately, Tom was approved. Dr. Pienta said regardless of how it goes, the likelihood is high that after the trial is over, Tom will still need to be on some type of intravenous chemotherapy.

During the trial, Tom had a cystoscopy with Dr. Jerilin Latini at the University of Michigan (which we MSU grads refer to as MSU's east campus) to check on his kidneys and bladder, along with a "FUDS"—fluourourodynamic study, which also looked at his bladder, urethra and prostate (and which necessitated the insertion of two different catheters). Nothing unusual was noticed in the FUDS, but the cystoscopy showed a red area, "carpet-looking," that could be cancer. Only a biopsy could determine that. No nodule was found on the sphincter in either of these two tests.

Tom went through the trial with flying colors, but his PSA continued to jump by leaps and bounds. It went from 29.77 in October, to 54.08 in November (the U of M's PSA was 76.5; remember that different labs can use different processes which can impact the score). Tom started Taxotere on November 29, 2010, and a referral was made for him to a doctor in Grand Rapids, MI, to see whether Tom qualified to take Provenge. If Medicare doesn't cover it, Provenge will cost more than $100,000. The same day, after digging for 45 minutes to try and find a vein in Tom's arm or hand, it was decided for future chemotherapy, Tom should have an infusaport. Tom is scheduled for outpatient surgery on December 22. The status now, at the close of 2010, before sending this tome to the editor, is that Tom will discontinue the Taxotere until the Provenge issues have been settled. Tom's PSA has come down in December, but apparently there is allowance for this, and Tom may not have to wait the full three months to demonstrate a rising PSA in order to receive the Provenge treatments. Tom did learn when he went in to have the blood work done for his PSA that Medicare is now considering not paying for Provenge, and that at some point in time, Medicare will only pay for Hospice, not the palliative treatments, which have kept Tom alive for nearly six years.

It bears repeating: we have much for which to be grateful. Tom's original prognosis was for three to five years, or as little as six months. We are now into his sixth year battling this disease and until November of 2009, he looked and felt very good. Every day we have brings us one day closer to a cure, or to more accurate and quicker diagnoses and to better medicines and improved protocols. We are hoping and praying for Tom to still get another few years of relatively good health.

On the research front, more good news is reported relating to prostate cancer: men are being diagnosed earlier than in the past. In addition, the "race gap" (which should actually be referred to as "ethnicity gap") is being narrowed. In the past, blacks were diagnosed not only at a later date with prostate cancer, but also at a later stage, and were consequently more likely to die from it. In a study cited in the *Journal of the National Cancer Institute*, the average age of diagnosis dropped from 72 years of age to 67 years (2004–05 data). Late-stage diagnosis fell from 58 per 100,000 to 8 for whites, and from 91 per 100,000 to 18 for blacks.

Alexis continues her good health. She participated in the DAL-MAC bike run (from Lansing to Mackinaw Island, a distance of almost 400 miles) just six months after her double mastectomy, and in May, 2010, graduated Magna Cum Laude with a Bachelor of Science degree in nursing (all while working full-time, going to school full-time and after undergoing chemo). Alexis has decided to continue her education and obtain her doctorate in palliative care. Shortly after Alexis graduated, Andrea gave us all quite a scare—she almost died from a viral infection in late spring. On her birthday in September 2010, she was tentatively diagnosed with Cushing's disease and with COPD. However, in 2011, she was diagnosed with a frontal brain lobe damage due to the oxygen deprivation she experienced last spring. Some of her memory may return but other pieces won't. We keep them in our prayers.

Likewise, this section for Linda has been rewritten nine times now, primarily due to all the changing circumstances in her journey with the big C. In the earlier versions of this section, she had done so well! A year into her treatment, the tumors in her lungs and brain had all disappeared—every one of them. Initially, this was a glowing paragraph about Linda playing with her grandchildren, enjoying her mother's cottage at the lake, and her annual participation at the Lungevity Fundraiser in September in Grand Blanc, MI (in 2009 and 2010, the event happened to fall on her birthday). Initially, this paragraph was closed with the statement, "Miracles, the miracles brought about by modern science, still do occur in this day and age," and they occur for those we love.

Then a CT scan showed a "nodule" on her adrenal gland, which had doubled in size from one three-month period to the next; it also showed "suspicious" shadows on her lungs. Linda underwent five more months of chemo. Like a lot of chemo patients, her red blood cell count plummeted, necessitating four pints of blood to be infused. The tests after the five months of chemo came back fine. The scan was clear; we celebrated. Then another CT scan was done—this time, the tumor on her adrenal gland had grown.

March 30, 2010, started out a glorious day, even though Tom was in the hospital for the second time in three months. Alexis was celebrating her 35th birthday. That she reached 35 and in such good health was cause enough for another celebration. Then Linda called mid-morning. In a heartbeat, the day iced up completely. Linda had been told the previous week, there was nothing more that could be done for her. She had only two to four weeks to live. During the next couple of days, Linda spent most of her time on the phone with a cancer institute in Chicago and trying to get Blue Cross/Blue Shield to give permission for her to enter their treatment program. Another huge chunk of time was spent filling out hospital paperwork, appointments with her attorney to update her will, getting her home insurance company to finish the work on her house that needed to be done, making sure her investments were in proper order to leave to her sons—just in case that became necessary, making sure her bills were paid up to date and then, trying to find flights to Chicago.

I found myself calling Linda just to hear her voice, just to hear her laughter, although those first few days we had little to laugh about. I wanted to cling to her, to shield her from having to go through this, to rage against someone, anyone for taking this life far too soon. I was desperate to find some way to help, denying that someone who had fought so hard and had been winning, might now be losing this battle. Linda, sister of the heart, in so many ways a soul mate, my confidante, was entering a state where all anyone could do was feel helpless and angry, desolate. Powerless to DO anything! She was not only at the mercy of "the system," but also this insidious disease that just would NOT let up, would NOT let go, would NOT let her survive, that was determined to WIN at the cost of her infinitely precious and singular life. I asked if I could go to see her in Chicago, and she said, "Yes."

She entered the cancer institute in Chicago on April 5. They had told her the previous week that she should ignore the two to four week limitation, that they had had other patients who had received the same news and were still alive seven years later, that they were on the cutting edge of cancer research and technology, and that local area doctors did not have the knowledge and expertise of the staff at their cancer center. Linda underwent three to five days of testing. The original plan was for Linda to have these tests, come home, and then go back to Chicago for two to three weeks of additional chemo and radiation. She never made it home. Linda began chemo and radiation on April 12. By April 14, Linda's Mom, Pat, had been telling the doctors that Linda's lungs were filling up, that that had been how her lung cancer had been diagnosed in the first place, because of pneumonia. Pat was ignored. On Friday, April 16, Linda was rushed to emergency where the doctors debated on whether to do a biopsy to find out what kind of pneumonia she had. After a couple of days, they decided not to do one. I spoke with Pat on Wednesday, April 21, and was told that Linda was not doing well. Then I had this sinking feeling of dread, and April 25 kept resounding in my brain. Something inside me was telling me this date was bringing disaster, and then I knew I was being told it would be Linda's last day.

Linda was placed, and remained, on oxygen while her family gathered around her. Her daughter-in-law, Lisa, Linda's granddaughter, Faith, and Lisa's Mom (another Linda) drove down to see her on Thursday (Linda's two sons, Jeff and Scot, along with Linda's Mom had not left her side since she had been admitted). Linda snuggled close and was in great humor with Faith on Friday, April 23. I called on Saturday, April 24 to see if I could go down to see her. The answer from a family member this time was "No." On Saturday, Lisa went in to say good-bye since she had to leave to drive back to Michigan, and later related that Linda's eyes had a "sadness" in them, a sadness that was both deep and otherworldly. Sunday, April 25, Linda was put on life support. Within the hour, her blood pressure dropped and she slipped away. The irony of it is that the cancer did not kill her, but the pneumonia did. She lived four weeks and three days after Dr. Rapson's last office visit, the local area office, the one that didn't have the knowledge and expertise of the Chicago cancer center, the one that gave her the life expectancy timeframe that ultimately came to pass.

Linda's death has created an abyss in so many lives. Life has now become divided into two parts: one, which had Linda in it, and the other, without her. That brief spark of hope flared up for an instant, and then was cruelly extinguished far too quickly. As this is being written, seven months after Linda's death, my tears still come, unbidden, at all hours of the day and night. A few days after Linda died, I went to a store to buy sympathy cards for her family; as I read different cards looking for appropriate ones, cards that really conveyed how I felt, tears kept streaming down my cheeks. I was missing her so much. Through the tears, my hand reached out—in a different section than the sympathy cards, and I picked up one with this inscription by American Greetings:

> *I miss the old days and simpler times*
> *When we were able to get together*
> *Whenever we wanted, or*
> *Pick up the phone and talk for hours,*
> *or spend entire days laughing, and*
> *Sharing, and planning our lives . . .*
> *But even though we can't talk as much,*
> *or see each other as often,*
> *You are still a part of me,*
> *. . . My Forever Friend.*

Thank you, Linda, for guiding my hand to this card.

Linda finds other ways of letting us know she is still around. A few hours after Linda died, I was in the kitchen in the evening getting a little snack for Tom and me. Tom wanted ice cream. My initial reaction was to say "no" because I was thinking of his high triglycerides and cholesterol, and because the drugs he was taking put him at increased risk of diabetes. Clear as a bell, Linda's voice came into my head and said, "Remember the time we stopped at Steak and Shake and you weren't going to get him ice cream then, either?" Tom got his ice cream—both times, thanks to Linda. Two weeks after Linda's death, Ricardo and I went out to lunch, our usual monthly lunch, the lunches we have done for over 30 years, at which Marc and Linda always attended (Marc couldn't come because he was taking care of his Mom who was dying of a form of ALS). As we left, parked right behind my car was . . . Linda's car. Not her actual car, but the same make, model, year and color. What are the odds? Was she trying to let us know she was still there with us? Then on Friday, September 10, just before the Lungevity walk, Jeff and Lisa had asked if I would watch Faith and Jack while they cleaned out Linda's house. Linda had lived a couple of blocks from Island Park in Eaton Rapids, so we (Tom, Faith, Jack and I) all walked down to the park. I know Linda's grandkids, but not that well—we don't see each other as often as we would like. On the way down to the park, I was saying over and over in my head, "O.K., Linda, help me with these kids. What do I need to be doing or saying?" The kids were playing and running around, and all of a sudden, Linda's voice came out of my mouth. It was her voice—her speech patterns, intonation, cadence and I found myself doing all kinds of goofy things with the kids that are definitely NOT a part of my persona. Within a heartbeat, Faith started calling me "Grandma." On Sunday, we went to participate in the Lungevity Walk. I had thought that Faith would have forgotten all about it, that she would go back to calling me "Terrymc." As I walked in the door, Faith called out, "Hi, Grandma." Thank you, Linda, for this special additional gift.

And yet, there is much for which to be thankful:

Pat is as close to remission as you can get. Her husband, Ricardo, just happened to sit next to one of the developers of Gleevek, the medicine Pat is on, while travelling to California. It is a wonderful thing to be able to thank the researcher who worked so hard to develop a life-saving drug—one that has saved your wife's life. If the Gleevek hadn't worked, Pat's only other option would have been a stem cell transplant. Pat is of Hispanic heritage, which means her odds of finding a donor are pretty remote. (If you are Caucasian, you stand about a 70% chance of success in finding a donor; if you are of an ethnic minority, your odds drop to less than 25%.) At this point in time, only people with leukemia and lymphoma are eligible to have stem cell transplants and stand a good chance of success. People with Myeloma can have a stem cell transplant, but right now, it really doesn't do them much good; they still have to continue with the chemo for the rest of their lives. On September 9, 2009 Pat e-mailed that her three-month checkup at the oncologist showed that her blood work had "0" "wacko" cells (Philadelphia Chromosome) and she did not need a bone marrow aspiration, plus she didn't have to see her doctor for another six months. Truly, that makes 9/9/09 a lucky day for her. Score one for the survivor team—it is growing, not cancer.

Nicky has had a few scares health-wise but is doing fine. She is now pregnant and expecting twin girls. Survivors—4 (plus 2!!!).

Rita's treatments were going very well, but have now had to be started all over again. The best news for her is that there are new medicines and protocols they can use now to help her which were not available when she was first diagnosed. She is far more tired this time than during the first round, and she has lost her hair. The doctors have decreased the dosage by 25% to help with the tiredness, so she can still work at Karmanos as an oncological nurse. She will be on a "maintenance" dosage of chemo every three weeks, probably for the rest of her life. Rita, Tania and I got together in December 2009, to have lunch and plan to do the same again in December 2010. We three share an unbreakable bond, the three of us and the survivors 6.

Rose is doing magnificently. She has this little device that she carries to hold conversations. Only in noisy restaurants does she have to resort to using a pen and pad of paper. She looks good, feels good, is gaining weight, can participate in many games and activities with her grandchildren, and really enjoys their cottage at the lake in the summer. She still has to go to her doctor to have her esophagus stretched every three months and to get checked, but that is a small price to pay. Survivors 7.

Erica, the apheresis technician, was diagnosed with breast cancer not long after I met her. She is currently undergoing treatment. It must be much more terrifying for someone working in the medical field to be diagnosed with cancer, simply because they have so much more knowledge than the rest of us when we undertake this journey. All the education and all of your knowledge don't help you in those first few months of diagnosis. Fear is still fear. Body changes are still body changes. Isolation is still isolation. Life style changes are still life style changes. I saw Erica during my first visit back to Karmanos. Her first question, with tears in her eyes, was "Will my hair grow back?" "Oh, yes, Erica, mine has grown back twice now." I stopped back to see her at my two-year post-stem cell transplant. She was in another building, but the staff in the apherisis unit said she was doing very well. I stopped again in September 2010, and actually got to see her. Her hair has grown back, her eyes were all aglow, she looked really great, and then, what a blessing it was when she told me she really feels wonderful! Survivors 8.

Our editor, Karen (also one of the Lansing School District gang), learned that her daughter, who is in her mid-30s, had been diagnosed with cervical cancer in July 2009. Along with her new husband of only two years, her daughter decided to take the risk and try to have one more child of her own before undergoing treatment. A baby boy was born at the end of July 2010. As a very spiritual woman, she had trusted her faith to allow her to give her husband a child. She survived the pregnancy without cancer complications. The baby, a son, was born and has a few medical problems, which specialists are addressing. After the birth, Marya followed up as expected, and had the additional tests her doctor ordered. To date, there has been no sign of the cervical cancer that had been found. Where did it go? How did it just disappear? Is it hiding somewhere deeper inside? Was it ever really there?

This brings us to a record: Survivors—9, and Cancer—2. We can hold it at that. As I have discovered, the human body and our faith can miraculously carry us through many storms; storms through which, if we will just look and surrender ourselves, we can see our lives as we want them to be, and it will happen.

And if my cancer recurs, . . . which it can do, simply because it has metastasized once already? Well, I am reminded of a saying:

> *"Just when the caterpillar thought the world was over,*
> *it became a butterfly."*

(Sure wish I could meet the people who think of these things.)

We will take it one day at a time. There is no sense in borrowing tomorrow's troubles today. Every day is a new adventure, filled with endless possibilities, endless joys (and some sorrows, which help us appreciate the joys). As Ralph Waldo Emerson said, "Write it on your heart that every day is the best day in the year." Here is one of the mottos by which I now live my life:

> *Learn from the past, plan for the future, but live, fully*
> *live, today.*

LIFE IS GOOD !!!

Now What?

How do you define what a survivor is anyway? For some, it's from the second they were diagnosed until the day they die. For others, being a cancer survivor means they die of something else. Everyone who surrounds you—family, friends, colleagues—are also cancer survivors, however you choose to define it. The word "survivor" implies there is life after cancer (AC), and that it is a worthy goal, something for which to aim. While cancer is a horrible diagnosis to get, it can also be a life-changing experience, and, if you will let it, be a force for good for you and those who surround you.

There is so much that doctors don't tell you about what happens after you survive cancer. That's probably a good thing in the short term, because you will have had enough to deal with in just getting past being diagnosed, and then, getting through treatment. Neither you, nor your doctors, will have had the time or energy to even begin to think about what will follow treatment.

But afterward, you begin to have many questions about all that you are beginning to experience. Is this behavior or feeling normal? Do other people who have survived cancer experience these symptoms? Could this symptom mean my cancer is returning? How long will these symptoms last? Do these symptoms ever go away?

Yes, and No.

What follows in this book are descriptions, along with potential solutions, for some of the most common changes and conditions that you may confront as a survivor. Some you will experience, others not. Some of you may never have any of them (lucky you). This list is not meant to be totally inclusive or exclusive, by any means. Along the way, we offer what we refer to as "truisms," short statements of ideas we have come to accept as "truth" now, because of all we have seen and experienced. The symptoms are listed in alphabetical order, NOT in the order in which you may experience them or according to the frequency in which they may appear. And even though there are so many things that can happen to you AC, we would still go through chemo, radiation and a stem cell transplant all over again. These symptoms are negligible in comparison to the other alternatives you might face without the existence of these treatments. Another resource you might want to access is provided by the National Cancer Institute entitled "Facing Forward: Life After Cancer Treatment," http://www.cancer.gov (search under "survivorship.")

Allergies

We have discovered that we have become more susceptible to spring and fall pollen. Neither of us had allergies prior to getting cancer. It hasn't gotten to the point yet where we have to take medicines for it, but we definitely sneeze much more and get more stuffed-up. A few other survivors have mentioned the same thing.

Some people, however, have developed some pretty severe allergies, such as an allergy to latex or relating to the sinuses. If you develop an allergy for latex, be sure and write it down on your list of medicines/ treatments that you bring to the doctors. In the case of sinuses, remedies include some over-the-counter products, the administration of steroids or surgery. If you use an over-the-counter inhaler or other nasal medication and you get nosebleeds, stop taking them immediately (this sounds like common sense, but there are a lot of people who would still continue to use them just to get the relief they provide). If you are all of a sudden snoring at night, you might have to lose some weight to alleviate that, or use some of those breathing strips (they don't work a darn for Tom, but other people have had some good success). Another option is a CPAP (continuous positive air pressure) machine. You will have to go through a sleep apnea study and then find out what is best. Check your insurance first, to see if they cover the cost. Sometimes the runny nose can be directly correlated to the level of activity in which you are engaged. Keep a diary for a month or so to keep track of when your nose runs the most. It is also possible it could be dietary (either food or supplements), so keep track of what you ingest.

Some people have developed an allergy to dust and pets. If you find you have developed an allergy to dust, you will have to be hypervigilant about keeping your house clean. A filter on your furnace that is especially treated to trap dust and pollens might be an option for you, as are air purifiers (you might need more than one). Be sure you change the filters regularly. The air purifiers may have to be checked daily, especially in the spring and fall when pollen is highest. If you have pets, and neither medications, nor constant sweeping or vacuuming up the hair is working, you may seriously have to look at giving your pets to someone you know would give them a good home. (You might want to initially make arrangements for the return of your pet in the future should your allergy eventually improve.) Some people develop continually watery eyes. Sometimes it will simply take time for the chemo drugs to work their way out of your system, which might clear up your runny eyes. We would strongly suggest you work with your oncologist, optometrist or ophthalmologist to solve this problem. A very few people have developed an acute sensitivity to light. Headlights on cars at night, as well as neon signs and the glare from TV screens, can cause discomfort. Some of these conditions may go away (or return to "normal") after a period of time, but sometimes you will be stuck with any or all of them forever.

Alternative Medicine and Strategies

We have explored several types of alternative medicines or practices while undergoing treatment for cancer. What we discovered, as with most things in life, is there are no magic treatments, no simple answers and even fewer miracle cures. But some of the alternatives work extremely well with some people and with others, you might just as well save your money. (This is also true with the prescriptions you may take; some are more effective with men than women, as an example. In any case, always follow your doctors' directions but keep track of how the medications are affecting you and then talk with him or her about it. Do not assume you know more than they do and begin to monkey around with your medications or dosages.)

One that Terry explored was Ayurvedic medicine. Pat had also done some research into this when she was first diagnosed, so it made sense to at least listen and learn. In the interim, however, it got shunted off to the sidelines while trying to learn about prostate cancer and later, lymphoma, lung and other cancers. While in the hospital in January 2008, for more chemo, Terry had a nurse from India who talked to her about Ayurvedic medicine, so the topic was revived. Ayurvedic medicine probably dates back to 3,000 B.C. "Ayurveda" can be roughly translated as "knowledge of life" or specifically, "knowledge of long life." Ayurvedic medicine incorporates a philosophy that impacts physical, mental, social and spiritual harmony. There are eight branches or areas of Ayurvedic medicine: internal medicine; surgery; the ears, eyes, nose and throat; pediatrics; toxicology; purification of the genital organs; health and longevity; and spiritual healing, which can also include psychiatry. It is holistic in nature. There are references to diseases, herbs and herbal cures in the Vedas dating back to between 1200 and 700 B.C. Ayurvedic doctors believe that most plants, animals and certain minerals have value as medicines. These treatment capabilities have been documented over centuries, and are used to not only to cure illness, but also to maintain good health. In doing research on this topic, we found several American and Japanese companies are taking out patents on many native Indian plants to scientifically explore their efficacy. However, you must be very careful in exploring Ayurvedic medicine. There are few qualified doctors in the United States who practice or understand Ayurvedic medicine. There is a formal course for doctors in India, but it lacks the normal rigors of training required in other countries. Sometimes the medicine contains urine as one of the ingredients. Check it out thoroughly before embarking on this venture.

If you would like to explore other alternatives, a website that describes some of the strategies to fight cancer is http://www.cancer fightingstrategies.com. This website contains eleven "natural" strategies or supplements that have been examined and, according to the website, determined to be helpful in fighting cancer. There are hundreds of pages here to read. Several products are recommended for you to take. Most of the stories citing success in treating cancer are anecdotal in nature. Some of the studies they report are effective with mice or in the laboratory, but have not been tried on humans. One thing we do concur with is that apart from possible genetic causes of cancer, we are exposed to a variety of pesticides, hormones and additives in our food that expose us to toxins. Our lifestyles are stressed to the breaking point at times, and we also fail to get enough sleep at night. The website alleges that often doctors are prevented from mentioning "holistic" or alternative medicinal strategies, because the insurance companies don't look favorably on non-drug treatments for cancer. In addition, the website alleges the medical industry makes tons of money from people's illnesses, so there is no real incentive to change this practice. We have not investigated these claims, but question the allegation for one reason: doctors, other health care providers and researchers also have friends and family who are going through cancer treatment and it's unlikely they would prevent any kind of "cure" or improvement in cancer care. On the other hand, the one who has the gold makes the rules (and since pharmaceutical companies are now funding a huge chunk of research at universities, it makes sense). If you decide to read this website, please do so with the idea of gathering ideas for future discussion with your doctor(s). However, this website would say that regular medical doctors would probably look askance at this because of their medical training. That might be true enough. It is possible some of the supplements this website recommends could be used in conjunction with chemotherapy and/or radiation. Some, however, may be toxic, taken in combination with the treatment(s) you are receiving. Not all supplements or "natural" herbs are beneficial. We do believe a healthier lifestyle is in order for most of us, but particularly once you have been diagnosed with, and treated for, cancer. This means increasing fruit and vegetable intake, limiting or eliminating meat consumption, purchasing meat and poultry that is grass-fed and free-range, and increasing your intake of whole grains. These dietary changes make sense whether you have cancer or not.

As with many alternative strategies, you need to check with your doctor about starting anything new. This is true whether you are in perfect health or have been diagnosed with a health concern. When Tom was first beginning his treatments, 100% of the supplements he had been taking, all of which he had gotten from the six alternative medicine newsletters he gets, turned out NOT to be beneficial at all. He had taken these supplements to prevent certain illnesses (which occurred anyway), and had potentially caused him harm; they all had to be discontinued because they conflicted with the medicines being administered to treat his cancer. A lot of these alternative medicine newsletters actually lie (or for sure, stretch the truth a distance that would measure equal to that from Bangor, Maine to San Francisco, California), so you must be careful. They are written in the most lurid manner to try and sucker everyone into buying their products. The vast majority of what they report is not based on scientific trials, but rather upon anecdotal stories. Because everyone is different, one alternative health strategy might work with one individual, but be potentially harmful or even fatal to another. As an example, Alexis's Mom was diagnosed with breast cancer and opted to do a holistic regimen instead of chemo. She is alive fourteen years later and doing well. She has also become a total and complete vegetarian, which may be the reason she has done so well. In another case, the mother-in-law of a businessman we know had traditional chemotherapy for her type of cancer, and that, too, was successful. Treatment ended and then a few years later, her cancer came back. This time she tried alternative medicines and, once again, had great success. But now, her cancer has come back again and she is currently trying to decide whether to go back to chemotherapy (with which she will feel awful during the treatment), or whether to try the alternative medicines again. Frankly, she felt better overall with the alternative medicines. It's truly a horrible position in which to find oneself. Whichever way she goes, should it turn out not to help, she and her family will always second guess themselves and play the "What if" game (again, a little like life itself).

The other reality to consider is that different strategies outside traditional Western medicine can be effective. Whether or not this is due to a belief in that other process, perhaps a sort of "placebo" effect, is, as yet, undetermined. You could certainly say we believed, really believed, the chemo would be successful—and it has been. It has been successful beyond our wildest imaginations (and we're both great in the imagination department). Both of us have inquiring minds and are always exploring other alternatives (which has helped in writing this book)—but we do so with the guidance and counseling of our doctors, as well as double-checking sources for validation. That is simply common sense. We also now try to do things that make sense from a health perspective: we try to eat real food, not the food that has been grown with pesticides or in the case of animals, have been fed antibiotics and steroids. We are switching to a more vegetarian diet. We stay away from products that contain sugar and high fructose corn syrup. We exercise fairly regularly, but are not slaves to routines and pain. We try to maintain a positive attitude about life in general. We are spiritual in our feelings about a Creator. We try to get a good night's sleep, but that can sometimes be unrealistic; the usual worries that accompany you to bed, whether work-related or family stressors, fears of illness or of the treatments, can often preclude one from getting eight hours or more of restful sleep.

The National Institutes of Health (NIH) has an office called "National Center for Complementary and Alternative Medicine," which actually was started in 1991 under a different organizational name. Its purpose is to investigate what is outside the mainstream of western medicine. To date, there have been no "magic bullets" discovered, no herbs, no harnessing of energies that will cure cancer (please read the section on diet and nutrition in this book for some recently discovered news). However, there have been promising developments that will help the patient. Acupuncture has been found to relieve the nausea that often accompanies chemotherapy. If you have head and neck cancer and have had radiation treatment, which has destroyed your salivary glands, acupuncture has restored some of the salivary gland functions. Self-hypnosis can ease the symptoms of hot flashes. Support groups appear to not only improve the quality of life for cancer patients and for survivors, but there is also some suggestion the groups can increase the lengths of survival times. Massage eases stress. Yoga may help fight fatigue. Reiki might help with prostate cancer, but is still undergoing analysis. Some vegetables and herbal supplements might help with lung cancer. M.D. Anderson is exploring how effective curcumin is (used in Ayurvedic medicine) for multiple myeloma and for rectal cancers. The Osher Center for Integrative Medicine at the University of California at San Francisco is exploring the effectiveness of mushrooms, long used in traditional Chinese medicine.

Another type of strategy you might want to consider is meditation. Memorial Sloan-Kettering (MSK) is using meditation with patients who have undergone surgery for cancer. There are always fears that remain after you have had cancer. The biggest is: Will it come back? Meditation can calm your mind and help loosen that tight feeling you get in the pit of your stomach when you become too mired in the dark and gloomy parts of your mind. There are several DVDs, tapes and CDs available on meditation. After reading a few books, we have discovered there is no right or wrong way to meditate, but you should select one that makes the most sense, or feels most comfortable and effective for you.

But be cautious—not all strategies will work for every person and some, such as herbal supplements, may actually cause you harm while you are undergoing chemotherapy and radiation, or as you survive, may interfere with the maintenance medications you are taking. A few to mention specifically are St. John's wort, which can impair liver function by not processing medicines properly; gingko is an anticoagulant and can lead to severe bleeding, particularly if you are taking Coumadin or about to undergo surgery. Please don't fall victim to every alternative magazine or health brochure that comes to you in the mail or that you see on the Internet. They are designed to feed on your fears. Both MSK and M.D. Anderson have websites that can help you negotiate between what is safe, and what could be potentially be harmful for you (http://www.mskcc.org, http://www.mdanderson.org). Two other websites to check on alternative therapies or strategies are as follow: first, http://www.annieappleseedproject.org and then, http://www.bulletin.aarp.org. We believe every cancer patient, whether current, a survivor or especially those with metastatic cancer, are looking for hope. As Terry's Mom used to say, "Where there's life, there's hope." Hope, along with a positive attitude, the faith that survival is possible, and the will and commitment to fight, may prove to be exceptional partners in your battle with cancer, giving you the hope you need both during treatment, and AC during your survival.

Is there bias in Western medicine regarding alternatives to health care? Yes, because some of it is well founded and should be heeded. There are others, however, such as acupuncture and perhaps Ayurvedic medicine, which have had a hard struggle to gain any acceptance in Western nations or with insurance companies. What is ironic about this is that American and Japanese companies have tried for decades to get patents on the plants that have been used by Ayurvedic doctors for centuries, a sort of bio-piracy.

So where does that leave us? Sharon is currently exploring an alternative diet (gluten-free) for her MS, and is experiencing great success. Her MS symptoms have abated (just as an aside, you might want to check a website Sharon sent to Terry: http://www.dogtorj.com. It is from a veterinarian who had been having some health problems himself and noticed a connection between his animal patients and what he had been experiencing; the diet he recommends is similar to the one Sharon is following. Look under "Food Intolerance.") Deb, Debbie and Nancy are each trying different food diets for their fibromyalgia. One of them was moderately successful; the other two weren't, even when it was the same diet. Tom tried the "blood" diet, which takes your blood type and then determines which foods you should and should not eat. It didn't do diddley for Tom, but for Alexis, it was wonderful.

We're not advocating one form of alternative health strategy or therapy over another (such as the CML diet, acupuncture, homeopathic medicine or Ayurvedic medicine). What we are advocating is that you learn as much as you can about different strategies, and then explore those that make the most sense to you, whether traditional Western medicine or an alternative, or a combination of the two. In this process, you also have to learn to trust your *self* and your body. Quite often your body will tell you what it needs (aside from pepperoni pizza and BLTs every day). If you suddenly crave bananas or are experiencing leg cramps, your system may be low on potassium. If you are craving beef (and remember, only a serving that fits in the palm of your hand), your body may be low on iron. If you live in a northern region with little sunshine, consider increasing your intake of citrus (unless you have an allergy or sensitivity to it, or are taking a medication that negatively reacts with citrus) and calcium with a lot of vitamin D in it. What is key is that good communication has to occur between you and your doctor(s) about what your body is craving and what you are thinking of ingesting. A nutritionist would also be helpful in this area.

Aromatherapy and Essential Oils

During our research, we accessed several websites and studied a couple of books to find information on this topic. We believe the National Cancer Institute website, http://www.cancer.gov/cancertopicspdq/cam/aromatherapy/HealthProfessoinal.com, has better, more recent, and more accurate information and suggest you access it for detailed explanations and the institute's referrals to associated research. The studies provide scientific information regarding efficacy.

Aromatherapy and Essential Oils are sometimes promoted for the improvement of the quality of life for cancer patients. Aromatherapy, an offshoot of herbal medicine, is used as supportive care for general well-being. There are some people who use these techniques and are quite successful. The practices learned while undergoing chemotherapy and radiation are continued once a person becomes a survivor. Aromatherapy is used as a compliment to traditional therapies, massage and acupuncture. Most studies regarding aromatherapy and essential oils focus on their psychological effects, rather than physical effects.

Practitioners of aromatherapy and essential oils contend that the approach has been used for thousands of years, and that the practice was mentioned in the Bible and in ancient Egyptian writings. Aromatherapy and essential oils were also used during the Middle Ages and the Renaissance. Then, aromatherapy and essential oils went out of vogue until the latter half of the 20th century. As a result of increasing awareness and acceptance of alternative medicines and treatments, aromatherapy and essential oils have gained new credence. Cosmetic companies have also gotten on the bandwagon, but tend to use synthetic ingredients rather than the natural substances used historically. Purists in aromatherapy and essential oil believe these synthetics are inferior to natural products.

The theory behind aromatherapy is that it works on the limbic system, the brain's emotional center. The essential oils may have antibacterial, anti-inflammatory and analgesic (the reduction or elimination of pain) effects. Studies on animals have shown that essential oils can have positive effects on behavior and the immune system. Functional MRIs (fMRI) on humans show certain odors in essential oils can have a positive effect on the limbic system. There is usually low toxicity, if inhaled, or if a diluted topical application is used. The biochemical experts and psychologists tend to refute these claims because there are no scientific studies to support these assertions. The FDA (Food and Drug Administration) does not need to approve plants (trees, flowers, herbs) and oils used because there is no claim made that certain diseases will be treated and cured.

The other reason it is hard to determine the effect of aromatherapy and essential oils is that different practitioners use different products for the same illnesses. Training in aromatherapy and the use of essential oils is available throughout the United States and the United Kingdom, but no professional standards or licensing procedures are required of practitioners. There are two organizations currently working on this void: The National Association for Holistic Aromatherapy and the Alliance of International Aromatherapists.

Articles have been published which describe the use of aromatherapy and essential oils when patients are critically ill. Aromatherapy and essential oils have been used as palliative care for stress, anxiety, pain, depression, nausea, HIV-positive children and terminally ill people. Since these have not been controlled studies, outcomes are more subjective in nature, and offer only anecdotal evidence in support of observed outcomes, as opposed to scientific analyses.

One recent study conducted in Australia was placebo-controlled, double blind and randomized, in order to ascertain the effects of inhaled aromatherapy on anxiety with people receiving radiation. There were no significant differences in depression, except in the group whose subjects received carrier (massage) oils; in this group, a statistically significant decrease in anxiety was found. In another controlled trial, those that received massage showed improvement with decreases in anxiety, but it was not statistically significant. In a U.K. cancer center, a study done to determine reduction in anxiety and depression in cancer patients showed no evidence of psychological benefit, but for patients' blood pressure, pulse and respiratory rates, all three were reduced.

The good news is there appears to be minimal adverse effects by using essential oils if inhaled or used topically. Ingestion is not recommended. Caution should be used if you decide to try using essential oils. As examples, massage with camphor oil can cause skin irritation and citrus oils can cause sensitivity to the sun making you more prone to sunburn. Make sure all essential oils are freshly made, because the chemical composition changes over time. Prolonged exposure to lavender and some tea tree oils that are topically applied may be harmful for women at high risk for hormonally sensitive breast cancer.

Attitude, Attitude, Attitude . . .

As an introduction to this section, a little story for us to reflect upon, especially those of us with cancer or who have survived it, is offered below.

> There once was a woman who woke up one morning, looked in the mirror, and noticed she had only three hairs on her head. "Well," she said, "I think I'll braid my hair today." So she did and she had a wonderful day.
>
> The next day she woke up, looked in the mirror and saw that she only had two hairs on her head. "Hmmmm," she said, "I think I'll part my hair down the middle today." So she did and she had a grand day.

The next day she woke up, looked in the mirror and noticed that she had only one hair on her head. "Well," she said, "today I'm going to wear my hair in a pony tail." So she did, and she had a fun day.

The next day she woke up, looked in the mirror and noticed that there wasn't a single hair on her head. "Hooray," she shouted, "I don't have to fix my hair today!"

—*Author Unknown*

And a little something else to consider:

"If there is no struggle, there is no progress."

—*Frederick Douglass*

The Parable of the Young Warrior:

A young warrior asked a wise man to tell him how to deal with the beasts within him who were at odds with each other (the good and the evil). The wise man told him, "The one that you feed is the one that will survive."

(Thanks, Pat, for this insight.)

And James Allen, a little known philosopher (1864–1912) who pre-dated Norman Vincent Peale's *Power of Positive Thinking*, says,

". . . Where we are today is because of our thoughts, for we are the architects of our own futures."

We recommend reading James Allen's *As a Man Thinketh*, for insights that can lift and carry you through the challenges life puts into your paths.

Throughout this book, you will find that 'attitude' keeps coming up as a recurrent theme and resource. We have, so many times now, been witness to its power and the vast differences it makes for people in many kinds of difficult situations, that we are not only believers, but also advocates. You may discover for yourself as you experience seri-ous illness, that the medical professionals you encounter consider attitude a critical component to the practice of medicine and a significant variable as to whether people recover.

If you ever go to Seattle, go to Pike Place Fish, where you will see Attitude with a capitol "A." There is even a book and video out entitled *Fish!* which documents their attitude. Sharon and Terry used this philosophy, along with an assets-based approach, in the early 2000s when they worked with middle and senior high school kids to try to help them in school. There are four basic lessons, which can be applicable to your business, your relationships and your health:

1. Choose your attitude
2. Play
3. Make someone's day
4. Be present

We have shown you several ways to choose your attitude at various points in our stories. Alexis and Terry decided early on that there was to be no pity party, that we would be upbeat, confident, believe we were going to be back in good health, that we deserved good health, and that we wanted to be around to see our grandkids become adults and have children of their own. There was the gift of that great expression—"I have cancer, but cancer doesn't have me!" We deliberately, consciously, with full intent and purpose, decided we would find a way to adopt and maintain a positive experience.

We have also shown you how to play—we laughed, joked, and found humor in every day events and even in our conditions. One website we really like is Drew Olanoff's "Blame Drew's Cancer." Olanoff was diagnosed with lymphoma at age 29. He has linked up with The American Cancer Society and Make a Wish Foundation. Every time someone accesses his website on Twitter and Facebook, sponsors will donate a dollar for every participant. A couple of years ago, there were well over 14,000 things that could be blamed on cancer—losing your keys, forgetting to feed the dog, your home sports team losing the Big Game, not remembering your anniversary, that greedy vending machine swallowing your money, the sun not shining on your birthday . . . Drew has found a way to Play—and make it pay at the same time. When you play, time goes faster, you are actually healthier, creativity is sparked, and people treat each other better and with more respect, something this world could really use.

All of us who have cancer (or other debilitating disease) could be forgiven for occasional lapses into "Woe is me." But the best way out of this is to find a way to make someone's day a little better. This not only means finding something positive to say to someone, or to help them in some way, but it also encourages them to play along with you. Help people become animated, to really feel alive, to explore their own creativity and their many blessings. Have people join in on your fun. Terry has a refrigerator magnet (the several she has are what's holding the refrigerator together) that says, "You never know when you're creating a memory." (Her personal favorite, however, is the one that says, "Save Earth. It's the only planet with chocolate.") What you get in return is this tremendous flow of positive energy, one that flows both outward and inward—it is infectious, the greatest infection you could ever get or give! If you've never seen the movie *Pay It Forward*, run out right now (walk if you must) and either buy it or rent it. There are countless examples in that movie for making someone's day. Sharon and Terry also used this concept when they were working with kids. You wouldn't believe some of the stories we got back from those young people.

We all have tendencies to live in the past ("Boy, did she ever have to go way back to dredge that up!") or in the future ("Tomorrow I'll get out the good china and use it" or "Next week I'll go see my aunt" or "This weekend I'll take you to the park and go on the rides—if it doesn't rain"). Figure out a way to really be present, in the "now" of the moment, to be fully engaged with the person, or the work situation, or wherever you find yourself. Talk with friends and family to focus on what is truly important, both *to* them and *for* them, and then make it a practice to take those examples and apply them to people, even strangers or coworkers, you meet during the day. Focus on how you can make every encounter a positive experience for that person, as well as for yourself.

Even after you survive cancer, you will always need to stay focused on the positive. Sometimes you will have to look for things, really look. When the basement is flooding or there has been excessive rain and your yard is flooded, or your child is in the hospital, it's hard to find positives, but they're there. "Look, honey, we won't have to wash the basement floors for a *long* time!" or "Gee, if this rain keeps up, we will soon have lakefront property." (O.K., these are really stretching it.) But it's not a stretch to say to your child, "This might be the opportunity to make new friends" or "This person has the exact same thing you have, and is someone with whom you can talk." Studies have repeatedly shown that the friendships you make while undergoing cancer treatment can have a healing effect. Cancer can be quite isolating on an emotional level, especially during those long periods of time you cannot be exposed to any germs. (There actually were times when Tom and Terry had to stay away from each other in their own home—talk about a difficult caregiver role. Come to think of it, there were times when that would have been a good idea before either of them ever had cancer! Just kidding, love.) Anyway, these feelings of isolation are why the friends you have had since the beginning of time, as well as the new friends you make, actually support your immune system and help you fight this disease. *You need to have a life outside cancer* and not live your disease.

There is probably no greater advocate for a positive attitude than actor Michael J. Fox. His latest book is entitled, *Always Looking Up*. He has taken Parkinson's disease and made it his life's work. He is an inspiration to millions of us. He gives credit to Lance Armstrong, testicular cancer survivor, for helping him realize he was bigger than the disease, that this could, in some way, benefit people. He also relies on a greater power, which gives him inner strength. He does not define what this "greater power" is, nor does he allow others to define it for him. He is surrounded by constant, unconditional love by his family and friends, including the new friends he makes while speaking about Parkinson's disease, which for him is a reflection of who and what his greater power is. He chose to change his perspective as a person from 'one with a disease' to '***one with a mission.***' He could either focus on the disease and what he couldn't do, or focus on his life's meaning and what he could do. He could either face things with a sense of humor, or allow himself to be caught up in the drama of the disease. He could either be Michael with Parkinson's, or Michael with a cause. He could very easily change our motto of "I have cancer, but cancer doesn't have me" to "I have Parkinson's, but Parkinson's doesn't have me." He uses his sense of gratefulness as a dedication to his greater power. In the long run, he chooses to believe that everything gets better from the first time he puts his feet on the floor in the morning to the end of the day when he goes to bed. He looks at Parkinson's as a way to learn new things, to travel paths he might never have taken, and meet incredible people all along the way. It's not how far you get that day on the path, but how far you travel in your lifetime and how much you can benefit others. His is a true life of service, a true example of living in the "now" of the moment.

Or look at the example of Peng Shulin (thanks, Pat, for sending this). In 1995, a truck sliced his body in half. He spent two years in a hospital in China recuperating (and to think, Terry complained about three or five weeks—why, she's an amateur!). Every major organ and system in his body had to be rerouted. Amazingly, doctors at the Beijing Rehabilitation Center have devised a way that would allow him to walk, called an RGO—Reciprocating Gait Orthosis. And now, after ten years, he has learned to walk and has opened his own small business called—"Half Man—Half Price." (His humor is remarkable!) He also uses a wheelchair that makes it possible for him to travel and give lectures on recovering from a disability. His secret? Cheerfulness. According to doctors, he never lets anything get him down. With this man as a role model, we too, can get through anything!

Another example of a positive attitude is a video (http://www.cmu.edu/randyslecture) and book, *The Last Lecture*, published by Hyperion and written by Dr. Randy Pausch, a Carnegie Mellon University computer scientist. Randy was diagnosed in August 2007, with pancreatic cancer, which has about a 15% five-year survival rate. He was originally given three to six months to live, but died after just about a year later on July 25, 2008. As a legacy, he had founded the Alice Project, which allows youth to tell their stories in three dimensions. He has also written "A Lesson on How to Say Goodbye" and "Keeping Priorities Straight, Even at the End." They are both available at http://www.blogs.nytimes.com.

There is another book you may wish to read called *On Pilgrimage*, by Jennifer Lash. This is the story about her mother's trip through cancer. Jennifer's mother was diagnosed with cancer in the 1980s; it was caught too late and was extremely aggressive. Her way to deal with this was to put on some sneakers, pack what today would be called a backpack, and set out alone. She went to France and Spain. She didn't want any of her family to go with her. This was her pilgrimage. This was her own personal conquest about meeting people, learning about others' faiths, her own journey to discover and understand how people from other places approached life in all its fascinating variations. It was a means of her having her own conversation with cancer, of putting cancer in its place, and taking some control of her own destiny, finding what she wanted from life. Our favorite, and perhaps the best line in the book? "Poor cancer!"

Stephen Jay Gould, evolutionary theorist at Harvard University, wrote *The Median Isn't the Message* (among other books). In 1982 he was diagnosed with incurable abdominal mesothelioma. Being a researcher and familiar with statistics, he sought information on his condition, which said that the median (average) survival was eight months. Being unwilling to settle for that, he decided to do more research. He discovered that for this type of cancer, he was young when diagnosed, even when considering his diagnosis occurred in the early stages of mesothelioma. He had access to the best doctors and medical protocols, and he knew how to read statistical reports. He also discovered that if you have a positive attitude, if you have a strong will to live, if you have purpose for your life, if you are willing to fight, and if you take an active role in your treatment and diagnosis rather than sitting passively and accepting whatever you hear, you will live longer. He eventually died at age 60 in 2002, fully twenty years beyond the original projected survival. And he died, not of mesothelioma, but of a new, secondary and unrelated cancer. The question is not whether he was merely an unusual case, but rather to what extent was his attitude a contributing factor to his longevity way beyond that of the expected or norm? If you are interested in statistics as they relate to various types of cancer, and want to learn more, please go to http://www.cancerguide.org/scurve_basic.html. A Truism:

> *"Choose your attitude, play, make someone's day, laugh, look for the blessings, be present in the now, go on your own form of pilgrimage, give joy, take back your life, and make of it what YOU want."*

And our thanks, to Pike Place Fish, Michael J. Fox, Peng Shulin, Dr. Randy Pausch, Jennifer Lash and Stephen Jay Gould. You each serve as inspirations to all of us.

Balance

There is no good way of saying this. The odds are, you will have trouble with your balance for a long time after receiving chemo—it could take up to six years to get it back. If you stand up too quickly, you will likely need to grab onto something to keep from falling. You can simply be standing quietly somewhere, turn to move, and lose your balance. You can be making the bed, bending just slightly to tuck in that last corner, then straighten up—and lose your balance. If you wake up from a sound sleep to go to the bathroom and haven't quite figured out yet how to open your eyes to make the trip there—you might lose your balance. If you're planting flowers in the springtime and are on your knees, then stand up—you might lose your balance. You can already be ambulatory and lose your balance (if you have chocolate in your hand, make sure to save that). It seems anything can trigger it.

We have found a couple of stretching exercises that might help your extension and strength, thereby helping you improve your ability to maintain balance. Our thanks to Audrey, a personal trainer we met, now in Virginia, for her help and with the following exercises. Again, please be sure to check with your physician(s) before starting any kind of exercise program.

Put your hands on a bed or countertop, bend your right leg at a right angle, and stretch your left leg behind you with your other foot flat on the floor and lean forward, sort of "into" your arms. What you're actually doing is stretching your calf muscles. Hold that position for between 15–30 seconds *while closing your eyes*. You might feel a little swaying, but you are already holding onto something to prevent falling. Then switch positions.

A good warm-up that joggers do before a run is also good for balance. Make sure you have something to grab onto that is very close by—a bed, chair, countertop, *something solid*. Standing upright, with your right foot flat on the floor, grab your left ankle with your left hand and pull your leg up toward your left buttock. Use your right hand to steady yourself. You are now working on your thigh muscles. After a few seconds, close your eyes and remove your right hand from the bed or whatever is supporting you. As you feel yourself sway, which should only take about a milli-second, reach out with your right hand to steady yourself. Try to do this several times, and then repeat with your right leg. And for heaven's sake, if you feel yourself really begin swaying, open your eyes and grab onto something quickly to prevent falling. Keep in mind that if you have low blood pressure, you will have more difficulty with this, so be careful.

Another stretching exercise is to stand with your right foot flat on the floor, and then stretch your left leg to the left as far as you can. Make sure both your feet are pointed straight out, at right angles to a wall or whatever you are using as a support. This time, you are actually stretching the muscles in your inner thigh. Again, you will want *something solid* nearby to grab onto if you feel yourself swaying or about to fall. Hold that position for a few seconds, and then close your eyes. If you feel yourself swaying or falling, open your eyes and grab onto the wall or countertop to prevent falling. Do this a few times, and then switch legs.

Another good stretching exercise is to have your feet close together, arms down at your side. Bend your knees until your buttocks are perpendicular to your knees. Try and keep your knees directly over your feet. Again, have something solid in reach. Hold that position if possible, for a slow count of five; then slowly stand up. This works the top of your thighs. The next time, go down and close your eyes. If you feel yourself beginning to sway too much, open your eyes and use your hands to balance yourself.

There is nothing magic or scientific about this. These are exercises Terry has been doing to try to help stabilize her balance. There has been some moderate success, but in reality, only time will fully restore her balance. If you are at "that age" where balance is beginning to become a factor in your life anyway, these exercises can't hurt and may actually help.

Tai chi is also a great exercise with many health benefits. Tai chi can help improve balance (maybe even helping to prevent falls), flexibility and muscle strength. It may also help people with high blood pressure, Parkinson's disease, and rehabilitation if you've had knee replacement surgery. It can reduce stress, arthritis and overall joint stiffness. One study has shown that cardiovascular health was improved by increasing the amount of oxygen in your system, and may slow the rate of heart disease. It may also help those with insomnia. (See the posting in *Healthy Living* on June 16, 2010.)

As we said earlier in this discussion, before you begin any exercise program, <u>talk with your doctor first</u>. If you have high blood pressure or any other condition, your doctor may prescribe different, less stressful, exercises and stretches for you to do.

Boogers (or "Bogies" in the Harry Potter Books)

First of all, does anyone really know what boogers are? Or how they are formed? Or how the name came into being? In our never-ending quest to make this a useful book, we have looked all this up for you. First of all, no one really knows where the term originated or how it came into being, but it has been around since the late 1800s. "Boogers" have had numerous meanings over the years, but now it mainly refers to the hardened, solid stuff in your nose. Boogers are actually mucus. We usually call the slimy stuff "snot." About a quart a day (yes, really!) of snot is made by our bodies. Mucus helps to protect the lungs by sorting out the pollen, dirt, germs and dust we inhale every day. Inside the nose are tiny hairs called cilia. When there is too much stuff stuck inside the nose, mucus forms around it and the cilia. The cilia keep moving this stuff toward the front of the nose. When it clumps and dries, we get boogers. (We were so sure there must be a scientific name for it, but as it turns out, there really isn't. One person, however, said it was called "candy." We did find out there is a scientific name for picking your boogers—it's called "rhinotillexis." If you eat them, it's called "mucophagy." And if you're reading this and are a boy 10 years old or know a 10-year-old boy, there is a rather neat website that explains the "ins and outs" of making boogers: http://library.thinkquest.org/J0112390/Boogers.htm.

As delicately as this can be said, chemo destroys your boogers (the hard, crusty, clumpy kind), or "bogies" if you are living in England. You might not have any boogers for months after you stop chemo, but you will definitely have snot, which drips uncontrollably at the most inconvenient times (like when you're brushing your teeth or are on a walk and two miles from home—note: take extra tissues with you on the walk and make sure the pocket you stuff them into doesn't have any holes; this is the voice of experience). This has happened to both of us and countless others of our acquaintance. In Terry's case, it was 17 months after her last chemo and the stem cell transplant that she actually got boogers back. It lasted about a week, then they disappeared and the clear liquid returned. About a month later, she got her boogers back, and they are still "sticking" with her.

There's always something to which we can look forward.

Brownouts

This is a temporary condition that manifests itself by a perception that light is dimming, colors may change, and is usually accompanied by a loss of vision, especially around the peripheries. Sometimes it can lead to fainting. It is caused by *hypoxia* (low brain oxygen level) and is quite often due to a drop in blood pressure. If you stand up quickly, sometimes you do more than just lose your balance—you feel like you are going to pass out and everything around you turns brown or into dark sepia tones everywhere. You lose your vision for a period of seconds before it begins to gradually return. It is usually over quickly, and doesn't cause permanent harm to your eyes, although Terry once did "pass out," and "woke up" to find herself on the floor. She has no recollection of gently sliding down the wall and didn't hurt herself in any way (she assumes it was a gentle slide because she didn't hurt anywhere and could not find any bruises). One way to address the condition is to lie down immediately when a brownout begins. This way your blood flow doesn't have to work against gravity. Another recommendation is to drastically increase your fluid intake, particularly water. It hasn't helped Terry much, but others have reported lower frequency of this state. If you have low blood pressure, you are more likely than others to experience the condition.

Cataracts

Cataracts can occur at any age but it is most common when people reach their 60s or later in life. At this point in time, there is nothing that can prevent cataracts, but certain behaviors increase your risk, such as: cigarette smoking, exposure to sunlight, diabetes, eye injuries, obesity and certain drugs, including chemotherapy drugs. According to a Johns Hopkins Health Alert e-Newsletter in July 2009, about 75% of people over the age of 60 have some degree of cataract formation. It has been predicted by 2020, more than 30 million people will have cataracts. In the US, cataract surgery is the most commonly performed operation, with more than 1.5 million performed every year.

Cataracts (from the Latin word for "waterfall") are a cloudiness (or *opacification*) of the eye's lens, which is usually clear. In ancient times, it was believed that "evil" liquids somehow flowed into the eyes of those perceived as undeserving, creating shadowed and unclear vision.

Two factors associated with aging contribute to the development of cataracts: first, a "clumping" of proteins in the lens promotes a disbursement of light, which then causes the transparency of the lens to decrease. This breakdown of the lens proteins causes an accumulation of yellowish-brown pigments that lead to the clouding of the lens.

Some of the changes in the eyes of people who have cataracts are a reduced level of oxygen by the lens, then a rise in the water content, then dehydration at some later point. When cataracts form in your eye, there is usually an increase in calcium and sodium, in conjunction with a decrease in potassium, vitamin C and proteins. In Terry's case, after chemo, her eyes have become increasingly dry, necessitating nightly eye drops to keep them moist. This was not the case prior to chemotherapy. She has also had to take additional calcium because of *osteoporosis*. During chemotherapy and the stem cell transplant, she received supplemental doses of potassium and vitamin C.

There is no pain associated with the formation of cataracts. They usually form gradually, over a number of years, and then in what appears to be "all of a sudden" things become cloudy, blurry and/or dimmer. Usually both eyes are affected, but one eye might be worse than the other. Common symptoms are: increased sensitivity to glare, the appearance of a "halo" around lights, especially on cars at night, increasingly poor vision when driving at night, objects might appear yellowish, the need to have more frequent changes in glasses and/or contact lens prescriptions, and you might also notice a need for brighter light while reading or doing other close work. In some cases, "double vision" may even occur. In Terry's case, she was what is known as "pre-cataract" (the cataract developmental stage) for many years, but after chemotherapy, in the course of less than one year, she saw (no pun intended) a dramatic increase in her left eye of the development of the cataract. There was no cataract in her right eye, but now there is. Her optometrist, Dr. Ken Marton, said the cataracts might stay the same for years now that the chemotherapy has been discontinued, but they could also grow quite quickly again, and would need removal to maintain her vision.

If you've had chemotherapy, or a stem cell transplant, odds are you will develop cataracts sooner than later. Fortunately, there are now incredible laser procedures to treat cataracts. Terry is legally blind without her contacts. Once she has the cataract surgery, she will most likely not need contacts at all. For further information, see *Vision* magazine, July 24, 2009.

Chemo Brain

"Chemo brain" is a very real condition. One theory is that the cytokines the body produces to fight the cancer may contribute to this condition, but in general the causes are unknown. Doctors and scientists don't know what triggers it, nor do they know how to prevent it. Possible causes are, of course, the chemotherapy regimen chosen (including the ancillary drugs to combat nausea, as an example), but it may also be related to the patient's age, stress level, lack of sleep, or depression. The projections show that perhaps as many as 70% of people, both men and women, who are fighting cancer will experience chemo brain.

Previously, it was thought that chemo didn't cross any barriers within the brain, but that assumption is now being reassessed. Some chemos do, in fact, cross the blood-brain barrier, but what happens is that the brain is weakened just a little bit. One possible side effect of the weakening of the brain is that, as we age, we might not handle the aging process as well as we might have under more normal circumstances.

Chemo brain is characterized by a number of emerging deficits, including the lack of concentration, inability to focus, inability to multi-task, inability to process problems (comprehension and reasoning) and an incredible ease in being distracted. These all probably sound like the same symptoms, and perhaps they are. Some people also find that it takes longer to do an every-day, ordinary project, because you are thinking more slowly and it takes longer to process what you want to do. Outsiders (family, friends and colleagues) may not notice any difference, but those of us taking chemo notice a definite difference in these areas. Sometimes inhibitions can be reduced during and after chemo. Only you and those closest to you will be able to determine if this is a problem (if you find yourself wanting to mimic Lady Godiva, but with short or no hair, we suggest you seek professional help.)

It is the production of neurons in the hippocampus in the brain that is derailed during chemotherapy. Chemo precludes any cell division that would generate new cells. This will lead to difficulty in learning new things or remembering those things you already knew. This does not mean you can't function quite well in "normal" circumstances—driving the car to the grocery store, getting dressed, being able to socialize with friends and family. However, different kinds of learning involving different cognitive processes will have been disrupted and scrambled somewhat. For an interesting discussion and more in-depth analysis of this and a process called "neurogenesis," please refer to "Saving New Brain Cells" by Tracey J. Shors, in the March 2009, issue of *Scientific American.*

One of the most frustrating occurrences is to be deep in discussion about anything, and have your mind all of a sudden go totally and completely blank. You can be in mid-sentence, have a brilliant observation or even a solution to a problem at work or quick-witted response to make, and, suddenly—whamo, it's gone. Wiped out. The memory banks have been erased. Sometimes the observation comes back—in a minute or an hour, or a week. Most of the time, at least initially, it's gone forever. It's as if you never had the thought or response at all, and you become very unsure of your abilities to usefully contribute in most every setting. You may even find yourself interrupting people, just to assure that you can get your thought out before it becomes lost.

It can also be quite difficult to learn something new and retain it. Repetition becomes the norm, which is frustrating for the person on the receiving end. Simple concepts are magnified in complexity. Nothing "sticks" in your mind.

If you are reading a technical journal, or something that requires some thought or new learning, you will re-read it over and over and over to try, not only make some sense out of it, but also to retain it.

If you have been concentrating on something, and get interrupted, you have to go back to the beginning and start all over. It seems your short-term memory just simply cannot kick in, so interruptions of any kind become costly in terms of accomplishing anything.

You can only do one thing at a time, and no more. If your spouse or roommate or parent puts three things on a list to do, you might get one done. It's hard to focus on more than one task or activity, even when they are attempted in some kind of sequence.

And sometimes, you will find that trying to think something through from start to finish, even tasks as simplistic and critical as taking your medications, for example, become impossible to do for a period of time.

We have had our sporadic moments with chemo brain and have learned to tolerate them, but for about eighteen months after our last chemo, we both experienced more than a month of total memory-wipeouts, which is more than the norm. We once again went through a shorter-than-is-now-normal attention span deficit. When we were doing something we had done a million times before, we found that all of a sudden, everything was gone—sometimes even the memory of what it was we had been doing. We found ourselves turning around in circles sometimes, trying to figure out why we were in a certain room or where it was we had been going. Under normal circumstances, we probably would have thought the situations were laughable, but when it is you who is experiencing total blank-out moments, it does not feel quite so funny; it can actually feel rather scary.

In Alexis's case, if she were working with a patient or her new supervisor, it truly was a scary thing. Would the patient be patient while Alexis searched her memory for what she wanted to say or do? Would the supervisor understand that Alexis really did know her medical stuff, but was experiencing a chemo moment? Would she have a lapse that could impact a patient's treatment? For Alexis, chemo brain was a serious condition to have in her career. For Terry, crunching numbers and keeping track of where things went on the spreadsheet didn't coexist harmoniously. Simple computer keystrokes were forgotten and led to requiring inordinate numbers of hours to accomplish the same quantities of work that, prior to chemo brain, had required less than two thirds of the time now needed. In addition, our abilities to work long hours became seriously truncated.

And the good news is, this condition can go on for up to ten years!!! For up to a whole decade now, we have something upon which we can blame our oversights and mistakes, if we so choose.

And the bad news is, this condition can go on for up to ten years!!! For a whole decade now, we will have to continually question our abilities and worthiness.

How can you cope with chemo brain? There are several strategies: the first is key—a DETAILED, DAILY planner. This should include any medical appointments, to-do lists, birthdays or other special events in your life, schedules of meetings you have to attend whether professional or personal (taking the kids to soccer practice or going to the barber/hairdresser or going to the movies with your significant other), and names, addresses, telephone numbers, e-mail addresses. If you've never been a planner before, if you're a "spur-of-the-moment, let-things-fall-as-they-may" type of person, this is a horrible time to start, but start you must if you don't want to further exacerbate the situation. Along with this is setting up a routine. Yes, it's dull and boring, not spontaneous, but there can be room for side trips, as long as the rest of your life is managed while you are going through chemo brain. It's easier for your spouse/partner and kids, too. There's enough going on in their lives without having total chaos reign. And as much as kids grumble about their routines, they need them to feel safe and secure. And now, so will you.

Other strategies include getting enough sleep at night, take a class that challenges you to do something new, work crossword puzzles (there was a study done with nuns several years ago; those that worked crossword puzzles did not present early symptoms of Alzheimer's), exercise, eat properly (including additional fruits and veggies in your diet), and try to do one thing to completion (we can hear you laughing). If you have to, make lists to help you remember what you need to do. Stick post-it notes around the house. It's also helpful if you can focus on something other than your having chemo brain. If at all possible, laugh about your condition, make jokes about it, but please remember to go easy on yourself. As someone somewhere once said, "This, too, shall pass."

As time has gone on, these symptoms have become more sporadic, but still occur. You simply have to "put yourself in neutral," accept it, and move on. Some days, that is ". . . easier said than done." It's still frustrating, aggravating, annoying, distressing—the list could go on and on. Just remember, it does get better! Recovery can and does take time, and you have to allow yourself the time to get through this. Really, you have no choice, so you might as well adjust. To be sure those around you do not begin to think you have lost your mind completely, you should alert your friends, family and colleagues about these recurring lapses, so they can be patient along with you. Remember—you are not crazy. You are simply experiencing one of the side effects of chemo, and will need the understanding of family, friends and colleagues to get through this. If you are particularly worried about it, ask your oncologist or other health care provider to refer you to someone who specializes in assessing memory loss.

It is important to mention not to discount the small stuff. "Chemo brain" is a large part of cancer patients' lives and can take on a multitude of forms. Many blogs have been written as cries for help to see if anyone else is experiencing these same things. It's amazing to find the collaborations online, the stories shared, the education that has been gained from these blogs. Alexis had started looking at potential meds that might help Andrea with her frontal lobe brain injury to help Andrea focus better. In one of those serendipitous events, she discovered information about Adderall. Adderall is one of 3 drugs, including Ritalin and Concerta, which are used with ADHD patients to help them focus. For those whose chemo brain was negatively impacting the daily functioning of cancer patients' lives, Alexis found that as part of "standard operating procedure," Adderall was being sparingly used with cancer patients to alleviate chemo brain symptoms. If chemo brain is a factor in your life AC, it might be worth your while to contact your oncologist about the feasibility and advisability of taking Adderall. Three websites to check out (the first two are forums, the third is a study) are: http://www.apps.komen.org/forums, http://www.csn.cancer.org, and http://www.cancer.gov (March 24, 2009, Volume 6, number 6—very interesting read!)

The American Cancer Society provides numerous helpful books and materials at: http://www.cancer.org, or 1-800-ACS-2345. For more help, you can also refer to the resource section we have provided at the back of this book.

Control Issues

What are the symptoms indicative of developing control issues? It can be as horrendous as physical violence and domination, or as insidious as how we speak to each other, or how we focus on another's insecurities and figure out how to manipulate them. Have you ever been in the grocery store and watched how parents treat their kids? The tone of voice?

The language used? The physical punishments? It can be absolutely scary observing them, and anticipating what those kids will inflict on their own kids in a never-ending cycle of verbal and physical abuse.

What causes these control issues? Deep down inside, there are probably multiple causes: the inability to trust, a weak sense of identity whether individual or group, low social status (the need to feel successful), how one was treated in childhood (these behaviors can be generational), persistent fear, feelings of inadequacy, feelings of being ignored, always feeling the need to be "perfect," shame, the feeling that one's life is "out of control" and the need to do something about it. Kids are masters at learning how to control and manipulate; it's a means to help them survive within their adult-centered environment. While manipulation is cute in an infant (being "wrapped around one's little finger"), it is hardly cause for joy in little kids or in adults. Really good manipulators can even make you think you came up with an idea, so you will feel responsible for them. Control and manipulation can also be a power trip. To see evidence of that, just look to our political, religious and advertising gurus. Worry, especially about financial issues, can lead to controlling behaviors.

People want deeply to be admired, respected and completely influential in another's life. The need to control can dominate one's life and have a lasting impact on those you are supposed to love. We can justify it as making sure our kids have enough to eat, but becoming overly stressed if dinner is 30 seconds late in getting on the table, or the kids come home a little late for dinner, goes beyond the assurance of a proper diet. We can say that planning a vacation is a good idea (and it is), but becoming stressed when the people going on the trip have other ideas about what they'd like to see and do, makes everyone involved uncomfortable or worse. And yet, the more we control, the lower our own self-esteem becomes. At some point, we must realize the only person you can control is—yourself.

Probably the biggest needs we have are sex, food and the need to control. Rituals give us the sense of control. Schedules give us another type of control. Long-established social rules help us feel safe because they provide a sense of control. Loss of control, a feeling of powerlessness, helplessness, the sense our lives are no longer our own, and that we have little or no command of our destiny, can be an even deeper emotion than the fear of death. Diagnosis of an illness gives us a horrendous sense of not being in control, leading to the need to control everyone and everything in our lives.

Being diagnosed with cancer can be devastating. One of the most difficult pieces of this diagnosis is the sense of the loss of control. Your body has betrayed you or you realize that with the life style you have lead, you have in some way(s), contributed to contracting this disease. In any case, you are now captive to a system. Your life has changed; you are under a physician's control; you are under the control of the medications; your days are under the control of treatment schedules, and you are no longer in control of events that impact your family and friends. Hobbies or events you used to enjoy are now not feasible. You fight to regain control; you fight to gain knowledge to help you conquer this disease; you fight for the strength to continue the fight, and you fight to survive.

Then one day, you do! You are now a survivor!

But it's hard to let go of the behaviors you learned, the behaviors you experienced on the road to becoming a survivor. There have been so many roadblocks for you to overcome while going through treatment. You have had to fight physical conditions (nausea, vomiting, pain). You have had to battle the health insurance companies. You have had to battle health care providers. You have had to battle fatigue. You have had to battle feelings of incompetence and failure when you couldn't do things for your friends and family. You want everything to go back to what was your normal life, but normal isn't there anymore. If you were a quiet, shy person before cancer, perhaps that's changed, and you are now more vocal about what your needs are. This can be disconcerting to your friends and family who had come to expect their own levels of what was normal. If you were mouthy before cancer, you may find this endearing characteristic has now quadrupled. No more Mr. Nice Guy. You find yourself being more short-tempered, more impatient with things—with all things. And no one hates these changes more than you do.

What can be done about these issues of control? In large part, it depends on how much you deep down inside dislike the "new controlling you." There certainly can be benefits to becoming more assertive, if you were quiet and shy before. However, power and control are illusory at best, and can cause quite a bit of damage, sometimes irrevocable damage, in your relationships with people over the long run. And yet, a Truism:

*"It is only when you learn the "give and take" compo-
nents of real communication that you can make your
viewpoints known, and have any hope to achieve
understanding and, if you are really lucky, acceptance."*

Here are a few steps that might help you help yourself and by
extension, those around you. You will need a lot of determination to
uproot these newly learned behaviors, and to evoke the ability to focus
on what you want your relationships to look like.

1. *Identify those areas of your life in which you actually have
   some measure of control.* This may mean life style changes
   (such as stopping smoking or eating a more healthy diet), where
   you live (if you're tired of doing yard work, can you afford a
   condo and the monthly assessments which keep going up every
   year?), where you work (if you've always hated your job, can
   you afford to make a change?), or what you do to help you feel
   productive and useful (is this the time you decide to work as a
   volunteer at Hospice, or maybe satisfy that itch you've always
   had to be an artist by taking classes?). You can't control people,
   nor should you. (And yet, we all try.) This is not to say you
   don't try to steer your kids or grandkids or nieces/nephews into
   a happy, healthy, sane lifestyle, or provide them with career
   choices (listening and suggesting are not controlling, as long as
   you aren't manipulating or forcing them to do what you have
   always wanted to do or think is best). When Andrea was a
   teenager, she and Terry used to talk about what she wanted to
   do with her life when she became an adult. Andrea wanted to
   go into law enforcement and asked Terry what she thought.
   Terry asked Andrea if she was asking her as an aunt or a school
   counselor. Andrea thought a moment and said, an aunt. Terry
   responded that she would prefer it be someone else's niece being
   put in harm's way. Then Andrea asked what Terry's advice
   would be as a school counselor and Terry responded, "You
   have to follow your heart's dream. And no matter what anyone
   says, it's your life and you have to live it according to how you
   see yourself, not in terms of the expectations or demands of
   others." What we are talking about are manipulative behaviors
   that are detrimental to others. If deep down inside, you are trying to control people to meet *your* needs, to help *you* live *your*

life the way *you* want, then maybe you might want to consider therapy to help you come to terms with your control issues.

2. **Once you have discovered what you can and cannot control, develop a plan to work on these areas.** Make a list of what gives you pleasure and what doesn't. Then pick one—ONE— and begin to work on that area. It won't be easy and could require a lot of time to resolve. Be patient with yourself, and recognize that there will be days or even weeks where you don't seem to make any progress. Be persistent. Another strategy is to give people choices, one of which is more beneficial to you, but no more than two choices. Quite often, once a person begins discussing the choices, they will begin to have fun with it and feel a part of the process. It's a little like giving people enough information at work to make good decisions. The more knowledge you give them, the more they rely upon you and your advice. If you give them a choice, they will also feel in control, which puts both of you in a win-win situation. This is especially beneficial when you repeat back to them what you have heard them say, and it may give you a clearer picture of the situation in the process.

3. *Treasure, honor and cherish all you have that is good in your life.* As the old saying goes, "Don't sweat the small stuff." You may find the one area you selected is one about which you can do nothing. Really, honestly and truly, you cannot change. It's not a matter of laziness or lack of persistence. If that's the case, then learn how to develop acceptance of that situation. Try to focus on those things that empower you in your life, and celebrate all that is good. We are no better than the rest of humanity—we do try to control, not only our own lives, but the lives of others as well. It's hard to give up.

What are some of the potential benefits of giving up control? Deepak Chopra lists eleven reasons, some of which are among the following. You no longer have unrealistic expectations of people and stop criticizing them; you begin to learn how to care *for* people, rather than taking care of them; you develop better listening skills; you begin to experience true emotions (for those of you who have bottled up your emotions all your life, this is admittedly frightening at first); you begin to listen to your body; you allow spontaneity in your life, and you learn tolerance and patience. (See Deepak Chopra, *The Path to Love*, Three Rivers Press, 1997.)

You have more than enough going on now, just being a survivor. Focus on what is meaningful in your life. Focus on how lucky you have been and how you might be able to give back. Relinquish control as much as you can in order to live fully and in the "now" of each moment. Let life open up for you and just happen. A Truism:

> *"Joy is hiding everywhere; you cannot make it appear; it will—when it will—how it will—why it will; just close your eyes and breathe, it will find you!"*

Dating

Dating is a time to get to know people who might possibly be a potential mate, or if not, to meet someone who will become a good friend, an integral part of your life. Sometimes we meet people in religious settings, through family members, from within professional or social organizations and associations, at school, bars, political rallies . . . the list is endless. We start to find things we have in common and begin to see how they might fit into our lives, and whether the relationship could be of a permanent nature.

Cultures and ethnic groups can define dating in very specific ways. For example, in Jewish culture, there is strong encouragement to date for marriage, rather than just a casual encounter. In other cultures, notably the broader American culture, a wider circle of dating is permissible and in some cases, encouraged (after all, when you buy a new car, you take it for a test drive).

Being diagnosed with cancer, however, changes the whole scenario. There are not only the physical changes, but also the emotional changes that come with the cancer territory. These changes impact long-standing relationships, including those with people new to your life. Your old "self" has disappeared and a "new you" has arrived. It may take some time for you to become comfortable with the "new you." In cultures or religions that encourage dating for marriage for the purpose of having children, this can put additional pressure on people. If you are a woman who has had either a breast removed or a hysterectomy, this may preclude you from marrying the man you desire. If you are a man who has had testicular cancer or penile cancer, and didn't preserve your sperm prior to treatment, you may also be precluded from marrying. In both cases, these concerns revolve around fertility issues. In most cultures or religions, adoption is a perfectly acceptable option, and marriage could occur. After all, even without cancer, both dating and marriage carry risks. You really don't know a person until you are with her/him a long time, 24 hours a day (Ricardo once said he spent a year in Cleveland one night), 7 days a week, 365 days a year (if it lasts that long).

Before you begin dating after you've had cancer, it's important to focus on what hasn't changed about you. You have talents, skills, abilities, and a sense of humor, which may all have changed somewhat AC, but you have a set of values or code of conduct you treasure, and you now have a new zest for life, a new appreciation for all that life has to offer, and perhaps, an even greater capacity to both give and receive love. You have courage; you have demonstrated an enormous measure of inner strength, and you may even have learned to have more patience ("Lord, give me patience, and I mean right now!"). You have gained a great deal of knowledge through this cancer-fighting process, and most likely, you will have developed compassion for human foibles. A Truism:

> *"These are all positive changes you now possess and can bring to any relationship, changes that will unquestionably make all interactions deeper, and more meaningful and long-lasting."*

But there are also a whole lot of unknowns.

First, for you single guys (although some of this can also apply to single women), if you were not in a long-term relationship BC, it is possible you did not have the family and friend support you needed to help you fully develop into a person ready to embark on a committed relationship. But now, it's likely all kinds of questions might be coming into your mind: How will the future somebody react when s/he learns I had cancer? When do I tell someone I've had cancer or do I even tell someone I've had it? What if I have to use a prosthetic device—will s/he be disgusted or afraid of it, or me? What will happen if s/he has to deal with my colostomy bag? (Similar concerns arise when you have had an ileostomy—the attaching of the small intestine to the abdominal wall, thereby creating a temporary or permanent opening, called a "stoma," to excrete waste.) If I have only one testicle, will that significant other find me less sexually attractive? And if surgery has left me quite disfigured or with a lot of scars, will anyone else ever be able to overlook them in a tender moment? And if I'm thinking about entering into a long-term relationship, because I've had cancer, will I live long enough to make it worth anyone's time to become involved with me? If we decide to have children, whether biologically or through adoption, will I live long enough to see them grow up? These questions are applicable whether you are a heterosexual or a homosexual. And these questions are significant, life changing issues that can leave you not only feeling insecure, but terrified of even trying to move forward in developing any kind of relationship.

You've been brave throughout cancer treatment. Now you wish it would all simply go away. As mentioned earlier, you want to be "normal" again, but AC, there is no such thing. *You are a different person now—a better person, one with more to offer another than ever before.*

We suggest you tell any person you are becoming serious about that you have had cancer. In this case, silence is NOT golden. Most of the time, when you tell someone you've had cancer, s/he will usually react by asking questions. Where kind of was cancer it? What treatment did you have? Will you have to have more treatment? Is your cancer now at a manageable stage? And what does *that* mean anyhow? What care do you have to exercise for the future? And if you've really picked a winner, s/he will say, "I'm glad you told me," followed by "How can I help?" If this person says, "Ewwwwww, I can't deal with that" it may be difficult for you initially to accept, but at least s/he was honest with you. And cancer *is* difficult for many people to wrap their brains around. It doesn't mean s/he is a bad person—it simply means, no matter how devastating the rejection can be, you will have to keep looking. It may be the person is already stressed with other life events and knows s/he can't add even one more thing to his/her life. Wish them the best and tell them you hope someday s/he will find someone to love and cherish. And, most importantly, you need to find someone who will love you for who you are, who you are deep down inside, not the physical shell we present to the world. A Truism:

"You deserve no less, and probably, a whole lot more."

We don't suggest you start every conversation with "Hello, my name is X and, hey, guess what, I have cancer." However, as the relationship deepens into something more serious, the time to say something becomes very clear. Is that the first date? Fifth date? One-month anniversary? You will have to decide when it feels right, and you will know when that is. It may occur quite naturally: for example, if you are continually going to keep doctors' appointments, this new person might likely ask you why you are going so often. If this doesn't occur and you have to schedule a special time to discuss your health, you quite possibly might need to give her/him some time to digest the news. That could take a minute, an hour, a day, or a week—it will depend on the person, and how far along in the relationship you are. Be sure you are prepared for this conversation, because it can go many different ways; anticipate the possible outcomes, and make sure you can handle the alternatives. You know she/he will have many questions, and you need to address them openly and honestly. You can honestly say something to the effect that you have been concerned about bringing it up, and have been hesitant because some people might NOT want to be with someone who has a history of cancer. That's a legitimate concern and needs to be discussed. You will need to be sure this person really cares about you as a human being, before delving into the topic. Make sure you are able to be to supportive of her/him, so the whole thing does not become hurtful for either of you.

We believe in rehearsals. Terry likes to rehearse her presentations about cancer or for presentations in the educational field by standing in front of a mirror and saying the words. Ask yourself: What is the expression on my face? Am I slouching or standing erect? What is the tone of voice? Am I speaking too slowly or not slowly enough? Another effective way of rehearsing is to ask a trusted friend to hear what you have to say and offer feedback. Ask them to role play the "Ewwww—that was awful!" role, and the "Woweee!" approval/acclaim role.

If you still need time before getting into the dating scene, do something else at first—get more involved with your family and friends, spending much desired time with them. If you have something you enjoy doing, like painting, biking, hiking, cooking, woodwork, learning a new topic or learning more about something you already know, join a club or take a class. You will meet people and ease yourself, first into the social scene, and then, as you become more comfortable, into the dating stage.

If you are homosexual, you may be at special risk for cancer, simply because you may not have asked for cancer screening. AIDS/HIV and hepatitis might seem to be more likely to occur than cancer. You may also not go because of homophobia on the part of medical staff, the lack of health insurance, your fear of discrimination, or you don't know where to go to access information about cancer and homosexuality. There are several websites at the end of the book you may want to access.

Regardless of the reason you have not talked about it, if you have been diagnosed with cancer and are in a long-term relationship, you and your spouse/partner need to speak with a medical representative (a trusted doctor, nurse, other health care provider) and discuss what special health care issues you could incur. As will be mentioned below, it is especially critical you have advanced care directives in written form somewhere. This is important so not only you and your partner know what you want, but also so your family, friends and doctors know exactly what your wishes are, as well.

Suggestions for a few other things you can do to help yourself, whether heterosexual or homosexual, are:

1. eat healthy foods (sorry, the bacon, sugared donuts, refined white flour in pizza, high fructose corn syrup and caffeine have to go, except on rare binges; you must increase your intake of non-sugared fruits, vegetables and grains and buy meats and poultry that are grass-fed with no antibiotics, hormones or steroids administered);

2. exercise consistently; current recommendations call for a hard 30–60 minutes *a day* (you should have started an exercise program when the recommendation was 30 minutes 3–5 times a week); or

3. find a hobby or do something that gives you pleasure. These suggestions are also confidence boosters, which can improve your frame of mind, help lift your spirit if you are depressed, and even help you in the bedroom.

And now, the ladies . . .

Single women may face many of the same issues and concerns as men. But most women, however, have a stronger support system in place, whether family or long-term friends. Women, as a rule, have closer relationships than men seem to have. Clearly, the same concerns apply if you are not in a relationship with that someone special. You are still wondering how that person will react when you tell him you either are undergoing treatment for cancer, or have had cancer and are in remission. All survivors, men or women, have their public scars (limb removal or a laryngectomy, as examples) and private scars (mastectomy, removal of a testicle), and possibly psychological scars. All of us will face insecurities about our appearance and the changes that have occurred to our bodies—our outer self, our shell.

Women face the additional pain of possibly not being able to bear either their first child or have another child. They will possibly also face the inability to breast-feed their child, which is so important for the child's future health and well-being. If they've never had children BC, and are in a serious relationship that may lead to a permanent commitment, how will the partner accept this? How do you approach the subject? What if the person is angry and feels like you have "strung him/her along all this time"? And what if you know for a fact that your life has been shortened? Now what? Do you still get married? Still stay in the relationship? And if you are able, do you still try and have a child knowing you might not be around to see him or her grow up?

Just as with men, we feel it's better to talk about it as soon as your relationship starts to become serious. Otherwise for you, it becomes the elephant in the room. Frankly, some men will react negatively. They may be angry. They may even leave you. As we said to the men earlier, wish him well. Be grateful for the time you had with him, and the many things you learned from him. Remember, that person may already be dealing with some serious problems in his own life, and simply can't take on one more thing.

Most men (or if you are in a lesbian relationship, most women), however, will react supportively. Most men who care for you will want to know how they can help. For example, early one morning while Terry was out grocery shopping, wearing her "cancer hat" because she had no hair, a man stopped her and said his girlfriend had just been diagnosed with cancer. He said he had so many questions, and would Terry mind if he asked her. Then he began. How could he help her? How should he talk to her? What should he say and what should he avoid saying? What could he do to make it easier for her? Would she resent him accompanying her to the doctor's office? How much time would he have to take off work to take her to the doctor's appointments, the hospital, the radiation treatments? How long do the chemo treatments last? How long does radiation last? What side effects could she have? Will there be any personality changes? Should he shave his head as a gesture of support when she loses her hair? Should he tell his children? How should he tell them? *What* should he tell them? The questions just kept spilling out.

Ladies (and gentlemen), we hope you find someone as compassionate, and as supportive, as this.

Terry and this gentleman chatted for about half an hour, with the bottom line becoming clear; he needed to talk with his girlfriend about each of his questions. If after they have spoken in depth, she is comfortable with it, he should go with her to all the doctors she will need to visit, and ask his own questions of them. A Truism:

> *"Throughout the entire experience, it is most important to keep the channels of communication wide open.*

Terry told him they should both put in double doors, instead of single doors, to their souls and to their hearts, to make sure feelings and information enter and exit freely.

Whatever you do, focus on all that is positive about you. What is good about you? What skills, talents or abilities do you have that can be a gift to others? What do you have to offer another person? Please don't give up dating, or decide you have nothing to offer. Although we've never met, we know you have a great deal to offer. If you think you don't, ask one or two close friends or a family member what positives they believe you have. Terry had always felt she had been too aloof with her nieces when they were growing up, until one day they had a chance to talk, and she discovered the one word they used to describe her most often was "safety." The other words were "fair" and "dependable." (They also mentioned "strict," but let's not go there!)

Once you realize you <u>*do*</u> have a lot to offer, and that special moment has come when you decide to talk about your cancer, please be open to many questions. Answer them as honestly as you can with whatever information you have. Realize it may take a day or months for all the questions, let alone all the feelings, to come out. If you do have some kind of prosthesis that has to be taken into consideration during sex, talk about it. And suggest, in your own way, how much fun you might be able to have exploring different ways to work around it.

Lesbian women face many of the same difficulties that single homosexual men have: delayed diagnosis for cancer, homophobic medical care staff, lack of health insurance, and the lack of knowledge of general health concerns for women. It is likely lesbian women have a stronger friendship support system than homosexual men do. (And, since we both are women, perhaps this is a sexist and stereotypic viewpoint. Point taken. If we are wrong, forgive our mistake, please). If your biggest concern is homophobic medical staff and finger-pointing because of your lifestyle, talk to other gay friends who have medical care staff they know and trust, and request a referral. As time passes, these issues will be of little or no concern for you or with the medical professionals you encounter. There are places online you can access for referrals for all types of services; some are listed at the end of the book, as well.

Dental Concerns

Oral cancer includes the pharynx, part of the throat and other cancers of the mouth. One-third of these cancers are found in the pharynx and two-thirds in the mouth. For men, it's the 6th most common cancer; for women, it's the 14th most common. Oral cancer is most often found in people over the age of 40, with men contracting it twice as often as women. Oral cancers are mostly preventable. They usually arise from smoking and alcohol consumption. One thing that might help either prevent or delay lip cancer is the use of lip balm that has sunscreen. Caught early, survival rates of more than five years can approach 59 percent.

If you have had head and neck radiation, you are at risk of side effects in your mouth that may be serious. You may find difficulty swallowing, talking or eating; you are at increased risk of getting an infection. If these are not treated in a timely manner, your treatment for cancer may have to stop. Side effects, even after chemo, may be: dry mouth, a lot of cavities, loss of taste, sore mouth and gums, infections, jaw stiffness and jaw bone changes. After chemo/radiation treatment, the most common are dry mouth and huge amounts of cavities.

Simple strategies to help cope with these symptoms are: drink a lot of water, suck on ice chips, use sugarless gum or sugar-free hard candy and use a saliva substitute to keep your mouth moist. If you feel you need to use a mouthwash, avoid those that contain alcohol, as this will add to your problem, causing even more dryness. A couple of mouthwashes that contain alcohol are Listerine® and Scope®. Instead, use a mouthwash such as Biotene, and Crest makes one that is alcohol-free. Use a toothpaste that has fluoride in it, such as Prevident®, as it will help keep your mouth moist.

Flossing becomes even more important than before you had cancer and had chemotherapy. Hanan says that flossing is almost more important than brushing. Floss gently—if your gums bleed or hurt, avoid those areas, but continue flossing. Flossing helps to eliminate all the bacteria that remain after brushing, which can also increase the risk of heart disease.

Even after chemo and radiation, continue to brush with an extra-soft bristled brush. Your mouth will still be quite tender and extremely susceptible to infection for the first several months after cancer treatment stops. The soft bristles will also protect the enamel on your teeth, which could prevent future cavities. Change your toothbrush quite often. If you find them on sale, Dr. Lynne Moseley recommends you buy a bunch, so you can change your toothbrush often without having to make special trips to the store. In the July/August 2009, issue of *Discover* magazine, there is a picture of one—one!—used bristle of a toothbrush covered with dental plaque biofilms. You would NOT believe it! Once you see that picture, you will want to change your toothbrush daily. Dr. Moseley has also heard of people using their dishwashers to disinfect their toothbrushes, but she doesn't think this is a good way to use the appliance! She also says there are toothbrush sterilizers for sale and can be found on the Internet. When looking them up, you will find a myriad of products available, along with a wide range of prices. We have not yet tried any of the products we found, and therefore offer no recommendation.

It also helps to rinse your mouth quite often during the day. You can make up your own mouthwash by combining 1/4 teaspoon of baking soda and 1/8 teaspoon of salt in one cup of warm water. After swishing with this solution, rinse with plain warm water.

If you have a child who has had head and neck radiation, there could also be other side effects. The most common are problems with the teeth. Permanent teeth may come in slowly and/or look different when they do. Teeth may fall out. Especially for children, a dentist should be an integral part of the cancer team of doctors, before, during and after treatment. All of the recommendations listed above regarding brushing, flossing, etc., are also applicable to children.

Oral oncologists are a rarity in the United States, but can usually be found at major comprehensive cancer centers. In order for the National Institutes of Health to designate a cancer center as "comprehensive," they must have an oral oncologist on staff as a part of each patient's team. Internationally, you may check The International Academy of Oral Oncology (The IAOO) (http://www.internationacademy oforaloncology.org/). Their website will provide you with several links for data sets, journals, online information sources, oral cancer specifically, organizations, patient support, professional associations, and a summary of the clinical trials currently underway. Members are also listed; the ones in red (as opposed to the ones in blue) can be accessed directly from the IAOO website.

For other information related to oral care, you may contact the National Institute of Dental and Craniofacial Research, at the National Oral Health Information Clearinghouse, 1 NOHIC Way, Bethesda, MD 20892-3500; 301-402-7364; www.nidcr.nih.gov.

Depression

Depression is feeling blue, miserable, sad and/or unhappy. We all experience these feelings at one time or another in our lives. It is when these feelings are present every day for an extended period of time that you need to give it serious consideration. Depression can be mild, moderate or severe. If you are continually fatigued, you find yourself withdrawing from normal activities, have difficulty concentrating, find you are either gaining a lot of weight or losing it, have trouble sleeping, have sudden bursts of anger, feel hopeless or helpless or have thoughts of death and suicide, you need to talk with your doctor or other health care professional. If you have five or more of the symptoms listed above that have lasted for longer than two weeks, you could be classified as incurring a major, or even a "clinical," depression. Children express depression much differently than adults. Watch for changes in sleep patterns, in behavior and changes in how they normally do in school. There is also something called agitated depression, characterized by inner tension, visible physical agitation, racing thoughts, continuous verbalizing, emotional outbursts and wringing of hands.

It has been estimated that up to 50% of cancer patients experience some form of depression. It is complicated by cancer being all pervasive for patients, encompassing family problems, pain management, work, financial issues, and child issues, to name a few. Further complicating these issues is the fact that oncologists have a difficult time diagnosing depression because of everything else that's going on with the body. The type of cancer you have can also be a determining factor as to whether or not you experience depression. Some of the medications you have to take, such as steroids, may also contribute.

Even after you survive cancer, you may still feel depressed. Depression is quite common among cancer survivors. You are continually going back for follow-up appointments, you are worried about a relapse, there are still home and work issues to deal with, including your quest for things to return to "normal," along with your efforts to rebuild some form of social life. You are still fatigued, and you may have changed your beliefs or values which may be in conflict with the rest of your family and friends. Sexually it may take a great deal of time to return to the way things were before cancer, leading to further frustration, both for you and for your partner. All of this may lead to feelings of anger and sadness; anger that you went through this, and the physical and mental toll it took on you, your family and friends; sadness that your body has changed so much, that you still don't have hair or it's coming in too slowly, that you either gained weight because of the steroids, or you lost considerable weight, and now all the wrinkles are showing up on your face, and your body has all these sagging parts (unless like some of us, you already had those sagging parts BC). And there is the possibility that the actual cancer drugs used in treatment may have contributed to a (temporary) change in your brain chemistry. Left alone too long, all of this can become overwhelming and degenerate into depression; you may need professional help even to begin to deal with it.

As mentioned earlier, it is normal to experience depression while undergoing chemo and radiation. Part of the depression is undoubtedly due, in part, to our loss of control over our lives (not that any of us really have any control at any time, but the illusion is nice). We have no control over what is happening to our bodies or our minds, and we live with the uncertainty of "What next?" when it comes to fighting this disease. Alexis didn't seem to have much problem, but about 18 months after the last chemo, Terry went through an intensely bad period. She still functioned "normally" in terms of day-to-day stuff, didn't have to be hospitalized or miss work, and refused to take any kind of medication, although in retrospect, she should have. Part of her hesitancy was based upon the belief that doctors tend to drug women more than men, and never really isolate or address the root causes of the depression.

Descending into the depths of depression was a horrific experience, especially to one who approaches life as an adventure, as something to look forward to, and believes that every day can be a blessing—a new and exciting opportunity. It was hard getting out of bed in the morning. There was a "what's the use" attitude that was alarming in and of itself. A negative attitude like that was intrinsically foreign to her, almost frightening. She slept more during the day than ever before in her life, but paced at night—all night long, every night. Exhaustion, bone-weary exhaustion, was the order of each day, and night.

At that point, Tom's PSA was increasing, but none of the doctors felt it was time to "do anything." It was a constant balancing act to find positives and yet deal with the pressures of the reality of Tom's condition. On top of that was Tom's need to jump off the deep end and to try any new "medication" or "procedure" available. He would sneak around and take stuff without telling either Terry or his doctors. He felt as though he was ten feet tall and bulletproof, that he could do anything, or eat anything he wanted. This was all done out of fear— fear of death, and in reality, Tom's cancer is still virulent. He is still on a short leash in terms of life expectancy.

The reality is, at some point, for him (as it is for all of us), there will be no more options. While it is understandable that he would want to try anything to save his life, in the long run, these behaviors have ruled the day, and in some instances, have made his condition worse (the supplements conflicted with his cancer meds).

And yet, our lives are no less stressful than that of many other people. A Truism:

> *"If one looks, there is always someone else out there whose life is infinitely more stressful or worse than yours."*

Truthfully, knowing that didn't help much. But of course, it never does when it's happening to you. The depression had to run its course. It took a couple of months before she felt she had returned to her "normal" life, at least one as normal as it could possibly be, when both people in a relationship are battling for their lives.

Specifically, if any five of the symptoms from the list below last more than two weeks, you need to talk to a professional trained in the area, because you could be clinically depressed. Those symptoms include, but are not limited to: sadness or anxiety that won't go away; feeling overwhelmed; feeling emotionally numb; feeling hopeless; refusing to get out of bed; being short-tempered all the time; feeling moody; having difficulty getting thoughts out of your mind; feeling like killing or harming yourself or others; avoiding friends and family; crying uncontrollably and/or frequently, unintentionally gaining or losing weight not related to cancer treatments or medication; having difficulty sleeping through the night; experiencing excessive fatigue; lack of energy and/or physically slowing down.

A study done in Canada with people who have metastatic or advanced cancer and depression showed that the depression appears to become worse as the end of life gets closer (you're reading this and thinking to yourself "Duh"). This is especially true if the person is young, has a history of anti-depressant use, has low self-esteem, does not have any kind of spiritual or religious base upon which to fall back, feels hopeless, and has physical and/or financial burdens associated with the disease. It may be the feelings of depression have been so prevalent, the person may not even be cognizant of how depressed s/he has actually become—depression may have become an every-day fact of life—"the new normal." Oncologists, as well as the other doctors in a person's life, need to, first of all, communicate with each other so everyone is aware of all problems that exist. Each doctor could quite possibly have a different viewpoint. Secondly, if the patient will allow it, find some kind of treatment that will help with both the physical and emotional aspects of depression.

Caregivers quite often find themselves depressed also. Caring for someone who has any kind of long-term illness or who is disabled in some way requires a great deal from the caregiver: stamina, patience, a variety of levels of understanding and an innate ability to keep encouraging the one who has the illness. Caregivers are advocates, organizers, financial wizards, nurses, record keepers, medical liaison, physical therapist, counselor, nutritionist, pharmaceutical dispenser, and quite often—the breadwinner, childcare provider, and the one who also has to maintain all their household responsibilities. In Denmark, a study was conducted to look at the partners of women who had breast cancer. Among men, a whopping 39% were more apt to be hospitalized because of depression, or other serious mental conditions, and these were all men who had never been hospitalized previously for any of these conditions. Perhaps one of the things that should be considered by oncologists when working with patients, partners and families is to offer a depression screening and support service for spouses/partners, parents, siblings or other caregivers. The screening could/should be done initially after diagnosis, before treatment begins, and continue periodically throughout the course of treatment, especially if the duration of treatment for the cancer will be lengthy. (Insurance companies, please note: this should be an allowable coverage; it will be cheaper in the long run in terms of lost productivity.) Once you have become a survivor, intervention for depression should continue as an option, but one you may have to pursue on your own, including the screening, if no diagnoses are available and current. Perhaps if the depression was caught early enough, the lives of cancer patients and survivors would not be so demoralized and ruptured.

If you find yourself depressed, whether you are in the process of becoming a survivor or are faced with metastatic or advanced cancer, or are a caregiver, what follows are some suggestions you might want to explore:

1. *Learn something about your cancer,* if you haven't done so already. The more you know, the more you feel in control, or at least, the more you can be an active, informed participant in any treatments that ensue to help your depression.

2. *Acknowledge your feelings.* Sometimes when you admit them, you are more able to let go of them. As in the section on emotions, if you are uncomfortable talking about your depression, write your thoughts and feelings in a personal journal. Even just writing them on a scrap of paper and then throwing it away or burning it up can psychologically have a positive impact, simply by seeing it disappear or "go up in smoke." There is an Asian culture (sorry, which one it is escapes us right now) that deals with grief by putting little candles in boats,

lighting them and then releasing them into the water. This is done at night when the candles really show up and you can literally see your grief setting out on a journey. One of the tricks Terry used in dealing with her depression was mentally constructing the little boats, mentally lighting candles and placing them in the boats and then sending them out to float away on an imagined lake.

3. *Find things relating to yourself about which you feel positive.* Look how far you've come! Look at what you have learned. Look at how you can help others who are going through the same thing. Helping is a two-way street—you get as much out of it, and maybe even more, as the person you help.

4. While this step may seem to be a contradiction to the previous statement, it really isn't. Sometimes you have not only a bad hair day, but you have a bad cancer day as well. *Simply tell people you are having a bad cancer day and then go to your room.* What you have to be cautious about is whether this begins to become a lifestyle pattern. If you are having more bad cancer days than good ones, please seek professional help immediately. If that is financially impossible, then talk with your best friend, your partner, your spiritual advisor, somebody—one who has your best interests at heart.

5. *Identify activities that you enjoy and provide you stimulation.* What helps you relax and take your mind off things? Music? Art? Dancing? Imagery? Yoga? Games? Walking in the woods or by water? Listening to the sound of your children's laughter? Taking a sledgehammer and breaking up stones? And what about those trees in the back yard that need cutting or trimming? You can say to yourself, "Take THAT, cancer! Take THAT, depression!" with each hack or cut you make.

6. *Find physical activities that are positive and throw yourself into them.* You will find this repeated again under "Emotions," but the idea here is to become as active as you can while doing something you like. Establishing an exercise regimen, regardless of how strenuous or NOT it is, will assist you mentally, emotionally and physically. Exercise of any kind provides your body

with a mechanism for releasing all kinds of stress, while simultaneously lifting your spirits.

7. *Realize you can't control everything.* You aren't supermom, or superdad, or supergrandparent or superfriend. If you are feeling stressed or depressed because things seem to be coming apart, when they should be coming back together, identify what you can impact, do that, and then, leave the rest for another day.

8. *Find humor in your life.* Laughter releases many endorphins in your brain, which can help muscles relax as they relieve the sensations of pain. Smiles, whether you do it yourself or see it on another person's face, can reduce stress. Find something funny in the newspaper, clip it out and tape it to a door. If someone sends you a funny card, tape that up and put it on the door, too. If someone sends you a joke or funny story on the Internet, run it off and tape it to your door. Ask friends to loan you some comedic books if you don't have any, or go to the library and look in their humor section. Instead of watching "heavy" movies, put in ones that are comedy based. While we love "CSI" and all its spin-offs, you might be better off watching old videos of "Laugh In," "I Love Lucy," "Gilligan's Island," and/or Johnny Carson tapes, at least for awhile. There is also a cable TV station that devotes itself entirely to comedy. If the dog has chewed on your wig or the cat has used it as a scratching post while you're waiting for your hair to grow back, wear the darned thing anyway and have a big laugh on yourself. A Truism:

"Laughter truly is the best medicine!"

This short section is being added literally at the last minute, moments before going to the formatter. We weren't really sure where to put it in the book, but it's such a great idea, we didn't want to lose it; to us, it seems to fit best at the end of this section on depression. Many times when a person is diagnosed with cancer, friends and family just simply do not know what to do or say. As a consequence, these well-intentioned and loving people avoid contact with the person they love to avoid causing any feelings of awkwardness to either person. Sometimes, the person with cancer has undergone treatments, which have left his/her immune system compromised, and s/he isn't allowed to have visitors. Other times, the resulting isolation and depression that can come with cancer become overwhelming, and even frightening. The cancer patient begins a longing for any kind of human touch or personal contact; feeling connected to others becomes not only welcomed, but also almost necessary for survival. As friends and family of one with cancer, you become a lifeline, a source or flash of sustaining energy to help lift the patient from the depths of depression, to a place where s/he has one little cord on which to grab, and receive the power from your life-saving touch to continue the battle.

You may ask, "What could I possibly do to make such a connection with anyone?" Ideas run rampant, but seem to fall short. And, yes, everyone knows funny e-mails are appreciated, but there is perhaps a better way to help. We offer this suggestion. Patty Leonard, by profession a mortgage closer, is a thyroid and cervical cancer survivor. Recognizing the need cancer patients have, she formed *Cancer Card Showers*, and has helped more than 100 people help those they know who have cancer. Her idea was for family and friends to go to the store and each buy six cards (or, if they are creative and talented, make six cards). Then, once a week, a card is sent to the cancer patient. If, hypothetically, there are six members of your family/friends team, and each of you send your one card per week, the patient you love will receive six cards every day for six weeks. Can you imagine how wonderful it would be when you are living some of your darkest hours, and every day some one of those you love let you know how much you are loved? The cancer patient benefits because s/he realizes how much others love and care for her/him, but also, how the friends and family members are in this battle, fighting along beside you. The cards give both the giver and the receiver hope, and a connection to each other that allows the sender to lift the one they love out of an isolated darkness, into the light of caring. If you would like more information about how to set up and organize your own Cancer Card Shower, you are welcome to contact Patty at 517-719-4697.

Diet and Nutrition

There are some books that have a lasting impact on you long after you have finished reading them. For Terry, in the 1970s, that book was *Atlas Shrugged*, by Ayn Rand, which dealt with the philosophy of objectivism. In the 1980s, any and all books by Joseph Campbell, perhaps the greatest mythologist that ever lived, resonated with her. And in November 2010, that book is *The China Study*, by T. Colin Campbell, Ph.D. and Thomas M. Campbell II. It has had such an impact on us, that this whole section has been rewritten (lucky you—and a whole bunch of other studies were discarded). (That's also why you should be sure to hang out with people who are smarter than you are—they will provide you with "brain food" in the form of books and information. Thanks, Sharon, for bringing this book to our attention and insisting we read it.)

We would like nothing more than to lift (copy, purloin, cite, steal, appropriate) about half of the content of *The China Study* (BenBella Books, ©2006; http://www.benbellabooks.com) and put it in our book. Instead we will try and do a brief summary of what is so important in the Campbells' book and also, urge you to go out right now and buy this book (we have never met the Campbells and have no monetary interest in your purchasing their book). This is a wonderfully written book, with very little technical/medical jargon; it can be easily understood, and everything is well explained.

Dr. Campbell became interested in how diet impacted cancer and found a number of interesting facts after over 50 years of research that spans the globe. *The China Study* focused on 65 counties in China, 130 villages and 6,500 people. There were more than *8,000* correlations in this study with findings that were *statistically significant*. The biggest discoveries made were that a diet high in animal protein leads to a higher incidence of liver and other cancers, and that a plant-based protein diet caused—ready for this?—Zero, zip, zilch, nil, nada cancers. Zero! *The more animal protein you consume, the greater the likelihood you will get cancer.* These findings were also borne out in studies conducted in India, the Philippines, Great Britain and Israel. If you have a diet that consists of 20% animal protein (the typical amount of protein affluent nations consume), you are more likely to get cancer than if you consume 10% or less animal protein (this is what the "developing" or "poverty" countries usually consume). The startling conclusion: cancer can be controlled through good nutrition. The more animal-based protein ("casein") you consume, the more likely you are to get breast cancer. The more animal-based protein you consume, the more likely you are to get advanced stage prostate cancer. The more animal-based protein you consume, the greater the likelihood you will get pancreatic cancer. The animal-based protein you consume feeds tumor growth. The animal-based protein you consume also leads to a huge amount of calcium that is excreted in urine, which impacts your bones. As income has risen in China and other countries, as people began to eat more "Western style" foods, the cancer, heart disease and other health problems also began to rise. In China, if your blood cholesterol decreased to below 90 mg/dl, cancers for the brain, breast, colon, esophagus, leukemias (both adult and child), liver, lung, rectum and stomach also decreased. What this ultimately means is that genetics are responsible for maybe 2% or 3% of one's risk for cancer. On page 84 of *The China Study* is an incredible graph that visually shows the relationship of fat intake and breast cancer; what you see is a clearly causally-related correlation between the two variables.

The other startling pieces of research show that with a higher animal protein intake, girls now as young as nine are beginning menstruation. This means that girls now have a longer period of time for reproduction, which in turn leads to increased risk of breast and ovarian cancer. Girls in countries that tend to ingest more plant-based protein generally do not get their periods until their mid-teens. This has the additional benefit of reducing teenage pregnancies.

Even autoimmune diseases (there are 40 different kinds) can be delayed or even stopped, by decreasing the amount of casein that is consumed. These results are true for rheumatoid arthritis, inflammatory bowel disease, Crohn's disease, Type 1 diabetes, rheumatic heart disease, lupus, multiple sclerosis (MS) and maybe even Parkinson's. Your geographic location may also have a bearing on what autoimmune disease(s) you may contract. The Campbells point out that the farther away you are from the equator the greater the likelihood you may develop an autoimmune disease (thyroid, arthritis, anemia, MS, Addison's, and others).

And wait until you read about the discoveries with obesity; heart disease; diabetes; and diseases of the bone, brain, eye and kidneys. His insights and experiences in government, industry, science, medicine and the media are mind-blowing.

As another piece of evidence, in September 2011, the World Cancer Research Fund issued a report that concluded that up to 2.8 million cases of cancer could be prevented each year if people were to adopt better diets and a healthier lifestyle. This includes reducing alcohol consumption, eating more fruits and vegetables, not smoking and increasing one's exercise.

Parents/Guardians, have you checked your child's school lunch program lately? Kids are getting sugared cereals for breakfast, pizza and other sugary desserts for lunch, plus cow's milk for the "protein"—to build strong bones (supposedly). This is happening at a time when children are becoming grossly overweight (actually obese), which could lead to diabetes at an earlier age. Very little is "health" food, let alone nutritious. Very little is plant-based. Ditto the WIC (Women, Infants and Children) programs. Secondary schools, and more amazingly hospitals, now offer "fast food" at their locations. Pops/colas/sodas are regularly offered at some schools now because they still fall under the "safe" regulation for sugar. And this is at a time when obesity is at an all-time high. Are the seeds for cancer being sown at an early age? The Campbells write, the ". . . most powerful weapon against cancer is the food we eat every day." They also cite a website you may wish to access: http://www.drmcdougall.com. Dr. John McDougall now runs a lifestyle program that has been very successful.

What you eat after cancer diagnosis and treatment is very important. A good nutrition program is actually something that oncologists and health care professionals should incorporate into each patient's medical diagnosis and treatment regimen. So often, the focus is on chemotherapy, surgery and radiation, but diet and life style factors should be just as important, both during treatment and after.

Many people believe the addition of nutritional supplements or other "alternative" health approaches will cover any gaps you may have in your diet. As we spoke of earlier, Tom is a staunch follower and reads the alternative medicinal newsletters insatiably, much to Terry's dismay. While we are not saying there are NO benefits to those supplements propagated in such publications, we are saying you need to read them very carefully, then do your own follow-up research, ask questions of qualified, licensed medical staff, nutritional experts or dietary staff, and then make a decision. That decision, however, should only be made after consulting with your doctor(s) FIRST, to ensure the supplements you are considering will NOT conflict with any medications you are already taking. Most of what these newsletters report are anecdotal in nature, and have no controlled studies to support their claims. Plus, dietary supplements (a multi-billion dollar industry in the U.S.) would become totally unnecessary if you were eating proper foods prepared in a healthy manner. Eating a wholesome, balanced diet conducive to good health will supply your body with the nutrition you need.

A recent study conducted in Korea, for example, has shown there are no conclusive indications that antioxidant *supplements* will prevent cancer. In four of those studies, results indicated the supplements may actually increase the risk of bladder cancer. Another study was conducted that monitored the meat consumption of 500,000 people over 10 years. The people who ate the most processed or red meats were from 16% to 36% more likely to die during the study than the people who ate the least processed or red meat. There was a corresponding link to a greater death rate of from 11% to 22% greater, from cancer. While this is not huge, when you consider smoking has been scientifically proven to raise the risk of lung cancer by more than 900%, it is still a significant enough difference to raise cause for alarm.

To the extent possible, it's best to eat fresh or frozen foods. If you prefer to buy canned vegetables, get the salt-free. There is usually enough salt that occurs naturally in fresh and frozen veggies that you don't need more. Also to the extent possible, if you can't make the switch to a vegetarian diet, and you simply HAVE TO HAVE animal protein, it's best to eat only grass-fed beef/pork/lamb, and chickens which have been outside pecking in the dirt for grubs. Many food packages, such as chicken, have labels which say they are "organic" and "free-range," but the chickens actually live and die in a building that has an itty-bitty door for the chickens to use *if they want to*, but because of their early life of restricted range of motion, pretty much stay "cooped" up (sorry; Terry's paternal grandmother was an inveterate punner; has to be genetic, since she died long before Terry was born) inside, and are NOT free-range. As was said in *The Omnivore's Dilemma*, by Michael Pollan, "If it wasn't food a hundred years ago, don't eat it."

What follows is a short list of foods and strategies you may want to consider, along with the reasons why:

- *Aspirin*—CancerConsultants, reviewing an article in *The American Journal of Epidemiology*, reports that regular aspirin use may reduce the risk of cancer in the lower part of the stomach. However, since regular aspirin use also carries risks in and of itself, you need to talk with your doctor(s) first before starting this regimen.

- *Bananas*—stimulates the production of dopamine in the brain, which, in turn, produces a "feel good" syndrome.

- *Berries*—blackberries, blueberries, cranberries, raspberries, and strawberries—contain quite a few polyphenols, which may help arrest the growth of tumors.

- *Brussels sprouts* (including other foods such as bok choy, broccoli, cauliflower and Chinese cabbage) contain sulforaphane and indole-3-carbinols (where do they come up with these names?). These molecules help to reduce some carcinogenic substances and may prevent some precancerous cells from becoming malignant tumors. One study reports these vegetables can help cancer cells commit "suicide," thereby preventing tumor growth.

- *Chocolate*—Terry has said for decades that chocolate was a health food, and now studies are actually supporting her theory. The flavanols, especially in dark chocolate, can increase the blood flow to your brain. This has also been shown to improve your performance on cognitive tasks. Eat the darkest chocolate you can tolerate, but no less than 35% cocoa. Chocolate with more than 70% cocoa contains both polyphenols and antioxidants, which slow the growth of cancer cells, and the blood vessels that feed tumors. A single square of dark chocolate is twice as good for you as a glass of red wine, and almost as good for you as properly steeped green tea. Be careful of weight gain if you begin to eat too much. (See the section on Obesity.)

- *Citric fruits*—grapefruit, lemons, oranges, and tangerines—all contain flavonoids, which help to detoxify carcinogens in the liver. One study has shown that the skin of the tangerine may help kill brain cancer cells. If you look to citrus fruits as a means of assuring you get your minimum daily requirement of vitamin C, you will find they probably only contain 1% or 2%. There are other foods that can provide higher percentages of Vitamin

C: broccoli, peas, papayas (which have four times more Vitamin C than one orange), peppers, and strawberries. Still, citrus fruits are healthy to eat and can provide health benefits as long as you make sure they do not interfere with your medication(s).

- *Fats*—yes, they taste good and they add flavor to foods, and for some people, they provide the best part of every meal, BUT you also need to skip them as much as possible. Omit fried foods from your diet. (Groan!) If you bake, broil, boil, grill or anything else except fry, chicken, remove the skin because it contains huge amounts of fat. If you love butter (as we do) try to eliminate it, but if you can't, limit it to one or two teaspoons a day and try to find butter that is made from grass-fed cows. Use olive oil or canola oil as much as possible, but use them sparingly.

- *Fish*—now also known as "brain food"; fatty fish, such as salmon, tuna or sardines may help ease symptoms of depression because they raise the levels of serotonin in the brain. These types of fish contain omega-3 fatty acids. These fish have also been shown to slow cancer growth in tumors affecting the breasts, colon, lungs, kidneys and the prostate. A tuna fish sandwich (made with whole wheat or multi-grain bread, not the white stuff) for lunch might help you in your cancer struggles. Try to eat fish at least twice weekly to get the most benefit— more often if you can. Smaller portions of fresh fish (not frozen) could also contain less mercury. Dr. Campbell suggests you minimize the amounts of frozen fish in your diet, and definitely limit 'processed' fish.

- *Fish oil*—supposed to fend off inflammation; also a few studies indicate possible cancer and heart disease prevention. However, the research behind this recommendation is inconclusive at this time. It's probably a good idea NOT to take greater than 3,000 milligrams a day. If you ingest more than that, it could impair the immune system, increase bleeding and the possibility of stroke. Instead, increase salmon and tuna in your diet.

- *Flaxseed*—contains lignans, which may help reduce your cancer risk. It also mimics the hormone estrogen and contains the omega-3 fatty acids. Research on animals shows that flaxseed may slow cancer growth in the colon, skin, lungs and breast, but results have not been confirmed in humans. It is better to sprinkle ground flaxseed on your cereal or yogurt, but it may cause an upset stomach. Drink plenty of fluids to prevent constipation. Flaxseed may also interfere with blood thinners, such as Coumadin (Warfarin) and may interfere with aspirin.

- *Folates*—increase the production of histamine (essential for both sexes to reach an orgasm). Asparagus and orange juice contain folate.

- *Garlic* family, including chives, leeks, onions and shallots—these are part of the alliaceous family and contain sulphur compounds that attack cancer cells in the breast, lung and the prostate. There is also a study that suggests if you eat a lot of garlic (Terry uses it on everything except ice cream), it may lower the chances of getting kidney and prostate cancer.

- *Ginger*—This is a powerful anti-inflammatory spice (like turmeric; see below), which reportedly slows the growth of tumors and may fight ovarian cancer cells. It may also alleviate nausea while undergoing chemotherapy and radiation. Ginger supplements are not recommended; increase the ginger in your diet instead. Ginger may also interfere with blood-thinners. In people with diabetes, it can lower blood sugar and interfere with the medications taken.

- *Greens* (arugula, asparagus, basil, beet greens, bok choy, Brussels sprouts, cilantro, celery, Belgian endive, all varieties of lettuce, parsley, rhubard, seaweed, spinach, turnip greens to name a few)—stimulates the production of dopamine in the brain, which produces that "feel good" syndrome; it is essential to the normal functioning of the central nervous system.

- *Lycopene*—this is a carotenoid and appears to reduce prostate cancer risk, but to date, research hasn't borne the theory out. Foods rich in beta-carotene, related to lycopene, seem to reduce lung cancer risk. However, *if you are a smoker, the cancer risk is increased, even doubled. DO NOT TAKE LYCOPENE SUPPLEMENTS.* Instead, increase your intake of tomato sauce, low-salt tomato juice, watermelon, guava and pink grapefruit. Lycopenes are especially recommended for men with prostate cancer; that is, lycopenes in normal amounts (do not megadose on lycopenes). In general, most, if not all, men will develop prostate cancer at some point in time as they age. Most men will die _with_ prostate cancer, NOT _from_ it. Prostate cancer is more prevalent in western nations than in Asia, where there are more plant-based foods as the main part of the diet. African-American males contract prostate cancer at higher percentages than other ethnic groups. No one knows why this is for sure, although a good guess for causes of contracting prostate cancer is the large intake of foods high in saturated fats (also linked to heart disease). If you have head and neck cancer, lycopenes may aggravate the sores that develop in your mouth.

- *Melatonin*—usually used to treat insomnia and may help to help the immune system. *DO NOT TAKE THIS SUPPLEMENT IF YOU ARE ON MEDICATIONS EVEN AFTER YOU HAVE SURVIVED CANCER.* Talk with your doctor or health care provider first. It may interfere with the medications you are taking, and if you have been depressed after cancer, it may worsen that condition.

- *Milk*—stimulates the production of dopamine, producing the "feel good" syndrome. However, beware that you are ingesting animal protein whenever you drink milk.

- *Pomegranate juice*—several studies have shown the juices of a pomegranate can reduce the development of even very aggressive prostate cancers, as well as a few other cancers. If you drink it daily, it has been shown to also slow the spread of prostate cancer by 50%.

- *Phytochemicals*—throughout this section, we have alluded to "phytochemicals." So what, exactly, are phytochemicals? First of all, they have no nutritive value; that means they have no vitamins or minerals. Some studies indicate they might help prevent blood clots, lower cholesterol and may block certain hormones that cause cancer. How do you get more phytochemicals into your body?
  1. CONSUME FAR MORE VEGETABLES than you do meat or poultry (try to eat animal-based foods only once a week or once a month). Each day you should have six servings of fruits and vegetables, three cups of legumes and six servings of grains.

(A serving is 1/2 cup.) If you feel you simply can't get by without some kind of meat or poultry, limit your portion sizes to two to three ounces a day (the amount that fits into the palm of your hand).

2. *USE HERBS AND SPICES TO SEASON FOODS* rather than just salt and pepper. (If you use salt, make sure it's sea salt or kosher salt, and not the bleached kind you find on the grocery shelf.)

3. *ADD TOFU, SOY PROTEIN AND SOYMILK TO YOUR DIET.* Substitute regular flour with soy flour (up to 1/4 cup of flour) and soy butter for regular butter and instead of peanut butter. But, as always, please check with your doctor first to make sure these dietary changes will NOT conflict with the medications you are taking. Also, make sure you DON'T have an allergy to soy products.

- *Protein*—You can probably have all the beans you want at any time of the day or night (unless your body processes them in a way that leads to excessive flatulence). Plant-based protein is the healthiest form of protein you can eat. Lean meat, poultry, fish and cheese in small amounts (two to three ounces) contain casein, which under certain circumstances, can be harmful, but they do contain norepinephrine and dopamine, which can help you get through some of those long chemo sessions, or a stressful day at work. Some studies indicate they can also increase alertness and concentration levels.

- *Resveratrol*—can act as an antioxidant but whether it slows the growth of cancer cells is only now being tested in research labs. Increase your intake of red and purple grapes. While red wine has been promoted as a health agent, drink it with caution. Alcohol consumption has also been linked with an increased risk of cancer. If you are a woman who is hormone-sensitive, you should avoid resveratrol supplements.

- *Selenium*—At one time, selenium was thought to prevent cancer, but this has been shown in recent studies to be untrue. In addition, selenium supplements may be potentially dangerous. As an example, selenium supplements may increase your risk for squamous cell cancer. The general recommendation is: *DO NOT TAKE SELENIUM SUPPLEMENTS.* In a study conducted to see how vitamin E and selenium might impact prostate cancer, it was discovered that there was a small increase in diabetes among those men who took the selenium supplement. Caught early, selenium may have a positive impact on lung cancer. Another study has concluded that if you have higher levels of selenium in your system, you may have a lower risk of bladder cancer, particularly for women. If your selenium levels are low, you probably feel grumpy and irritable, perhaps more prone to anger. To boost your selenium levels, eat more fish, liver, poultry, sunflower seeds, raisins, almonds, Brazil nuts and whole wheat.

- *Soda/pop/colas*—(SPCs) What can we say? From almost every resource available, not just from the Campbells' *The China Study*, but everywhere, only one recommendation regarding SPCs emerges. To put it delicately—*ELIMINATE THEM FROM YOUR DIET.* Not only are they NOT good for you, especially the caffeinated colas, but they simply don't help you when you have cancer. Sodas/pops/colas will also leach out the phosphate in your bones and destroy the enamel on your teeth (parents, please pay particular attention to this with your children). The amount of sugar and high fructose corn syrup in them can also lead to increased obesity. If you won't do it to help get rid of obesity then consider the reports of gout being on the increase in Canada and the U.S. In the August 17, 2009 issue of <u>Arthritis,</u> an article notes that over a twelve-year period, a study indicated that men who drank two or more servings of pop a day had an 85% risk of developing gout. For those who drank only 1 serving of pop a day, the risk was 45% for developing gout. While this is not proof, it is certainly a link. You don't need to totally eliminate them from your diet, but just drink them in moderation (once or twice a month). Diet colas have added chemical sweeteners which also carry risks if consumed in great quantities. The best SPC substitute is water with slices of lemon, lime or orange. Choose fresh fruit over dried fruits. As long as we're on the subject of gout, we should address alcoholic beverages, as well. If you "have" to have alcohol every day, see a counselor! If you simply want to have an alcoholic beverage once in awhile, check with your doctor first to make sure it doesn't conflict with any of your prescriptions. If you drink two or more beers a day, you will be 2.5 times more likely to develop gout. If you drink other alcoholic beverages, you will be 1.6 times as likely to develop gout. Moderate amounts of wine appear to have no effect on gout. You don't need to add gout to your list of ailments, especially when it is so easily prevented.

- *Soy products*—contain isoflavones and have been shown to prevent tumor growth and block the growth of sex hormones, such as estrogen and testosterone. (Remember, men, if you develop stage 4 prostate cancer, all the testosterone in your body has to be killed in order to treat it). Even more interesting are those studies among Asian people, who have eaten soy since their adolescence. The outcomes revealed significantly fewer instances of breast cancer among the women, and if they did develop breast cancer, the tumors were usually not as aggressive; there was a higher survival rate as well. The Asian men who consumed soy also showed positive results, recording reduced incidents of prostate cancer. Soy pills may aggravate some breast cancers but soy, eaten as food, appears not to have this affect. It's probably safe to eat one or two servings of soy foods a day. However, if you have been diagnosed with a hormone-dependent cancer, severely limit your intake. This is probably a good idea after you have survived cancer, such as estrogen-receptor-positive breast cancer, at least for a period of time after treatments have stopped. Check with your doctor or health care provider before increasing your soy intake. For other types of cancers, soy probably won't hurt you, but it may also not help you. The role soy products may or may not play in helping people with cancer is currently being investigated.

- *Tea—black:* helps people cope with stress. According to some studies, results indicate it may suppress the stress hormone, cortisol, after a stressful occurrence. (And chemo can certainly be stressful.) You could freely drink decaffeinated tea throughout the day.

- *Tea—Japanese green:* is rich in polyphenols that can reduce the growth of the blood vessels, which feed cancer tumors. It is also an antioxidant and stimulates the production of enzymes in the liver that extract toxins from your body. In one study, Japanese green tea appeared to play a role in helping cancer cells die, and has helped to increase the benefits of radiation on cancer cells. Drinking green tea may lower cancer risk, especially for cancers of the bladder, esophagus, ovaries, pancreas and maybe breasts. Drink up to three cups of green tea per day (preferably decaf). DO NOT take any of the green tea supplements.

- *Turmeric*—is a spice often found in curry powder. It has natural anti-inflammatory properties. In early lab studies, it was shown to stop melanoma cancer from spreading. Turmeric contains an antioxidant called curcumin, but to date, it has not shown any anti-cancer effects in humans. Turmeric may impede chemotherapy for breast cancer, increase gall bladder problems or slow the clotting of blood. If you are on a blood thinner such as Coumadin (Warfarin) or Heparin, restrict the use of turmeric in your diet. As a cancer survivor, however, if you aren't on Coumadin or Heparin for another medical condition, there are several websites to get recipes for incorporating turmeric into your diet.

- *Vegetables*—yellow and dark green leafy—contain lutein and have a lot of vitamin E in them. People who have had chemo run a much higher risk of developing cataracts than they would have normally. Studies of the benefits of these types of vegetables in preventing or delaying the onset of cataracts, or in showing they confer a degree of protection from developing cataracts are mixed. If you don't have cancer, it won't hurt to start eating more of these vegetables. If you have had chemo, it won't hurt to add several helpings of them to your diet to perhaps prevent a quick spread of the cataract.

- *Vitamin D*—is one vitamin definitively linked to reducing your risk of cancer. Recent studies have shown it might help prevent cancer, but nothing has yet been determined relative to how much Vitamin D you need to take for full efficacy. To increase your intake of vitamin D in your diet, eat oily fish (tuna, salmon), drink fortified milk (but beware the animal protein) and eat fortified cereals. If you are over 50 or have darker skin, ask your doctor if a vitamin D supplement would be beneficial for you, and get more sun without overdoing it. If you are between the ages of 51–70, the recommended amount is 400 IU a day. If you are over the age of 71, it is recommended that you take 600 IU a day. When you are out in the sun, continue to use a non-carcinogenic sunscreen and limit your exposure to avoid the risk of skin cancer. Now that you have survived cancer, there's no sense in being foolish and getting it again or developing a new type of cancer. Use caution to limit your risks and stay cancer-free!

- *Zinc*—is a mineral that increases sperm count. Some people say that taking additional zinc also helps make their colds easier to bear and go away faster. All it takes is one oyster (sure hope we find foods other than oysters) to fulfill the necessary daily requirement for zinc.

There are cookbooks available to help you not only during your journey through cancer and the treatments, but also afterward. Cancer Fighters Thrive recommends *Eating Well Through Cancer: Easy Recipes & Recommendations During & After Treatment*, by Holly Clegg and Gerald Miletetello, MD (http://www.cfthrive.com/recipes.aspx). The book contains recipes and suggestions (especially foods that are more likely to be tolerated through all of the nausea), to help develop and maintain healthy eating habits after treatment. Additionally, the Cancer Treatment Centers of America also have recipes available (http://www.cancer center.com/after-care-services/recipe-cards.cfm).

Dry Eyes

If you've had chemo, you will likely develop dry eyes and will need drops to help keep the eyeball lubricated. A couple of the chemo drugs that may cause dry eye are isotretinoin and tretinoin. If you want to get really technical, the official name for this condition is *keratoconjunctivitis sicca*. What this basically means is that your eyes don't produce enough tears. In some cases, your eyes may actually be producing enough tears, but your eyes may still feel dry. However, it is not always the chemo meds that cause dry eyes. Other factors may be aging, other diseases, the environment or other medications you may be taking. Check with your physician(s), an optometrist and/or ophthalmologist to find out what is really causing the condition, so it can be effectively treated.

To help with dry eyes, you may need to lubricate your eyes during the day and just before going to bed. In some drastic cases, surgery may be needed to alleviate the dry eyes. Whatever has to happen, please be sure to use any medications as prescribed and keep all your appointments as scheduled. In addition, please DO NOT share any medications you have! What may be beneficial to you may be harmful to someone else. If your eyes aren't improving after three or four days on the prescription, call your doctor right away. Either the dosage might have to be increased, or the medication itself might have to be changed entirely.

Dry Mouth

Like everything else, dry mouth has its official name: *xerostomia*. Dry mouth can be caused by radiation, especially if you have had radiation close to your salivary glands. Although the salivary glands can recuperate after radiation, they will most likely never return to your prior "normal," and you will need supplemental treatment.

Sometimes during chemo, but even long after, you will likely have dry mouth. Dry mouth leads to increased cavities in your teeth. Using a good fluoride toothpaste will help. One brand that has been recommended is PreviDent®, made by Colgate. There are two kinds of PreviDent® and odds are, you will need the one that is labeled "5000, dry mouth." It is recommended that it be used twice a day. The only difficulty with the scheduling is that you have to brush a half hour before you eat something, and you can't drink anything for a half-hour after you brush. You should also be very careful not to swallow the toothpaste. Other than that, it has sort of a pleasant taste and is not too bad.

In general, you should keep your mouth and lips moist during the day. If possible, try and rinse your mouth every two hours with a mixture of 1 teaspoon of salt or baking soda to 8 oz. of fluid (water). Biotene® mouthwash is available without prescription, but may be difficult to find; you may have to Google it to see where it is located in your area. You can also suck on hard tart candies, but watch out for the sugar content; while you are working with your dry mouth problem, you don't want to incur any additional cavities (you will likely have more than enough of those already). Another oral hygiene product you may want to try is called Oralbalance® moisturizing gel. Using Water-Pik® toothbrushes might also be helpful.

Use a soft-bristle toothbrush. You should brush your teeth after every meal AND every snack (yes, we are very serious). If you have dentures or a bridge, clean them after every meal and snack. Avoid mouthwashes that contain alcohol (such as Listerine® or Scope®). Drink at least 64–96 oz. of fluid, preferably water, each day, unless your doctor(s) tells you otherwise. Use only *unwaxed* floss, especially if your platelet counts remain low while you are recuperating. Limit your intake of caffeine and alcohol, both of which contribute to dryness in your mouth; this is true whether you have had chemo or radiation or not.

When you eat, try to eat more plant-based protein, and substitute fish for meats. Food should be lukewarm in temperature. Avoid dry foods (pastries, salty crackers, toast). If you want to have bread or rolls, soak them in milk or a sauce first before ingesting. For awhile, avoid citrus fruits, and other acidic foods such as tomatoes. Increase your intake of yogurt and make smoothies from other fruits. If you really are craving pops or sodas, let the fizz out of them and then drink them. Be careful how much milk you drink, even rice milk or soy milk. If your mouth remains excessively dry for long periods of time, you may need to receive intravenous fluids.

Again, please remember to first consult with your doctor(s) about proper oral care for dry mouth, before embarking on any of these suggestions. Your doctor(s) must always be your first point of contact before you make any decisions about what you put into or on your body throughout your treatment schedules. Don't ever be concerned about asking too many questions. A Truism:

"Questions are the mechanism of knowledge."

Emotions

So—once more—we celebrate with you! You have survived cancer. You have had an incredible team of doctors, nurses, technicians, physicians' assistants or nurse practitioners, secretaries, billing clerks, office managers, phlebotomists and receptionists (sorry if anyone has been missed). You have been doted on, pampered to the extent possible, sheltered, formed friendships with most, if not all, of them (and if you have been as lucky as Terry, they have become extensions of your own family), and now, you've survived! Congratulations to all, including you, who have worked so hard to get you to this point. You are now embarking on a new metamorphosis, from cancer patient to cancer survivor. But now you are faced with the irony that while you have wished to get to this place, what seems to be all of a sudden, there is a perceived drop in support by this team with whom you have spent so much time and have become so dependent. Your appointments start to be stretched out, at first three months, then six months, then yearly. All of the support and love this lifeline has offered you begins to diminish. Your friends and family are delighted because now their lives can get back to "normal." Why don't you feel the same way? For you, it's as if you have been yanked from your warm and safe world, and been thrown into the middle of an ocean without a life preserver.

Remember, each person's experience with cancer is different. Each person reacts to things differently. Values you had BC may have changed. You might be feeling fear, anger, loneliness, and maybe even bits of grief and guilt. But please remember one important point: recovery from cancer isn't just about your body; it's also about your mind. You will need to take baby steps in coping with your emotions AC. Let's take a look at them one at a time.

Anger . . .

It is normal to feel anger when you are diagnosed. We have yet to hear of anyone dancing out of the oncologist's office singing "I have cancer, I have cancer!" to the tune from *West Side Story*, "I feel pretty, oh so pretty . . . " During cancer, you lose your hair, you don't feel pretty, your body and mind change, you can't do what you have done in the past, the end of treatment might as well be in the next millennium, and sometimes friends or family abandon you. Perhaps a member of the health care staff may have been having a bad day that one day out of all the years you have gone to that office, but while you would normally be understanding, for some reason, it has hit you the wrong way and has impacted your feelings on subsequent visits.

Anger can serve as the means to take action. You don't feel pretty when you have survived? Go see a massage therapist. Get a makeover.

Your taste buds have changed and you no longer like a certain food? (Perish the thought that it might be chocolate.) Find another food, especially from an ethnic group you might not normally think you'd enjoy. It could open up whole new worlds for you. And that situation with the health care professional? Go talk to him or her and explain what happened and how you felt about it. The odds are, first of all, the health care professional won't remember the situation, secondly, won't have been aware of ever being anything except the consummate professional 24/7/365, and thirdly, will apologize profusely.

But if you are continually angry, holding onto anger as a lifestyle, it can get in the way of your recuperation, of getting back to a healthy way of living once you have become a survivor. Anger eats away at you inside. Try to figure out why you are so angry, what is triggering it, and then try to solve the problem. If you were an angry person before chemo, and you haven't learned yet how wonderful life is now that you have survived, you may need a professional therapist to help you deal with those issues at the root of your anger and to discover alternative response options. If part of your anger involves a formerly close friend or a family member, you may need an intermediary to work things out. But deal with the anger. Do what you can to lessen it. It may not ever totally go away, there may, in actuality, be nothing you can do about a particular situation, but find some way to make peace with it and LET IT GO! A Truism:

> Harboring anger is very much like having cancer; left untreated, it will grow, metastasize and perniciously rob you of your life's purpose, energy and joy.

Let your survival have some kind of chance for being the true rebirth you deserve after having fought such an arduous battle for your life.

Fear . . .

The fear probably stems from the fear of the cancer returning. Even if you have received a "clean bill of health," or you know you are in complete remission, or you have not had a recurrence in years, even decades, there still hovers in the back of your mind the fear that this will happen again. The fear fades over time, but it will never completely disappear. Acknowledge this fear to yourself, and even to your health care team and trusted family members and friends. Please don't think it will just go away if you ignore it. You can ask your health care team what steps you can take to avoid or delay a recurrence. Some of those steps are:

1. *Take preventive measures to keep yourself healthy.* This usually means—you guessed it—exercise and diet. With exercise, start slowly, and as your strength returns, increase the amount and intensity. Alexis started jogging a half-mile a day, then a mile, and then eventually three miles. Terry did the same with walking, but then tried to "beat" her previous times in the walk and walk faster. Diet is just as important. We really do believe increasing your intake of fruits and veggies, and changing the meat/poultry from the hormone- and steroid-ridden stuff you find in grocery stores that you know is harmful, to eating grass-fed animals instead, is vital for you. You can't always trust the labels on foods packaged for stores, whether animal or fruit/vegetable. Try to find local farmers who can show you their operations to make sure they are truly "organic." (Plus it helps the local economy.) Yes, it's more work and more time-consuming, but that commitment of time and energy in acquiring new knowledge is what is required to get you to have the healthy life you (and everyone around you) have worked so hard to achieve and enjoy.

2. *Attend and follow up with each of your appointments.* Following through with your cancer doctor(s) is an absolutely critical point in preventing a recurrence. Yes, you may only be seeing the oncologist every three months or every year, but the purpose of these visits is preventive and precautionary. Should your cancer recur, it will have been caught very early, which means the corresponding treatments can begin early. Although you may feel like a hypochondriac, make a list of all the aches and pains you have been feeling (especially if they resemble symptoms you had before you were diagnosed); describe where your emotions are, what questions have occurred to you in the meantime and discuss all of these issues with your physician. Your first three-month appointment after you think you have beaten cancer is scary (as will the six-month one be). At Terry's first three-month appointment after cancer, she was to be told

her cancer had metastasized. But it was caught early; over that short three-month period, some slight improvements in treatments had become available, the stem cell transplant was successful, and now entering three years later, all tests and scans are coming back *"no evidence of recurrence of disease."* KEEP THOSE APPOINTMENTS!!! AND LISTEN TO WHAT YOUR DOCTORS TELL YOU!!!

3. *Ask for a referral to a therapist.* If you are continually having trouble dealing with your emotions, and feel there has been little progress, it is important to take this step and reach out for help. If you are uncomfortable with seeking therapy, you might want to consider keeping a private journal where you not only chronicle your journey AC, but also your emotions and afterthoughts as you experience them. Alexis kept a journal and was amazed to go back two years later and see her progress, physically, mentally and emotionally.

4. *Get busy and stay busy.* Get back into that club you haven't been able to attend. Join a club, whether social, professional or health and take an active role, perhaps even holding an office or leading a group. Volunteer someplace, perhaps Hospice, where you are helping others and can be fully empathetic and sympathetic to what the person and their families and friends are going through. After all, you have been there, done that, but you have been lucky enough to survive. You will come away from your experience with Hospice feeling a deeper appreciation for life, and will have learned more than you could ever have imagined from the people you comfort. A Truism:

> *"After all, when you give, it's always a two-way street."*

Other possible activities include: Garden, once you can get your hands back in the soil. Take out season tickets to a local theater or sports event or concert. Become active in your place of worship. Spend more time with your kids, really getting in touch with how they are dealing with their emotions. Scrapbook. Do needlework. Take a class in wood burning or dry-walling. Take an art class. Think about what interests you. What do you think you would enjoy? And now, hooray, oh joy, all those household chores and repairs you have been putting off while getting treatment have been sitting there, just waiting for you to recover. Avoid stressing about them by taking them on one at a time. Remember the old adage that the Sistine Chapel wasn't painted in a day. While working on these chores and repairs, take your time and be sure to put in time for yourself, and the people and activities you enjoy.

5. ***Continue to be informed.*** Keep learning about your cancer; keep up with the research, new protocols and medicines for your type of cancer. Follow the new clinical trials and results of other cancer studies. Take time to search for possible support systems and services available to you, and find out if there are any survivor groups in your area. Find information about any new studies being conducted that might give you greater hope for the future.

Grief . . .

Even though you have survived cancer, you may still have experienced grief as you went through the treatment process, and now find that grief continuing AC into your recovery process. By definition, grief is a naturally occurring emotion of deep anguish that follows the loss of something or someone that has been of importance to another person. In a way, you have lost a form of innocence; you have lost part of your identity, and you may even have lost portions of your anatomy. Grieving is an emotional process and the length of time it lasts, as well as its intensity, depend entirely on the person and his/her own particular set of life experiences. Grief may be physical, mental, emotional or social. We will first talk about the four phases of a potentially fatal illness, then go into the phases of grief.

There are four phases you may go through once you have been diagnosed with a potentially fatal illness:

1. before diagnosis,
2. acute,
3. chronic and
4. either recovery or death.

Before diagnosis is when you begin to realize something might be wrong. This is the phase when you go to see several doctors, have myriad tests run, which may take weeks, then there is the actual diagnosis.

The acute phase is when the diagnosis is made and you have to face what kind(s) of care you will need, and learn which of the treatment options are available to you. The chronic phase is the time between the diagnosis and the ending of treatment. You are faced with trying to continue your normal lifestyle, going through treatment and any side effects as a result of that treatment. In the recovery phase, you deal with the financial aspects of treatment, and readjusting your physical, mental, emotional and social expectations. If your cancer metastasizes or recurs, then you might have to confront the likelihood of death. That brings with it a whole other set of issues, such as how long do you continue to fight? What financial decisions do you have to make? What about pain medication and its impact on your life and relationships with people?

Keeping those four phases in mind, we will now look at the three phases to grief. The first phase will present itself in the form of numbness or shock. You may feel cut off from the world as you know it. You may feel like you are simply "going through the motions" of everyday life. As you deal with cancer and perhaps losing portions of your body, you will begin to realize how this will affect the rest of your life. You will feel as though you are frozen in time, and cannot dare to move forward or backward, almost unable to breathe.

At that point, the second phase begins to emerge in the form of emotions—out of control emotions. The emotions you experience will run the gamut, from anger, to fear, to denial and disbelief, to name a few. Your feelings at this stage may be quite intense. While your head knows you are not the first person to go through this, it still affects *you* and nothing else seems to matter. Your grief may come in waves. You may become disorganized, or you may have trouble remembering even the simplest things. You may have trouble sleeping or your appetite goes away. You may feel continually fatigued, because grief is not only emotional, but it also impacts you physically. You may withdraw from those you love most. In some cultures, such as Middle Eastern cultures, there is often the feeling of being unclean, of being unaccepted, of fearing how this will impact your family, or whether the type of cancer you have will preclude you from having children. Try to stay focused and remember: you have gone through deep losses and have earned the right to grieve them.

The final phase is, perhaps, a grudging acceptance, a realization of the reality of what your new life has become, as you leave your old life behind. You feel the loss of the world as you knew it, and of the person you had always been. You truly have lost your "innocence" as you confront a life where death looms upon your days and nights. You begin to learn how to cope with your loss(es) and how your daily life will have to be adjusted. Adjustment does not mean that the pain of your loss of your old life BC will totally go away. It may linger for days, or even years. But eventually, the pain will fade. As it does so, your sense of grief will lessen. In some people, that pain will be replaced by the joy of having survived in this new challenging life, of finding they are alive, and of recognizing how much they have to live for and ultimately, of how much more they now have to give back to their new world.

Guilt . . .

Some people take on intense feelings of remorse, self-reproach and shame; they actually feel guilt at having survived cancer while others have not. There is an overwhelming sense they have done something wrong. You may have met people in your cancer journey who had the same type of cancer you had, and they died. Why didn't you? What makes you so special? Perhaps you are a single, life-of-the-party gal, and you meet a devoted mother of four children. You lived; she died. If life were fair, you could make the case that the devoted mother should have survived. You look for answers to the "why" questions in rationality and your sense of justice; you come away confused and wondering if is "right" that you survived.

There are others who feel no guilt, who feel they shouldn't have any guilt, that each of us must play the hand we are dealt in this life. This is often accompanied by a belief that God has plans for you, that there is some special reason or purpose for you to have survived, and you may never know what that was. Others feel survival means a celebration of life, of a renewed time to help others, to devote their lives to a cause that has meaning for them. Some feel we have to die of something; some will die from cancer and others will die of something else, but in the interim, live life to the fullest and be grateful you have it. Everyone has their own path, their own journey. This might be an opportunity to teach people about this disease. Some might ask, "Why me?" while others might ask, "Why not me?" They use the lesson of cancer to make a difference, not only in their own life, but also in the lives of others, to make each moment count. It is an opportunity to take a close, hard look at your life, and change your priorities if necessary. As one person put it, "Life is all about the journey."

Above all, find ways to stay positive. One of those ways is to focus on how you have changed, and changed for the better, that you are more than your cancer ("I have cancer, but cancer doesn't have me!"). Perhaps you have become emotionally stronger; perhaps you have become wiser, or you have become more realistic about life, and no longer fear death. You may have even found a whole new purpose and direction for your life, a real legacy, because of all you have experienced and discovered about yourself and others—the gifts from cancer. These lessons and gifts are worthy of being passed on to others, whether they are going through their own battle with cancer or not. A Truism:

> *"You have a unique and integral place in the world;*
> *there is no one quite like you, and the world would be*
> *an emptier, less wonderful place without you in it."*

Loneliness . . .

Throughout your treatment, you may have had to separate yourself from the people you love most, simply because your immune system has been compromised and you couldn't take the risk of even catching a cold or developing a fever. Hugs from kids or grandkids may not have been allowed because they each could bring home whatever was floating around their classrooms or the school that day. Your treatments have consumed the greatest part of some days, after which you have spent many days trying to get your strength back. Your life has revolved around the health care team and maybe a certain few family members and friends. You have spent the majority of your time alone, and now, you most likely feel isolated and apart from everyone.

And now, happy day, you have survived. But the safety net that was your health care team is now being pulled away. And the family and friends who have been isolated from you these past months or years are now afraid to come back. They don't know what to do or say, let alone how to help. They may be afraid that somehow or other, they might cause a relapse. And they may have found other interests or people in the interim with whom they have become involved.

So—how do you address this situation? There are several steps you can take.

1. Try to maintain contact with your health care staff, albeit on a much-reduced basis. They are, after all, trying to help people just like you were all those months or years ago. Maybe on the anniversary of your release, cater in (or fix it yourself to make it more personal) a breakfast or lunch for the staff as a way to thank them for their kindnesses and professional help. If you have gotten especially close to a staff member, see if you can't still continue the relationship on their days off. Have a movie night, go to a museum, have lunch, exchange birthday cards. E-mail each other as you have time.

2. If you are feeling really lonely (there's a difference between "aloneness" and "loneliness"), seek professional support services. Many are listed in your phone book or you can find some on the Internet (be careful, however, that you check them out first). Check with your physician, spiritual advisor or perhaps a family member or friend could recommend someone for you.

3. Find a cancer support group to work with. Quite often with cancer survivors, there is the feeling that the only person who could understand what they are going through is another survivor. These support groups may also work with your family as they cope with this next phase in their lives. Joining a support group can give you new meaning for your life, and increase your own chances for survival. Alexis has begun to get involved with the American Breast Cancer Society. Terry has worked on some stem cell drives and will continue to participate in the Lungevity walk every September in Grand Blanc, MI in memory of Linda. Regardless of the type of cancer you have had, the American Cancer Society is always looking for volunteers and has many services available to help you, as well as many areas through which you could become involved to help others. Because of all you have been through, you have learned so much that has equipped you to become an incredible resource for others. The important thing is to get involved! We know you will

feel better emotionally, physically, mentally and spiritually—been there, done that, feel that. A Truism:

> *"As you are helping others, you are also helping yourself."*

Are you the type of person who can benefit from a support group? Some people aren't. To be around people who have had the same kind of cancer you have had might be depressing to you. You may initially feel you don't need a support group, but over time, those feelings may change. The reverse is also true. Other factors may either encourage or discourage you from going to a support group; some of those factors include: size of the group, who attends, time of the meetings, how often and for how long they meet, how long people have been in the group (will you feel like an outsider or is the group a new one, just being formed, that will not have already established a group dynamic?), who will lead the group (a survivor or a professional?), what is the focus of the group (share feelings, solve problems?), and can you simply sit in and listen to see if the group is a "fit" for you or not? Other, more personal issues to consider are whether you are comfortable sharing your own issues, whether you feel you have something to contribute, whether the dynamic of the group indicates an overall environment of positive thinking, and whether your own personal goals could potentially be addressed by attending the group. Many organizations, such as Sharsheret, link you personally with someone who is going through some of the same things with which you are dealing. They also provide webinars, which are focused on young Jewish women with breast cancer, but there is a wealth of information that is completely applicable to women of other cultures and beliefs. Another website that might be helpful to you to locate support groups is The Association of Cancer Online Resources (ACOR), http://www.acor.org.

Fatigue, Energy Level and Naps

This is probably the most common complaint after receiving chemo or radiation. As high as 90% of the people who have had chemo or radiation report fatigue. Up to 65% of people who have had cancer report that fatigue can be more common, and more worrisome, than the pain. Slightly fewer than 60% of chemo patients have reported decreased ability to socialize with family and friends. Sometimes the ability to earn a living is taken away (up to 30% of people find they are unable to work, either full-time or part-time). And the strange thing is, doctors do not know why this fatigue occurs. Some potential causes are the cancer itself, the type of treatment(s) you received, side effects from the treatment (nausea, weight loss, pain, insomnia, anemia), your exaggerated and unpredictable emotions, poor diet, lack of exercise, and/or hormonal changes. Whatever the cause, your fatigue will be highly individual in nature.

The fatigue you experience is not always solved by getting extra sleep, and in fact, may be negatively impacted by too much sleep. It will feel overwhelming, and your whole body may feel tired. This is truly different than the fatigue others who have not had chemo or radiation have experienced. For those who have had a stem cell transplant, you may find you are always fatigued from that point on. Whether you have had chemo, radiation or a stem cell transplant, you may find you need to take an afternoon nap almost every day for the rest of your life. That is especially true if you are older; it may simply become part of your daily routine, so don't be surprised if that happens. For most people, however, after the first year or two, your former energy level returns or at least, very nearly does. It is very frustrating to feel this fatigue, and you should work with your doctors to make sure there aren't other factors, such as anemia, low platelet counts, or your immune system is still compromised in some way.

You may also be taking several medications after your treatment(s) ends. It is possible that some of these medications contribute to your fatigue. Check with your doctor(s) to see if the medications can be changed or dosages altered. Some drugs, such as vinblastine, taxol and Taxotere, have an impact on your nerves because of their toxicity, which may lead to fatigue. Additionally, a change in your diet may have to occur (you may need additional nutrients because the cancer has been competing with the rest of your body for any available nourishment); exercise may have to be increased (while on chemo, you may have ignored this area and your muscles have become weaker); you may need to drink more fluids, and, if your medications permit it, perhaps some vitamin supplements may help. You will need to work with your physician(s) to make most of these determinations. Ask for a treatment plan to help with fatigue. It may be something as simple as a blood transfusion, if you are anemic. It may involve physical therapy or strength training to help your muscles regain their strength. One thing to remember is that *unused muscles do not process oxygen properly.* Stress can also contribute to your fatigue and to the depression, but your doctor(s) could recommend counseling, self-hypnosis or other strategies to assist in alleviating your fatigue as much as possible.

You may find yourself becoming frustrated with this seemingly endless fatigue, and worrying about how this condition is affecting your family, friends and your job. In reality, some of these behaviors and activities might need adjusting. For example, rather than going out to lunch every day with your co-workers, maybe go once a week, and instead, use that hour the other four days to simply lie down somewhere. When you get home after work, simply say, "I am going to need a half-hour or so to rest" (unless the house is burning down). This could also turn into snuggle time with your youngest kids, a private moment for all of you just to close your eyes, relax or talk in quiet voices. In this day and age, as busy as everyone is, to have that half hour may seem impossible. And some days it will be. Kids have to be taken to soccer practice or band practice or the doctor or the neighbor's house for a sleep-over. But as critical as those activities may appear for your kids, you also have to make your health a priority, if you want to fully recuperate (or as fully as you will be able). If taking time to deal with your fatigue feels like it's bordering on hedonism or selfishness, just say to yourself, "So what? I deserve it!" (Read Ayn Rand's *The Virtue of Selfishness*.) A Truism:

> *"Taking care of yourself today will help you take care of all those you love tomorrow and in the future."*

You, too, will come to this realization as you learn to prioritize appropriately. Putting yourself first at this time is not only appropriate, but also necessary for your recovery.

There is no question, however, that fatigue *is* hard to deal with. It *is* frustrating. You *will* have to develop patience with yourself, and be willing to allow yourself the time it takes to resolve. Some strategies that might help you are: plan your day—develop a *realistic* schedule and set realistic goals: last week you walked 15 minutes a day, this week increase that to 20 or 25 minutes; change how you expend your energy (perhaps have a chair or stool handy to sit down while you are cooking or folding laundry); as mentioned earlier—take a nap (this is especially helpful as you recuperate from "chemo brain;" naps also help as you recuperate from memory loss); it's important that, to the extent possible, you wake up and go to bed at the same time every day—even weekends; if you have twenty hobbies, look at paring them back to five or ten, and also cut back the time you spend on them at any one stretch; pamper yourself—you have earned it; and the two biggest concepts—Let others help, you don't have to do it all; and—Let go of what you can, of things you cannot change. Terry's guidelines now are based on two criteria: if it won't change the course of history, or if 50 years from now, no one will know, then Let it go!

For additional ideas to help with fatigue, see the Fatigue Coalition, http://www.ncbi.nlm.nih.gov.

Financial Resources

Costs to treat cancer have almost doubled in the last 20 years according to an article in *Cancer* magazine in the May 10, 2010 issue. In addition, costs to both private insurance and Medicare were increased at about the same rate. In 2006, the estimated costs to treat cancer were $104.1 billion. It is projected that two up-coming events will have a devastating impact on the future costs for treating cancer:

1. the increasing rate of cancer diagnoses and
2. baby boomers turning 65.

Even though some expensive treatments have been implemented and are now considered standard, it seems, after analysis, the increase in costs were not so much due to increased costs per patient, but rather to an increase in the numbers of cancer patients treated.

Across the globe, cancer has a greater cost than premature death and death caused by disabilities. The World Health Organization (WHO) conducted a study to discover what the costs might be. They first estimated the costs of a year of healthy life. Next they analyzed 17 kinds of cancer and the 15 leading causes of death. Countries around the world were classified by income. Their findings were significant:

1. costs from premature death and disability (but not cancer) were $895 billion; heart disease had costs of $753 billion;

2. of all causes of death, cancer had the greatest costs from premature death and disability;

3. the largest financial drain from cancer on economies around the globe were lost productivity and a shortened life span;

4. breast, colorectal and lung cancers had the greatest costs worldwide due to death and disability;

5. in poorer countries, the greatest financial costs were associated with breast, cervical and head and neck cancers associated with death and disability.

These data point to the need for global strategies to deal with cancer, especially in cancer prevention and treatment in poorer countries. We are all interconnected; what impacts one country eventually has an impact on the rest of the world. To use Joseph Campbell's analogy, we need to think of ourselves as "earthians," not just as citizens of a particular country, but rather as citizens of the world.

The cost of treatment can be a burden on both the patient and family members, even with private insurance and Medicare. As mentioned earlier, Terry and Tom had well over $6,000 in out-of-pocket expenses in 2009, and for each of the prior two years. While they are both grateful for what insurance has covered, the total uncovered expenses each year place a huge burden on their ever-shrinking budget, as they incur life with the limited funds of retirement income concurrent with escalating medical expenses. There simply are NO funds available for meeting the rising costs.

If you are faced with increasing medical bills after you have survived cancer, where might you go to seek help in paying them? The sources will vary from country to country. In the United States, there are actually several places that might help, depending on your age and yearly salary. What follows is a thumbnail sketch. For more coverage of the potential financial assistance resources available, please call The American Cancer Society at: 1-800-ACS-2345, or refer to their website: http://www. cancer.org/docroot/mlt/content/mlt_1x_medical_insurance_and_ financial_assistance_for_the_cancer_patient.asp. Another helpful booklet is *Mapping the Maze, A Personal Financial Guide to Blood Stem Cell Transplant*, by the National Marrow Donor Program®, at 1-888-

999-6743, and the National Endowment for Financial Education®
website: http://www.nefe.org.

First and foremost, figure out where you can economize. Is that
new drill really necessary or could you get by with the old one for
now? Did you really need that fancy mixer to make your child's
birthday cake? If you have been saving for your children's college
education, they may have to work to help pay their own room and
board, tuition and/or books. While you may be loathe to do it, check
any pensions or tax sheltered annuities/IRAs you may have to see if
you can borrow from them. You might also want to check to see if
you can refinance your house (really a bummer) to pay for the out-
standing health care costs, or you may have to remortgage your
house to either get a reduced rate, or to spread the payments out
over a new 30-year period. Transfer your credit card debt to a lower-
interest card. Shop around for lower prescription costs. While it's a
pain to have to drive to two or three or more pharmacies to get your
prescriptions, the cost difference may not only justify your time, but
also the gas used to get to them. For one of Tom's medications, Terry
shopped around and saved over $200 per month on the cost of one
prescription alone. As you are recuperating, you might want to check
with the Registered Financial Planners Institute at 1-440-282-7176
or their website, http://www.rfpi.com, to help put you on the road to
a financial recovery.

Check with your state government to see if there are "health
insurance risk pools" for which you might qualify. These are created
by individual states and are non-profit associations. Under the new
health care bill, $5 billion has been earmarked for states to subsidize
health insurance premiums for those who have not been covered for
at least six months and/or have been denied health care coverage
because of a pre-existing condition. Some states have these funds
available; some others do not. Some states also offer better, more
complete coverage than others. The Health Insurance Resource Center at: http://www.healthinsurance.org/risk_pools has a list of the
states that provide this coverage. There are 34 states that currently
offer the health insurance risk pool coverage.

Check with the hospital in which you received treatment. Often
they will have special funds set aside to help pay for treatment, if you
are struggling. Some hospitals provide a financial counseling service to
help you manage the medical bills you will be incurring for the treat-

ment(s) prescribed at their facility. They may even know of other potential financial resources for you.

If you have exhausted all of your sick pay and benefits, check with your employer to see if extensions are available, and if so, find out how to go about being granted an extension. You may also want to check to see whether you can retire on a medical disability; this would allow you to draw your retirement ahead of your natural retirement age. But, if you do that, be aware you will most likely receive somewhat smaller monthly checks than if you waited to retire at the natural age for your birth date; that decreased amount will continue to be a lesser sum for the rest of your life.

If you have left the company which had provided you with health insurance, the COBRA (Consolidated Omnibus Budget and Reconciliation Act) of 1986 will allow you to temporarily continue your same health insurance coverage, although your monthly premium might be higher than your company paid. You can receive 18 months of coverage if you have had to either resign from your job, or have had to reduce your hours of work due to your illness. You may receive up to 29 months of coverage under COBRA if you, as the beneficiary, have become permanently disabled. Up to 36 months of coverage may be available to the spouse or minor child if there is a legal separation or divorce, if you qualify for Medicare, and in the case of your death. However, there are deadlines that must be met. They vary due to the circumstances, so you will need to talk with your employer. If you have been fired from your job, you are not eligible. As a piece of federal legislation, COBRA is managed by the U.S. Department of Labor, http://www.dol.gov/ebsa/faqs/faq_consumer_cobra.HTML.

If you have become permanently disabled, check with the Social Security Administration to see if you qualify for social security disability or for supplemental insurance (SSDI or SSI). You will need official medical records and physicians' statements in support of your disability claim, as part of the application process. Once you have been on disability for 24 months or more, you may then qualify for Medicare.

Medicare, a federally funded health insurance program, has already been mentioned several times. However, there is also a jointly funded federal and state equivalent called Medicaid. To qualify for this program, your assets and income must be at or below a certain amount based on your family size. Each state will have its own version of this plan. One real drawback with having Medicaid is that some physicians do not accept patients with this type of coverage. To find out about the coverage, use a search engine and type in something like "(name of state) medicaid." A plethora of topic options will pop up on your screen, areas such as eligibility, application, program and formulary. Or, look in the section of your phone book under (name of state) government, and then under your state health department. Your state may also have special health insurance programs for any of your children if they are the ones who have or have had cancer.

Women who have or have had breast and/or cervical cancer, and who are uninsured, are considered members of an underserved population. As such, if they also meet the criteria for being identified as low-income according to state established criteria, they may be eligible for financial assistance through the Centers for Disease Control and Prevention. Contact them at 1-800-232-4636 or http://www.cdc.gov/cancer/nbccedp.

If you are a U.S. veteran, contact the Veteran's Administration to see if you qualify for financial assistance. You can reach them at 1-800-827-1000 or http://www.va.gov/healtheligibility. If you are still in the military, contact TRICARE. This is a health insurance program funded by the Department of Defense for people on active duty, family, reservists, retirees and survivors. Like anything to do with the government, there are about a bzillion rules to qualify. To find out if you are eligible, contact http://www.tricare.mil.

The Hill-Burton Free and Reduced Cost Health Care Program was enacted in 1946 to help hospitals and some non-profit health care providers (those who were "obligated" to provide treatment) pay for services for those who are unable to pay. You cannot access this through Medicare or Medicaid. These funds are based on income and family size. The Program was basically discontinued in 1997, but there are still about 200 places that are obligated to provide health care services. Contact 1-800-492-0742 (1-800-492-0359 in Maryland) or for further information, visit the following website http://www.hrsa.gov/hillburton. The website contains a list of the medical facilities which are still participating.

For help with living expenses, you might want to look into "living benefits"—your health insurance policy may be able to provide you with immediate cash by accelerating the death benefit. This option may be accomplished by "viaticals" (selling the life insurance policy) or loans against the life insurance policy through a third party. Viaticals are usually intended for people with terminal ill-nesses; your physician must verify your eligibility or qualifying med-ical condition. The holder of the life insurance policy may sell it for from 60%–80% of the cash value, in return for immediate cash to help pay bills associated with the health condition. The drawbacks are that your heirs will not receive any potential inheritance from this policy; you may not get the best percentage rate from the cash value, and once sold, the policy is usually not reversible. For detailed information, refer to the American Council of Life Insurers, http://www.acli.com or call 1-202-624-2000.

Some community organizations might also be able to provide financial assistance: your own place of worship, Catholic Social Ser-vices, Jewish Social Services, the Salvation Army, and the United Way. The Alliance of Information and Referral Systems in conjunction with United Way have set up a 211-phone system (not available in all parts of the United States). Dial 211 to see if your state has this service or log on to http://www.211.org. Another great resource is the offices on aging in your city or state. To find out what is available in your state, contact the Eldercare Locator, 1-800-677-1116 or their website http://www.n4a.org. The American Cancer Society also has many resources: http://www.cancer.org.

There may also be financial assistance available through your county department of social services (DSS). That local service unit may be able to help with paying your mortgage or arranging for you to receive funding for government-sponsored short-term housing if you have become unable to pay your mortgage and lose your house.

For help paying your phone bill when you are low-income, contact the Universal Service Administrative Company to see if their program is available in your state, 1-888-641-8722 or http://www.usac.org/li/low-income (although, as quite an irony, if your phone has already been disconnected, you would have difficulty calling the company or accessing their website). Be sure, once you do reach them, to mention your health issues that have negatively impacted your ability to keep up with your bill.

For food assistance, you might want to contact your local school to see if your children qualify for free- or reduced-lunches while you are struggling to pay your medical bills. You might also qualify for the food stamp program (now called Supplemental Nutrition Assistance Program—SNAP). Other programs which might help ease your food expenses are the Farmers' Market Nutrition Program, the Senior Farmers' Market Nutrition Program, and a commodity supplemental food program in your community. To find out about these programs, log on to http://www.fns.usda.gov/fns/default.htm.

Friends and family can also help raise funds by doing a fundraiser. The social worker at the hospital or your physician's office can provide you with a list of organizations that specialize in this type of fundraising. Just recently, we have discovered My Friends Care Cancer Fund. This organization helps cancer patients with fundraising assistance. They provide expertise, support and information to help raise funds to pay your medical expenses. They also help educate and support the Be The Match © Registry. If you are searching for a way to do fundraising to help defray medical expenses, please contact them at 586-783-7390, or e-mail info@MyFriends Care.org or visit their website: http://www.MyFriendsCare.org.

For those who are uninsured, there are several options for possibly acquiring insurance coverage:

- Find an independent insurance broker or one that offers group insurance (usually cheaper by group).

- Try to become employed by a large company that offers health insurance (we wish you good luck with that in this economy).

- Check with your state government to see if they have subsidized health insurance coverage for low-income people, or if they have "guaranteed issue" (automatically qualified to receive health insurance, usually no medical questions asked) individual plans, which should be available to you, even with a pre-existing condition.

- If you were employed for at least one day and had health insurance coverage by your employer, or if you were employed one day past the initial grace period after which a new employee's insurance coverage becomes effective, you may be eligible for COBRA insurance.

- If you belong to a professional or fraternal organization, see if they have access to health insurance plans. Specifically, check to make sure it is what is referred to as "guaranteed issue."

If you believe your insurance company is not giving you all the benefits to which you are entitled, find out which governmental agency oversees insurance in your state. Talk with the consumer advocacy office. In addition to the state-level regulatory offices are several organizations which might be of help: the Kaiser Family Foundation at http://www.kff.org/consumerguide; the Patient Advocate Foundation, a national advocacy organization, which offers specialized mediation and arbitration services for those with insurance access issues who are experiencing medical debt crises at http://www.patientadvocate.org/resources.php?p=13; and another national organization, the America's Health Insurance Plan (AHIP), which is a sixty year-old association of 1300 member insurance companies. The purpose of the group is to represent the interests of the member companies through defined roles, which are to research, represent, monitor and ensure quality about health care financing and delivery; its service roles include educating, informing and assisting interested consumers and customers. You may contact AHIP at: http://www.healthclaimappeals.org/home.html.

In the event you have any legal issues that arise, the Cancer Legal Resource Center may be able to help; you may call them at 1-866-843-2572, or go to the website at: http://www.cancerlegalresourcecenter.org.

We have provided several website resources, but the reality is that if you are experiencing financial problems, access to the Internet can be expensive, and most likely, a bit beyond your budget. That may also be true for the telephone referrals we provided. Should this be the case for you, consider using your local or state library; they often have Internet access, and it is usually offered free of charge.

In the United Kingdom, one of the largest charities and resources is the Macmillan Cancer Support, a 100 year-old institution dedicated to the provision of health care, information, and financial support to people who have been affected with cancer. It not only focuses on the treatment of patients for the disease, but also on the social, emotional and practical impact cancer has upon its victims, thereby treating through the use of a more holistic approach—they treat the whole body. To get more information about the charity, go to the website: http://www.macmillan.org.uk/Cancerinformation/Livingwithandafter cancer/Financialissues/Financialissues.aspx or call 0808-808-0000. One of the unique features of the organization is that it has cancer support specialists to help you explore your treatment options once you have been diagnosed. Its services are designed not only for cancer patients and their families, but also for the patients' caregiver(s).

Other countries will also have their own financial resources. It's hard to know exactly how to help you access this information. When we did a web search, for example, "cancer atlas India" (India has one of the highest rates of cancer in the world), we found the National Cancer Registry Programme, but nothing on helping with finances. We looked up "financial help for cancer survivors in Mexico," but didn't find anything either. Given the nature of global travel today, we wanted to find something that might help if you found yourself in another country and needed some temporary financial assistance to cover the medical bills you are acquiring, or other costs you may be incurring, such as housing, transportation, prescriptions and telephone. We were largely unsuccessful in locating the information and suggest you check with the doctor, hospital or other state, county (shire), or other country governmental agencies to see what might be available.

Fingerprints—Loss of

Depending on the type(s) of chemo you receive, such as capecitabine (Xeloda), you might—MIGHT—lose your fingerprints, especially if you are on the drug(s) for an extended period of time. One case was reported in the May 2009, issue of the *Annals of Oncology,* and on CNN, the BBC and MSNBC. It appears this had happened to a man from Singapore who had been undergoing chemotherapy since 2005 for head and neck cancer that had metastasized. A side effect of this medicine is hand-foot syndrome, which causes peeling of the skin in these areas. Over time, fingerprints can be erased. The gentleman flew from Singapore to the U.S. to visit relatives. Citizens of countries outside the U.S. have to go through a mandatory screening of their fingerprints. Each person with a visa has two index fingerprints taken. They are matched against millions of other fingerprints to see if the person in question has entered the U.S. under any other name or has a criminal record. For those people coming from, or going to, a country outside the U.S., whose fingerprints have been eradicated, it is recommended a letter be carried from the oncologist or other physician, stating the condition for which you are being treated and the type of chemotherapy that has been used. The gentleman from Singapore was held for four hours, until it was finally determined he was not a threat to U.S. security.

It is common for people who are bricklayers, sometimes secretaries, people who work with lime, as well as senior citizens, to have their fingerprints erased. Bricklayers can have their prints worn down because of the roughness of the materials they handle. Paper handled extensively during the day can cause secretaries to lose the sharpness or definition in their fingerprints. Lime can dissolve the skin layers. In the case of senior citizens, elasticity of the skin is decreased as one ages; the ridges thicken, the height between the ridges and the furrows narrow, resulting in less distinction. The fingers of the elderly, especially older women, are often so smooth, no prints at all remain. For those of you tempted to try to "test the system" and destroy your fingerprints, the resulting scars become the identifiers.

Flatulence

There is no delicate way of putting this: if you have had a stem cell transplant, you will—will—have flatulence. It will creep out at the most inopportune moments; you won't be able to help it. It just appears from. . . . well, not out of nowhere (we all know where it comes from), but all of a sudden, there it is. Sometimes it will be a brief toot. Other times it will seem to go on endlessly, and for some of us, actually be quite musical in its tones ("b-sharp" or "c-flat" is usually the key). Once at the physical therapist's office, Terry could have taken first place in a contest—or at least, honorable mention, twice, maybe. . . . Changing your diet will not necessarily help to resolve it, because food doesn't actually have anything to do with it. It simply is. So, when it happens, just politely excuse yourself and continue with what you were doing.

Fungi (There's a Fungus Among Us)

Chemo destroys your immune system and leaves you vulnerable to many potential diseases and other conditions. One of these is fungus. It is common to find a fingernail or toenail discolored. There may also be an unpleasant odor. You may find a white or yellow spot underneath your fingernails or toenails. If it spreads, nails can grow back in a somewhat deformed shape. Sometimes the nail falls off and doesn't grow back at all.

The fungus more often occurs in toenails than in fingernails, because the fungus doesn't need sunlight to thrive, and toes are normally in a dark, warm, moist (and sometimes smelly) environment. In addition, because we are constantly washing our hands during the day, it would be difficult for the fungus to get a start on our fingernails. Another risk factor is that with chemo, your fingernails and toenails may be subject to reduced blood flow, resulting in tingling and numbness. This makes it harder for your immune system, which is already compromised from fighting cancer, to fight the fungus, as well.

Once you notice that your nails are discolored, have a little spot underneath them, you smell an odor, or you feel pain, contact your doctor right away. Left untreated, it can lead to more difficulty in getting rid of the fungus. It is not contagious, so you don't have to worry about passing it on. It is wise to be as clean as possible, in order not to exacerbate the condition. There are several medications available over the counter to help treat this condition.

Hair

After chemo, for the most part, your hair should grow back. If you have had radiation on your skull, those portions that received the greatest dosage might not grow back, or could be somewhat sparse, if it does. The good news is that for most people, hair grows back thicker and curlier. As mentioned earlier, you hair can come back in a totally different color. Terry is a natural redhead, but the first time her hair grew back, it was brown. The second time it came back, it was more red, and did not have as much grey (hooray!). Alexis is a natural blonde. Her hair has grown back in darker, but it is still a rich shade of blonde. Other people have had brown hair naturally (or black, as examples), but it has grown back totally grey or even white. There is no way to determine what color your new hair will be when it grows back; just wait and be surprised.

If you are unhappy with the color of your hair, you will have to wait several months after chemo before you can change your new color. There are many suspected carcinogens in the chemicals used to color your hair. Some people have put on a temporary rinse, but you have to be very careful about that, too. It is best to just give it some time –who knows, you may even grow to like your new color.

If your hair was naturally thick and curly to begin with, your hair will probably be the same when it comes back. However, in Terry's case, she has noticed that 18 months after her last chemo, her hair has now become thinner (her hair is falling out), softer (the hair strand is thinner, and not so thick, fewer strands per square inch on her scalp), and the natural curl is disappearing. These new changes in her hair this time may be related to the thyroid. She has no idea whether these changes are permanent, or will eventually be resolved.

Health Care Medical Bills

So—you've survived cancer! You have fought the good fight and won! And now you're possibly faced with huge medical bills. The viciousness of the cycle seems to be never ending. The Fall 2009, issue of *Thrive* magazine, published by the University of Michigan, offers these pieces of advice for those who are overwhelmed by medical bills.

1. **Public assistance** is there to help you if you need it. You have paid for this help through the taxes you paid during all the years you have worked, **SO USE IT**. It is not a failure on your part. You may also qualify for financial assistance, such as Medicaid.

2. **Ask for help as soon as you realize you need it**. Your doctor, cancer center or hospital often have people who are familiar with the bureaucratic mazes that have been established to prevent people from getting help. There may also be other programs, such as charities, either private or through the hospital, which can help.

3. **File a Power of Attorney** allowing someone else to manage your finances while you recuperate. Often after treatment, a cancer survivor can be exhausted for months and needs someone to make sure the bills are paid, and paid on time. You can make

this for a specified period of time and it can be rescinded at any time you wish.

4. **Stay well organized.** Keep all records related to doctors, hospitals, pharmacies, correspondence with insurance companies, etc. If you speak to someone over the phone, be sure to get their name, title if applicable, phone number, date and time of the call, and take notes of what was said during the conversation. Even after you have survived cancer, there will still be battles to be fought (just what you needed, right?), and you have to have the proverbial paper trail. Remember the "kiddie vacs" story earlier.

5. **Stay current with your mail.** Often forms or information come through that you have been too tired to deal with, but if you don't respond, your case may be closed, or interest can accrue, which leads to more expensive bills. It may also have a name on the return address with which you are unfamiliar. Open it anyhow.

6. **As often as possible, go in person.** This applies not only to Medicaid or Medicare, but also to the insurance company itself, or if you are retiring, the person in charge of getting your retirement in place. There is nothing like sitting eyeball-to-eyeball with that person; you become a human being rather than just a case or an account number. You will find the personal connection will make a big difference, not just in how you are treated, but in the time it takes to resolve issues, and in some cases, the outcomes, as well.

7. **If you don't understand** something, from a bill or a letter, **ask questions, and keep asking** until you do understand. If you are still too exhausted to go in person, ask whether e-mail communication is an acceptable mode of correspondence.

8. **Be nice** (at least, for the first three or four times you talk)! Caseworkers are often overwhelmed with the day-to-day grind, and the vast majority of them truly desire to help you. The laws and rules and regulations change as often for them as they do for you, but it's probably much worse for them, because of all the specificity and nuances they have to take into consideration. Realize this early and take action to make them an important

part of your team of caregivers in this battle with cancer. Remember how you like to be treated and as much as possible, reciprocate.

9. **If you can't pay your bills** in full and on time, **make arrangements for a realistic payment plan.** Even if you believe the insurance company will never reimburse you, pay on time and according to the payment plan. It *will* be difficult (not "*may* be difficult") to get your money back, but in the vast majority of cases, you will be reimbursed. And what a treat that will be, when that long-awaited reimbursement actually arrives—you might be able to go on that trip you have been postponing because of the battles you have been waging. Work with the staff at your doctor's office, the hospital, the cancer care center, with anyone who can help you. That's their job. Remember, they do want to help!

Health Insurance: The Good, The Bad and The Downright Ugly

In the United States, the fact is there are between 36–45 million citizens (depending on who is doing the reporting) who have no health care coverage at all. What is often underreported, is that there are an approximate additional 25 million people who are what is referred to as the "underinsured." These are people who spend more than 10% of their income to pay for out-of-pocket medical expenses. A Harvard study found that in 2005, more than 1,700 bankruptcies had medical problems and medical costs as the primary reason for the financial crisis, and about 75% of those had health insurance coverage of one sort or another. Most of these medically bankrupt people were middle class, had good jobs, a good education, and were buying their homes. Texas has the highest rate of totally uninsured people in the United States, at about 25%.

Medicaid programs in each state vary across the country in their coverage. Michigan and Tennessee, as examples, generally do well by the people who need their services. Parts of Texas, on the other hand, are parsimonious to the nth degree. If you live in a rural county, you are more likely to receive minimal services. The American Cancer Society has a national call center for cancer patients who are struggling with their bills. Some pharmaceutical companies have programs that help patients cover their pharmaceutical costs. Terry had to have three Emend pills for nausea from the chemotherapy, each of which was $600 (for a total of $1,800) every two weeks, or nearly $4,000 each month (no one she knew could afford that). At that time, she was without employment, and astonishingly, the drug-manufacturer helped with the cost. At the same time, Tom also had to take pills that cost $800 per month. Again, the drug manufacturer of those pills also stepped in to help pay for the costs. A Truism:

"Once blessed, twice blessed—thrice blessed you will be."

What all this means, is that for anyone, anywhere here in the U.S., it is possible you could fall ill, and if you have a deductible, you could exhaust your savings or your paycheck before meeting that deductible. If you think about buying a short-term policy to supplement your own health insurance policy, you should save your money. There are loopholes big enough to drive a semi-truck through. Even if you have been faithfully paying on private health insurance for several years, when you are faced with a catastrophic illness, or have had an illness within the previous six months, you might be labeled as having a "pre-existing condition" and denied health coverage. You, too, may be faced with either paying for your mortgage or having a biopsy done. Sometimes purchasing supplemental or short-term policies can disqualify you at a future date from comprehensive, long-term coverage. There are some doctors who still continue to treat their patients, even when it is apparent they will receive no remuneration. Those doctors are a rare breed, an unusually generous group, and much under-celebrated . . . one of the many unsung heroes you will encounter throughout this war.

The incongruity in all of this is that those who can least afford health care coverage are ultimately being charged the highest costs. Health insurance companies have the numbers of customers, which gives them the negotiation powers over how much they will pay for a procedure. If one procedure (say a mammogram) will be paid by the health insurance company in the amount of $1,000, an individual with no health insurance or limited insurance might be required to pay five or more times that amount. Some insurance companies (such as the one Terry is with now) will only pay for a 30-day supply of her medications—when it is actually cheaper to buy them in 90- or 120-day supplies. Sometimes, there is also a "cap" on hospital stays. If your daily care while in the hospital exceeds your allotment, you will most likely accrue horrendous bills to pay. If that happens to you, make arrangements to pay something on each of your bills—$10 here, $50 there, $12 somewhere else, to demonstrate your good faith in trying to meet your financial obligations. Keep up those payments until you can figure out where you can possibly cut your monthly budget, to pay more toward your medical debts. While bill collectors are notoriously unsympathetic, there are some who will genuinely try to help you find some kind of recourse or payment alternatives.

In the irony of all ironies, Medicare, the federal government program, will pay for medical treatments toward the end of life, when it is most expensive. In so many cases, if adequate treatment could have been accessed earlier in the illness, that end-of-life expense might have been avoided, or at least delayed. Once you reach that stage, you are no longer able to purchase any additional health insurance, even if you could afford it. If you have an illness that has been determined to be a "pre-existing condition," there is quite often a waiting period, sometimes as long as twelve months, before you could qualify for additional health insurance to help defray the ever-increasing costs of a serious illness.

As this is being written (November 2010, although it may be revisited at different points in the future), the debate has finally been settled about whether or not to have a national health care plan in the U.S. We do, or rather, we do until it gets voted on again, or is repealed. For better or worse, for richer or poorer, in sickness and in health, until death do us part, we have a national health care package. The supreme irony in all the debate about health care is, according to the AARP, what was eventually passed, was very similar to the health plans Republican Presidents Richard Nixon and Ronald Reagan had proposed years ago. The 2010 health care bill was passed with virtually no Republican support. The worst part of this story for our country and its people, however, is that the two major political parties were unwilling—not unable—to find common ground. Is this the time when we say that the two-party system has become outdated?

A huge problem with this bill is that many of the players who should have been involved with all of the discussions, such as public health staff, social service staff, health maintenance organization staff, staff from other medical health care organizations, people from businesses and our universities, were not allowed to participate in the process of writing this bill. In addition, the public (the tax-pay-ers—all of us) and others who have expertise in this area (what's the sense in having an educated public if the government won't listen to them?), were not allowed any formal decision-making role in what they wanted to see. As changes need to be made in the bill, this lack of representation will need to be rectified. Indeed, if public opinion polls are to be believed, the taxpayers were clearly saying they are dissatisfied with this bill, and that they don't want it in its current form. The bill, as passed, is cumbersome and difficult to read. In our dreams, we would like to see the health care bill be summarized in 25 pages, to clearly state what is being proposed, along with the expected costs for each section. A short addendum, say ten pages, could contain an analysis of why things are being proposed and who had input into that decision-making (if it was just lawyers and elected representatives and representatives of special interests, we are in serious trouble; let's not go there). Well, we can always dream. In reality, the issues are more complicated than that but the jargon or "legalese" is not really helping the citizens of this country to fully understand the bill, and that in itself opens the door for opponents to unleash scare tactics upon us all.

The fear-mongers raise the ugly specter of "socialized medicine." But how awful is socialized medicine? Has anyone bothered to check, or because fear is such a powerful emotion and motivator, have they simply decided that others know best? Let's look at "socialized" medi-cine for a minute. Under the previous (and still current) health system in the United States, Americans wait longer to get in to see the doctor than in any socialized medicine country. Americans rank last (along with Canadians, who do have a public health care system) to be able to see their doctor on the same day they call. This is likely because there are fewer primary care physicians in America than in other coun-tries, and fewer students are entering the primary care medical field. Americans do well, however, when it comes to elective surgery, better than in a country with a public health system. The fear-mongers say that socialized medicine (meaning "the government") will decide who gets medical treatment and who will not, based on your age, medical condition and whether or not your life is deemed worth saving. If that truly were the case, how is it that Stephen Hawking, the brilliant physicist who has ALS, and is a person who lives in a "socialized med- icine" country (Great Britain), consistently gets expensive medical care, and has for decades?

The other issue fear-mongers raise is their claim that the current health care bill provides for counseling so you can decide to pull the plug on your grandparents. NOT TRUE. The health care plan just passed allows older citizens to access counseling—*if they want it*—and it will be paid for, it will NOT come out of Grandpa's or Grandma's checkbook the way it does now. It also provides for annual preventive checkups, for which your grandparents will NOT have to pay. Another facet of "socialized medicine" is that, in Great Britain, for example, scientists conduct studies that ascertain whether a surgical procedure or a medicine is effective. Perish the thought we would continue to pay for things that simply don't work. (And how necessary are all the tests that are conducted? We suspect that if Americans weren't so litigious, those tests wouldn't be so prevalent.) The health care bill just passed is designed, in theory, to reduce spending over $1 trillion by 2029.

Under the current health care system, our insurance companies decide which doctors we see and what medicines we have to take. The health insurance companies also dictate how much doctors will receive for not only office calls, but in the case of oncologists, the price of the chemotherapy administered in their offices. Most health insurance companies do not fully reimburse the costs oncologists incur, leaving these doctors scrambling to pay their bills. At some point, oncologists will need to assess how, and to what extent, they will treat their patients, which could lead to a decreased quality of care. As one friend points out, perhaps it is the health insurance industry that needs to be scrutinized, and undergo a complete overhaul, rather than tinkering with developing a comprehensive national health insurance program.

Before any of us make decisions about national health care legisla- tion or make recommendations to our legislators based on our stances and issues, we need to ask ourselves a few key questions. The ques- tions are those with which we struggle today, and have continued to struggle for decades now. The questions are not easily answered, and we clearly recognize the importance of cultivating open discussion, and of finding resolution for both the ethical and the financial considera- tions inherently intertwined in the issues. As you contemplate the fol- lowing questions, try to put yourself in the shoes of the "Haves" and the "Have-Nots" as you answer.

- Is medical care something that humankind should feel they are guaranteed when he/she is born a citizen (or becomes one) of the United States?

- Does it make any sense at all that, in our country, one of the wealthiest on earth, any of our fellow citizens should be unable to receive the life-saving health care they need because of a lack of funds?

- Do you really want someone with your health insurance company, who has a high school education or a degree in business, making your health care and treatment decisions for you and also determining what medications you can and cannot have?

- Do you believe that the litigious resolve by the people in our country against those who care for us has led to the increase of 50% or more to the costs of health care, just in order for physicians and hospitals to protect themselves from the frivolous and punitive law suits filed against them?

- Would you support a systematized form of mutually acceptable agreements or contracts, countersigned by all parties involved—patient, doctor, hospital, that allows for the practice of "proactive medicine" at highly reduced costs, rather than the extremely costly form of "defensive medicine" that is currently practiced today?

If you will examine the policies you have now, you will notice the insurance companies will most likely only allow you to have generic medicines, and to only see doctors within their health group. If you go out of their health group, you will have to pay full price for medical consultations and surgeries. Who is there to assure that the doctors in your insurance group are the best in their specialty? Under the current system, you can't afford to quit your job because of the loss of health benefits, and the potential inability to get either comparable or better coverage in your new job. For those who are on a state-sponsored health care program (such as Medicaid), you can't afford to get a job because there is the possibility the company you work for can't afford health insurance as one of their benefits. And for those of you who are concerned about having to pay for providing health care for "them,"-the poor and currently uninsured—think about this for just a minute: what if you lose your job and health insurance and you become one of "them"? It is happening to more and more people in our country every day—"them" are "us" and we also need health care!

Under the current wording of the health care package, if you want to keep your own health insurance, you can. In Great Britain, as an example, people often carry additional insurance coverage as a hedge against the national system. Even older people here in the U.S. carry additional health insurance coverage that pays for things that Medicare does not cover.

One of our major mysteries in the U.S., is the oh, so famous "donut hole" in Medicare (federally-funded) prescription coverage for people over the age of 65. It's either a Rube Goldberg contraption, or else someone was on some serious mind-altering drugs when this was written, so grab your hats, and hang on for the ride to nowhere:

- Total out-of-pocket prescription costs between 0–$310—you pay the full amount—up to $310.

- If your total out-of-pocket prescription costs are between $310–$2,830, you pay $310 plus 25% of the costs over $310 (if you have $2,830 in prescription costs, you pay $310 + $630 for a total of $940).

- *Here's the donut hole:* if your total out-of-pocket prescription costs are between $2,830 and $6,440, you pay $940 plus 100% of the total cost over $2,830. This means that if your total out-of-pocket drug costs are $6,440 per year, you will pay $940 + $3,610 for a total of $4,550 for the year.

- If your total out-of-pocket prescription costs are over $6,440, then you pay $4,550 + 5% of the total costs over $6,440.

Please remember that these costs are true "out-of-pocket" expenses, and do not include what your other insurance might cover.

The health care bill, as passed, provides for the gradual elimination of the donut hole, which is currently scheduled to fully take effect in 2020. That is, unless it's changed in the meantime. Shall we take bets on this?

For people who are on a fixed income or who lost their savings in the stock market collapse, this is an untenable amount. The older we get, the more medicines we need, and the more expensive they are. Older citizens on a fixed income are often faced with either paying their rent or paying for their medications. Over and above that, you will find, quite often, the insurance companies have "deductibles." On Terry's BC/BS insurance plan, there is a $500 deductible for family and a $250 for "individual" deductible. In 2009, her medical and pharmaceutical expenses amounted to over $6,000 out-of-pocket, and yet, BC/BS said that only $250 of the family deductible had been used. Can someone, anyone, please explain that? It must be one of those elusive benefits hidden in the literature of the insurance benefits handbook, you know, one that is given in one place, taken away in another, given back, and ultimately cannot be offered because of a contingency specified in the description of a different benefit altogether. And if you don't understand that, don't bother to call the insurance company; they most likely won't either, at least not until you have spoken with the sixth or seventh representative. But, as said earlier (just in case we sound a little frustrated), they really do want to be of help to you!

As for paying for those 32 million or more people who currently don't have coverage, you are already paying for that out of a portion of your insurance premiums. Illegal immigrants? No, they are not covered in the health care package. (Speaking of immigrants, illegal or otherwise, another "hot button" for the fear-mongers, are you aware the immigrants generate more jobs than they take? The highest skilled immigrants create jobs in the fields of engineering and technology. According to a report prepared for the Cato Institute by Maureen Rimmer and Peter Dixon, two Australian economists, tighter border control "is unambiguously negative," primarily because the jobs that would have been created higher on the job chain, are eliminated.)

The good news is most of the health insurance plans, whether "socialized" or not, will cover a significant portion of costs associated with the treatment of cancer (or, likely, any other debilitating illness). If you are old enough to be on Medicare, the vast majority of chemotherapy, doctors' visits, lab work and other areas are covered at little or no cost to the patient. Other good news from the health care bill recently passed: your health insurance company can no longer deny you coverage because of a serious illness, or for any kind of pre-existing condition. They can't cancel your coverage if you get sick. Steps have been put in place to curb health care costs, so families won't have to go bankrupt, and businesses won't be penalized if they want to provide health insurance for their employees. Terry used to work for a school district where the fringe benefits package, of which health insurance constituted a huge portion, averaged about 30% of the cost of a person's salary. Small businesses can't afford to pay health insurance; even large corporations are faced with either cutting their employees, and/or eliminating or reducing the health care benefits they can offer.

You will still need, however, to be prepared to fight battles with your health insurance company (or the national health service) about what IS covered and what IS NOT, what they should pay for according to their policy handbook, and what they decide not to pay. While Blue Cross/Blue Shield did pay for the stem cell transplant (thank you!), they did not pay for the necessary dental work done prior to having the stem cell transplant, nor did they pay for all of the "kiddie vacs" that were required a year after the stem cell transplant, *despite copies being submitted to BC/BS from their own policy handbook that said they should.* Whether there is a national health care plan or whether you have your own insurance, you will need to be constantly informed and be willing to fight for the services for which you are paying and, in some cases, entitled. In Terry's case, it took months, several letters and several phone calls before the kiddie vac issue was finally settled. (Blue Cross/Blue Shield is not being singled out; it is simply the coverage both of us have and therefore, it is the company with which we are most familiar. And in fairness, the representatives encountered on the phone were courteous and tried hard to get this issue resolved.)

Having come down pretty hard on Blue Cross/Blue Shield, it is only fair to provide one area in which they are doing stellar work. On December 4, 2009, a meeting was held in Lansing, Michigan, to look at a plan to fight cancer and reduce medical costs. Dr. Michael Harbut, a cancer specialist at Karmanos Cancer Institute, in conjunction with Blue Cross/Blue Shield, is testing a program to work with people who are symptom-free and then, see long range, whether they will develop cancer or not. It is hoped this will not only stop cancer before it starts, but will reduce costs in the long run. They will push for early screenings, and try to find people who have been exposed to cancer-causing products. Part of the program will be preventative in nature, by showing people how to protect themselves from carcinogens. Blue Cross/Blue Shield will pay the doctors to conduct these tests. By treating cancer early, it would not only save lives, but also prevent millions of dollars in medical expenses for treating the disease. The program will focus on three leading causes of cancer—arsenic, asbestos and radon. (Well, they have to start somewhere.) We would like to see diet and exercise, from birth on up, added as variables to this study. As a further breakdown, look at those who tend to eat primarily fast foods, as opposed to "real" foods. For example, the Amish report far fewer incidences of cancers than that in the general population. Are diet and lifestyle factors? We would be tempted to say, "Yes" and should be included in this study.

One would think insurance companies would be vitally interested in prevention services, or at least early detection, which is why it's puzzling to us that health insurance companies are reluctant to endorse those types of expenses. Study after study has documented that prevention promotes healthier living, and that the onset of declining health can be delayed. Early detection also reduces long-term health costs. As an example, a recently published study conducted in Norway studied more than 40,000 women over a 20-year period. The results of the study showed that for women between the ages of 50–69, mammograms reduced the risk of death from breast cancer by 10%. Additionally, for women of all ages, there was just under a 33% decline in breast cancer mortality. While these numbers may seem small, would you or your daughter or wife or sister or aunt or grandmother want or choose to be a member of the group of women who went undetected?

Another piece we do NOT understand is, if *The China Study* is to be believed and acted upon, why aren't health insurance companies (and the national health insurance plan) insisting that, for people to be allowed full coverage, they must first fall within the "normal" or "desired" range on the Body Mass Index (BMI)? For decades now, studies have shown that people whose BMI falls within one of those two categories require less medical care and therefore, cost less to insure. Equally important to consider is if a person is a smoker, and/or who consumes more than (shall we arbitrarily say), four ounces of alcohol in a week, then s/he would be classified as "uninsurable." Under a hypothetical new preventative health program, an "uninsurable" would be a person whose life style choices directly caused or led to the development of her/his self-imposed disease or condition, one for which s/he will be held financially liable for all costs incurred in the provision of the medical care and treatment for the induced condition. Conversely, diseases acquired by the uninsurable NOT caused by the person's life choices would be covered by the insurance company. Perhaps some of the other questions we need to ask ourselves are: What are the goals of our health care plans and policies? Is it the achievement of good health in our country, or do we simply want to put band-aids in place to support and enable people with self-destructive life styles?

And yet, a Truism:

> *"Every curse has a blessing; and Every blessing has a curse."*

Returning now to the original discussion of health care, is Medicare and the corresponding end-of-life care bankrupting the system? Yes. Does something have to be done to contain the spiraling costs? Yes. The *Journal of the National Cancer Institute* predicts that cancer costs in the U.S. will increase to $158 billion by 2020,—assuming the costs stay the same between now and 2020; in Great Britain they are going to try and save an additional 5,000 lives by spending more over the next four years. Health insurance costs by the second quarter of 2010, in the U.S., were up 6% if you had insurance provided by your employer. Hospital care rose 8.2%, 5.5% for physician services and 3.4% for prescription drugs. Between 2002 and 2009, employer-sponsored health insurance costs were 53% higher. New drugs for treating cancer especially, are growing more rapidly than in other areas. In 2011, one estimate projects that employers will face another 9% in additional costs; if you also pay for a portion of the insurance costs, your share may also rise as high as 12.4%. Does the current health insurance system work? Yes—and No. Will a national health care plan work? Maybe quite well in some areas; maybe not so well in other areas—just like the current system. We suspect that the health care plan won't do half what the proponents think it will, and it won't do half what the opponents fear. We will be working on this for decades to come—and passing the costs on to our children and grandchildren. Is it a perfect bill? No. We will have to learn by trial and error as we do with all bills that are passed. Some pieces of coverage will be missed and have to be included at a later date. Other pieces will be overplayed and have to be reduced or eliminated. It's a little like a marriage or a long-term relationship—some days and years are better than others, but to be successful, both require dedication, work, commitment, persistence, evaluation and education (some strategies work better than others and you have to learn over the years which ones work best—until something changes, then the learning and strategizing have to start all over again to meet the new situation).

All health insurance coverage and providers are not "one size fits all." In the long run, you will be in the driver's seat, and have to make decisions to the best of your ability, given the knowledge you have at any given time, and that are best for you and your family. (This will become especially true if the insurance companies are able to implement the 80–20 plan—they will pay for 80% of costs, you will have to pay for the other 20%. If a stem cell transplant costs $150,000, would you be able to come up with $30,000 to pay your share? Or for Provenge: at the current cost of about $93,000, you would have to pay $18,600 out-of-pocket. (This is starting to make a national or "socialized" health care plan very appealing!) You will have to continuously educate yourself about health care, medicines, medical research, clinical trials, medical insurance providers, and the quality and competency of your doctors, nurses and hospitals—all of your health care providers. And that's the good, the bad and the downright ugly.

Hot Flashes

If you have been through menopause before you have chemo, and are done with hot flashes, sorry to tell you, but they'll likely come back during chemo. Usually about three to six months after your last chemo session, the hot flashes will begin to dissipate. However, in Terry's case, they came back again 17 months after her last chemo and stem cell transplant. They were quite frequent—about one every hour, lasting a minute or more. They were not debilitating, just uncomfortable and embarrassing when making a presentation in front of a bunch of men. In September 2009, the hot flashes were still taking center stage and quite relentless. By May 2010, they had started to be much less frequent. As someone wise once said, "This, too, shall pass." (She hopes.) While doing research for "Alternative Medicines and Strategies," we discovered that acupuncture has been shown to alleviate some of the experiences with hot flashes, especially for those women who have had breast cancer.

On the other edge of the age spectrum, if you are younger and have had chemo, you may experience early onset menopause. While undergoing chemo, you may have already experienced a few gynecological changes, such as irregular periods, a change in the number of days, and/or an increase or decrease in the flow. Whether your periods go back to "normal" or whether they will permanently cease is unknown, as this varies from woman to woman. The same holds true for your ovaries. Some women never ovulate again. This will depend on your age during treatment and the type of chemo meds you have been given. In Alexis' case, she never stopped having periods. She experiences the occasional hot flash, which she likes to compare to one of those cartoon characters whose face gets beet red just prior to blasting into outer space! (Although her feet have never left the ground, it's been close.)

What causes hot flashes is not known, but some triggers can be spicy food, the weather, being stressed, caffeine and alcohol. The other theory being explored is that there is a change in the part of the brain that regulates body temperature. (Hooray, pass the cayenne pepper and let's move to San Francisco!) Generally hot flashes will diminish over time, but you may experience them on and off for the rest of your life. Oh, joy!

Should you do hormone replacement therapy? Again, that is an individual decision, one that should be made in conjunction with your physician. Terry had been on HRT from 1989–1990, but took herself off when she began to read of some dangers of the medication. On the other hand, her Aunt Alma had been on HRT for 50 years and has shown no sign of damage. If you have had breast cancer, HRT is not recommended, because it could cause the growth of hormone-sensitive breast cancer cells. There are non-hormonal alternatives you can use, but none of them will eliminate the hot flashes entirely, either in terms of frequency, duration or intensity. There are studies being conducted now on whether soy is a good product to use. Generally speaking, if you have had breast cancer, it may be safe for you to use, but check with your physician first. Using soy as a food is probably better than pills. Black cohosh should be treated gingerly, but if you've had breast cancer, it's probably better to avoid it altogether.

The other strategy you may want to try to reduce hot flashes is something called "relaxation training." This may include deep breathing, guided imagery, and muscle relaxation. In one very small study, women who did the relaxing exercises twice a week for 20–30 minutes for up to three months reported a slight lessening in the intensity and frequency of the hot flashes. These techniques also reduced the level of stress, especially in women who had had breast cancer. The website http://www.breastcancer.org has a section called "Complementary Medicine," and contains an array of strategies you might want to use.

Infusaport and PICC Lines

Most people are quite ready to get rid of their infusaport and PICC lines. The length of time for the removal varies from person to person. In both of our cases, we were able to get the infusaport removed about six months after our last chemo. In part, the reason for the delay was to have one or two MRIs or PET scans to make sure the cancer was either gone, or apparently held in abeyance. There was a difference, however, in how they were removed. Alexis's infusaport had only been in a few months. Hers could be removed in the doctor's office. A little local anesthetic, and, pop, out it came. The only disconcerting thing Alexis found was the snipping sound as they cut it out. In Terry's case, the infusaport had been in for 20 months, necessitating outpatient surgery because of the likelihood that some scar tissue had formed around the port, making it more difficult to remove in the doctor's office. She was in surgery just a little over 15 minutes, was mostly wide- awake immediately afterward, and after a couple of hours of observation, was able to go home. She couldn't drive for 24 hours, but that was about it. There was no pain following the procedure. If there had been, the doctor said either extra-strength Tylenol or Ibuprofen could have taken care of it.

For the PICC line, the story was basically the same. There really was no need to continue to keep the PICC line implanted. To Terry, it became more of a liability in terms of preventing the development of an infection. During her stay at Karmanos, the dumb thing kept moving around, which meant that almost every day someone was coming in to fix it (usually between 1:00–3:00 A.M.). After she got home from Karmanos, the Nurse assigned to her case from the Visiting Nurses Association (VNA) came to check on her and to teach her how to clean and maintain the PICC line, and what to watch for as indicators of imminent problems. Terry had an appointment less than a week after discharge from Karmanos. Dr. Rapson gave her permission to have it removed the next time the VNA Nurse came out, which was a couple of days after the appointment. The nurse unwrapped the bandage, and, no pain, no nothing, the tube slid out. It was amazing how long that tube was, but if you think about it, it had to have been long to go from her upper arm, through veins and into her heart. Terry put it in her Christmas scrapbook, as a memory of all there had been to be thankful for that year; that book was overflowing with tokens of more blessings than she could count.

Intuition

This phenomenon has just recently come to our attention. We had gotten together with the family for a party and had the chance to ask the proverbial "Now What?" question to each other. Alexis said that since her chemo, she had developed more intuition about things. Terry responded that she had noticed it, too. We both can now walk into a room or stand next to someone in the grocery store or any other situation, and find we are picking up "vibes" of that person or that room. We are especially attuned to unhappiness, fear, anxiety or sadness. We don't think it has anything to do with facial expressions or "body language," because some people are pretty adept at having a "poker face," or even holding postures that belie their feelings at that moment. It is simply a sense that something is amiss. Perhaps it is because we have been through so much stress that our need for peaceful surroundings has become paramount. This does not mean if you are having a "bad hair day," that we won't be sympathetic (there is no-one more sympathetic than a cancer survivor for what you might be going through), but if you are making this bad hair day a lifestyle, we will move on. We will do so regretfully, but just cannot hang around. We have a lot of Life left to live, and being in less-than-peaceful surroundings is not conducive to our good health (let alone yours). A Truism:

> "*Looking down and inward at your storms, keeps you in one place, but Looking up and outward away from the storms, leads you to your dreams and visions.*"

Lymphedema

One of the more common possibilities that may occur after cancer and radiation is a condition called "lymphedema." Lymphedema occurs when there is inadequate or insufficient lymph drainage. The lymph nodes are responsible for transporting nutrients to all the cells in your body, and for removing waste products by transporting them back to the venous system near your heart. Lymph nodes also remove all the "gunk" that the capillaries don't remove. Lymph fluid is comprised of four substances: cells, long chain fatty acids, proteins and water. Lymph pathways occur all over your body, but the biggest channel is near and along the spinal column. This is called the thoracic duct and it moves lymph fluid from your legs and the pelvic region to the venous system near your heart. As the lymph fluid moves throughout your body, it goes through lymph nodes. Lymph nodes filter the lymph fluid and help fight infection. The lymph nodes also form cells, such as lymphocytes and plasma, to help fight infection. There are between 400–600 lymph nodes in our bodies.

"Primary" lymphedema may be caused by any number of factors, including lymph vessels that are either too large or too small; you may not have sufficient lymph vessels in your body, or you may be born with a condition in which the function of the lymph system is impaired. It is possible for you to develop lymphedema at any point in your life, whether or not you have cancer.

"Secondary" lymphedema may arise if you have had a tumor surgically removed and/or had radiation (through which scar tissue may have formed, which could prevent lymph fluid drainage). You could have had a trauma (from a critical car accident or severe cuts or scratches), cancer, some types of infections, or have had parasites. Secondary lymphedema may occur at any time, as well.

Lymphedema is usually found in the face, neck, abdomen, your trunk, or the genital area. It is most common in either the arm or leg. If you have had lymph nodes removed (such as in a mastectomy), or have had radiation given on or near lymph nodes, you are now at risk for lymphedema.

You will need to be fully trained by an accredited lymphedema therapist in order to properly wrap the pressure bandages that must be applied to help your condition. The training can be quite extensive depending on the severity of the lymphedema. The wrappings can be super bulky, necessitating the wearing of baggy clothes. Initial treatment can be up to four days a week for up to four weeks. Once you are discharged from actual therapy, you will return for reassessment either in six months or annually, thereafter. You want to make sure you keep these appointments. New and improved techniques and methodologies are continually being developed, which you will want to adopt as you progress through your survival.

As a suggestion, you might want to incorporate the following guidelines offered below to prevent developing lymphedema, delay the onset, or help you manage the condition if you already have lymphedema. Only a few of the numerous guidelines available are listed below; for a complete set relating to various sites affected, visit the American Lymphedema Institute website at: http:// www.health board.com/websites/Detailed/8321.html.

- The potential high-risk areas of your body should be kept scrupulously clean, especially the areas where you have creases in your skin, such as between your fingers and toes.

- Regularly launder your clothes. If you have already developed lymphedema, this also includes any wrappings and compression garments. Wrappings should be washed in hot water, in the washing machine, but do not use a fabric softener, Woolite or bleach. Do not stretch or wring the wrappings while wet. Lay or hang them flat to dry. If the wrapping is 5 meters long (about 5.5 feet), you may have to fold them in half so they don't stretch out. If you have to use foam wrappings, they should also be washed. Roll the wrappings tightly, either when you remove them, or after they are dry. Depending on the quality of the bandages you have purchased, you will usually get between three to six months use of them before they have to be replaced.

- We recommend the use of Eucerin to help keep your skin from drying out and creating other irritating skin conditions. Whatever lotion you prefer, make sure it does not have alcohol, dyes, perfumes, petroleum products or talc. If possible, get a lotion that has antiseptic ingredients, including a correct ph. Use the lotion after your shower, or when you take the wrappings off, and again, before rewrapping your arm or leg.

- Do not take hot showers (that also means no saunas or hot tubs); do not hand-wash your dishes in hot water.

- Avoid all extremes in weather. If it's hot outside, go someplace where it's cooler. If it's cold outside, go someplace where it's warmer. If you have to go out, make sure you are dressed appropriately for conditions (bundled up in the winter, sunscreen in the summer).

- If you have to have blood draws, blood pressure taken or any injections, make sure it is done on the arm or leg that does not have the lymphedema. If both your arms have lymphedema, as an example, these procedures can be done on the legs. Do not have acupuncture in any area where you have lymphedema.

- Be very careful when you cut or have someone else cut your nails; you should always avoid any puncture wounds.

- Try to avoid any kind of cuts, bruises, burns, and insect bites. If you have to go outside and your geographical area is loaded with biting insects, put on insect repellent, hopefully one that does not contain carcinogens.

- You must exercise, but check with your physician or lymphedema therapist before starting. Preferred exercising is walking and swimming. Your arm or leg should have the compression wrappings on them while walking. Do NOT exercise to the point of exhaustion. If your arm or leg even begins to ache or feel tired, stop immediately, elevate your arm or leg, rest a few minutes, then continue, only if you are able.

- If you live within a humid geographical area, use cornstarch to keep your skin dry in order to avoid developing any kind of fungus.

- Use the Body Mass Index (BMI) to find out what your ideal weight should be. If your weight is higher than the BMI indicates, lose weight. You should drink pure water—the recommended ratio is one ounce of water per 2 pounds of bodyweight. This means if you weigh 150 pounds, you should drink 75 ounces of water a day. Likewise, if you weigh 200 pounds, you should drink 100 ounces of water a day.

- Your diet should contain easily digestible proteins that make up between 10% and 30% of your caloric intake.

- Keep careful track of your swelling, especially in areas that have not previously been swollen. It is recommended you keep a monthly record. If you notice any increased swelling or swelling in new areas, get to your doctor or oncologist right away.

Women, who have had or will have a mastectomy, may want to refer to a lymphedema website just for them at: http://www.imaginis. com/breast-health/lymphedema. *Other websites with a wealth of information relating to lymphedema complications and treatments include:* http://www.lymphedemapeople.com/thesite/lymphedema_resources_ united_kingdom.htm (for Great Britain) and then at: http:// lymphoedema.org.au/index.html (for Australia). If you are travelling or residing outside the United States while experiencing your complications relating to lymphedema, this website may be helpful: http://www.lymphormation.org/associations.php.

Caught early, lymphedema is manageable. Can it be cured? No. You will likely have to wear wrappings for the rest of your life, and pay particular attention to your lifestyle by following the suggestions mentioned above. The primary goal of any lymphedema therapy you receive is to reduce the swelling as much as possible, and then to teach you how to maintain the reduction in swelling you have accomplished, and hopefully prevent any further complications. As with most things in life, success will rest on your commitment and follow-through, both during and after treatment. For additional information, please refer to Michigan State University's (MSU) Rehabilitation Medicine Clinic website at http://rehab.msu.edu. The information from the website and the videos should be used in conjunction with the lymphedema therapist who is working with you.

Multi-tasking

If you had been quite good at multi-tasking before chemo or a stem cell transplant, you can kiss it goodbye, at least for the short term. Your ability to concentrate and remember is the equivalent of a fish going around the bowl once. Every time the fish gets back to the beginning of the circuit, it's a whole new adventure. If you had to develop lists to remember what you had to do, you will now have lists for your lists. Sticky notes become *de rigueur*—they will appear on your laptop screen, the microwave, your coat, the trash-can, your calendar, any- and everywhere. If it weren't so utterly frustrating, it would be comical.

The ability to multi-task will usually start to return about six to nine months after your last chemo, depending on your age. Alexis was able to resume more complex activities in a shorter period of time, because she was in her 30s (at least that's what Terry would like to believe). But what a gift it is when it starts to return! It is such a helpless feeling while you are going through it. You feel so incompetent, so useless, and so dependent on other people to do even the smallest tasks. On the other hand, that is a good lesson to learn, that we are all inter-connected, and that there are people in your life who genuinely care about you and want to help. Don't let your independence become a blockade for you; accept graciously—or NOT—the help from others as evidence of their expressions of caring.

For those of you who work with someone who either is going through chemo or has just completed it, we ask that you please be patient with us. We will not initially be able to do what we did before, but we will work just as hard as we can to be a fully functioning team member again, so you won't have to do our work for us for any longer than absolutely necessary. The former co-worker we were is still in there, fighting to find the person we were. A Truism:

> *"Just as strongly as you want to be who you were BC, those who love you want it for you even more than you do.*

Blueberries have been found to be great for memory loss, even with people who have dementia. If you want to get your memory back more quickly, and to help make "chemo brain" a symptom of the past, it won't hurt to mega-dose on blueberries, although there are no guarantees. And of course, chocolate has been shown to improve cognitive abilities before taking a test. (Yeah!!!) So—why not make it a dark chocolate bar with blueberries in it, or on it, either way?

Neuropathy

One of the most frustrating things to have happen post-chemo is neu-ropathy. Neuropathy can affect three different groups of nerves in your system: peripheral nerves (the nerves that carry messages to and from your limbs), nerves that impact your bowels or other internal organs, and nerves in your head (nerves which connect your ears, eyes and taste buds, as examples). The most common kinds of drugs that can cause the neuropathy are: carboplatinum, cisplatinum, cyterabine, eloxatin (gener-ally not one used in chemo), Etoposide/VP-16, Hexalen, suramin, taxol, taxotere, thalidomide (generally not one used in chemo), vincristine, vin-desine and vinblastine. The type(s) of cancer you have may determine whether you will experience neuropathy. Some cancers may produce a kind of biological product that interferes with the nervous system.

While chemotherapy can affect any or all nerve centers, the most common is peripheral neuropathy—presenting with numbness or tin-gling in your fingers and feet, for example. In more severe cases, it can also be quite painful. It can come from out of nowhere. You can be driving down the road, minding your own business, doing what you normally do, and your fingers will become numb or feel as though they just fell off. It might take several seconds or minutes of shaking your hand, rubbing your wrist, and rubbing your fingers before it goes away. When you wake up in the morning, your toes can be numb, so numb that if you aren't quite awake, you will fall as you get out of bed. Word processing on the computer can sometimes be difficult—while your brain knows where the keys are, you can't really feel them, so it can take much more time to type a document. None of these symptoms are debilitating, and certainly people with diseases such as diabetes make the appropriate adjustments. Discuss this with your physician, who may ask you to see a physical therapist, particularly to help with your balance skills.

The other unusual symptom of neuropathy that can occur is that when your fingers are numb, they may turn a white-white-white color, (and we mean like a hospital sheet) and remain so for several minutes. This is called "Raynaud's Phenomenon" (formerly Raynaud's Syndrome and even Raynaud's) and can be caused by chemotherapy and/or emo-tional stress. Women tend to get it more often than men. It is caused by a lack of oxygen-rich blood getting into your fingers. If action isn't taken, they can then turn blue because of the lack of oxygen. Once oxygen is again flowing, the fingers can become red or "flushed" in color. This can also occur if you have been exposed to the cold for a period of time. It is potentially a serious condition; left untreated it can lead to tissue damage and gangrene, which can lead to the loss of the appendage. If you find yourself with this condition, run hot water (or as hot as you can stand) over the parts affected (fingers, toes, sometimes lips, the tip of your nose and earlobes), and massage the area until your fingers return to their normal color. If you live in a cold climate, double and triple layering of outer clothing becomes important, especially for fingers and toes. Wear two or three pairs of socks on your feet and the same for gloves and mittens on your hands when going outside for any extended period of time. You might want to go to a hunting and fishing store to get some hand warmers like hunters use to put into your gloves or mittens (thanks, Colleen, for this suggestion).

Air conditioning may also trigger this discoloration and the lack of oxygenated blood flow. Turn down the air conditioning and dress as skimpily as you dare, or the law will allow, if you're out in public. If you have to take something out of the freezer, wear a pair of insulated gloves. If you are drinking a glass of liquid with ice in it, you may also have to switch to using an insulated cup or glass. The important thing is to stay warm, take care of any sign of an impending attack immediately; do NOT wait and allow your tissues to become damaged. The other actions you take that may be helpful include: to quit smoking, to get regular exercise and to find new interventions to help you cope with your stress levels. You should consult with a doctor when the condition increases in the frequency and/or intensity of attacks and if the condition appears to be occurring on only one side of your body, or if sores or ulcers develop on the affected parts of your body. For more information, see www.mayoclinic.com/health/**raynauds**-disease/DS00433 or http://www.raynauds.org.uk.

It is hard to know how long these periods of numbness will last. For some people, it can be a lifetime. For others, it will be temporary. For the most part, when you have the numbness or tingling, it will only last a matter of seconds or at most, a few minutes. There are no drugs currently available to recover any of the nerve damage that has been incurred (but we can always hope for stem cell treatments in the future). Alexis hasn't reported any difficulties, but Terry has now had this condition for nearly two years.

Non-Carcinogenic Products (Sunscreens, Makeup, Etc.)

Now that you have survived cancer, you should really examine the products you use, whether for sunscreen (this could be especially important if you have young children and want to also protect them), bug spray, cosmetics or any other product you use on your skin. The number of reports of the inclusion of potential carcinogens in all these products is alarming, but with a little research, you can find "natural" products, which are non-carcinogenic. One report says that nearly half of the 500 sunscreens most used contain Vitamin A. Manufacturers use Vitamin A as an additive to sunscreen because it is an antioxidant, which supposedly slows the skin's aging process. However, some studies show that Vitamin A can hasten cancerous skin growths. This claim is actually in some dispute, since the study was conducted on mice only. Don't panic yet—the jury is still out on this theory, as further studies are currently in process. Find sunscreens that contain zinc oxide or titanium dioxide. These ingredients keep ultraviolet light out. Make sure your sunscreen **blocks both UVA and UVB rays.** As for SPF, as it turns out, these ratings don't really mean much, whether high SPF or lower SPF. If you have light skin, use the ones that have higher SPF, but make sure it **does block both UVA and UVB rays.** European sunscreens are actually better, so try to find those retailers who carry foreign products. For more information on sunscreens, and for specific profiles of other studies related to skin care products, please go to: http://www.nlm.nih.gov. Two American companies that make products we have used and have liked are Burt's Bees, which makes a sunscreen that is non-carcinogenic, and TilVee, which makes a variety of skin lotions that are made from all-natural products.

Obesity

In a September 2009, edition of the *Caring4Cancer* e-newsletter, an article appeared entitled "Number of Obesity-related Cancers Is Growing." It reports that in 2008, over 124,000 new diagnoses of different types of cancer were causally related to excess body weight. Obesity is known to stimulate increased production of the hormones insulin (the hormone critical for regulating the metabolism of carbohydrates and fat in the body) and estrogen; if the levels of the hormones rise too high, they can actually stimulate the growth of cancer cells. Excess body weight is not only recognized as a risk factor for cancer, but also has an impact on outcomes after you have received treatment. Obesity has been related to endometrial cancer, postmenopausal breast cancer, colorectal cancer and possibly to others as well: cervical, gallbladder, non-Hodgkin's lymphoma, renal (kidney), ovarian, and pancreatic cancers.

In a study conducted by lead researcher Dr. Andrew Renehan, for The World Health Organization and the International Agency for Research on Cancer, the following was noted:

- Excess body weight in Europe was responsible for an estimated 70,000 diagnoses of cancer in 2002.

- In 2008, the number was estimated at 124,000. Excess body weight in 3.2% of men and 8.6% of women were factors in all new cancer diagnoses.

- The most common weight-related cancers were uterine (endometrial), postmenopausal breast cancer and colorectal, with 65% of these cancers being due to excess body weight.

A similar report was made in the September 8, 2009, issue of the *Journal of Clinical Oncology*, in which researchers from the Seattle-based Fred Hutchinson Cancer Research Center reported that obesity, consumption of alcohol and smoking increased the likelihood of the development of a second breast cancer among those women who had had breast cancer first (remember, men can also get breast cancer). Alcohol is also strongly linked with breast cancer. If you drink more than one glass of alcohol a day, it may increase your risk of breast cancer by 7%–10%. The Women's Health Initiative conducted a study of more than 87,000 post-menopausal women. Of those, 2,944 developed breast cancer. In the women who were hormone receptor-positive for breast cancer and who drank seven or more drinks per week, their risk of breast cancer almost doubled. For lobular breast cancer, non-drinkers had a ratio of 5.2 per 10,000 women, but 8.5 per 10,000 women among drinkers. Non-drinking women who were hormone receptor-positive had a ratio of 15.2 per 10,000, compared to 17.9 per 10,000 among drinkers.

Quite often, when you have been on steroids during chemotherapy, you will experience considerable weight gain. Once the steroids are stopped, the weight should start to come off, but it will not just fall off without effort on your part. Diet and exercise will, once again, play key roles. This will mean not only portion control, but also changing your eating habits and incorporating healthier foods. Please don't say pizza is a health food because of the tomato sauce. Drink the tomato sauce; leave the rest on your plate, especially processed meats like pepperoni and the white processed flour in the crust. Cancer can actually be a lifesaver, if it gets you to alter your eating habits in order to become healthy again.

If you want to know what a healthy weight is for you, check your body mass index, or BMI. You should aim to have a BMI between 22.5 and 24.9, although this is at the upper end of the scale, as determined by the Centers for Disease Control (CDC) and the World Health Organization (WHO). There is some concern that the scale the WHO uses has people being too thin, which is not healthy, either. For men especially, your waist should be less than half of your height. If you are 5 feet, 10 inches, your waist should be less than 35 inches (wearing your pants below your belly button may help avoid the truth that you are overweight, but it does not make it any less of a concern. And, did you guys know that for every point your BMI is more than 25, your testosterone drops at least three points? And another little tidbit—for every 20 pounds you are overweight, you lose something like one inch off your most valued and cherished body part. Just FYI).

Percutaneous Endoscopic Gastrostomy Tube (PEG)

Neither one of us had to have this, but a friend of Alexis's has, so we've included it. Some cancer patients will be required to have a PEG tube (also known as a "feeding tube") inserted into their stomachs from the outside, and through the abdominal wall to the belly. This will be done if the patient is unable to feed him- or herself, or has something like head and neck cancer. PEG tube insertion becomes necessary when either eating regular food, drinking or swallowing are not possible, and nutritional needs have to be met. The tube is surgically placed and acts as a direct route to the gut. With a PEG tube, you need to watch for infection and practice general cleanliness. Depending on the patient, the PEG tube can remain for as little as several months, to as long as two or three years, before having to be replaced. The PEG tube is reversible. Depending on the length of time you have had the PEG tube, it may be endoscopically removed through the navel. Most often, this is done while the patient is under a local anesthetic, and the PEG incision heals with little or no problem.

Pills

Pills will have become, and will continue to be, a large part of your life AC, depending on the type of cancer you had. For Alexis, this has meant a constant stream of Tamoxifen. This little white pill is an estrogen receptor blocker. Since her cancer was estrogen receptor positive, meaning the cancer was using her body's estrogen to make more cancer, she needed to block all the little receptors on her estrogen so nothing else could use it. Sounds fun, huh? She has also consistently taken multivitamins, and been very watchful of her lab results. Simply being on top of which levels were low, and then combating the low levels, has made her immune system much stronger. For Terry, it meant Acyclovir for a year after the stem cell transplant to prevent Shingles, along with potassium and ferrous oxide (iron) pills until her bloodwork came to within the normal range. Because of the steroids administered during chemo, osteoporosis has become a risk for her, which meant calcium supplements. For the most part, pills should be <u>taken with water</u> (**not ever with juice**) in the morning, along with some kind of food. The calcium supplements may require a second pill during the day, but this is easily taken with lunch or dinner.

For those of you with a thyroid condition, it becomes a tad more complicated. Thyroid pills have to be taken on an empty stomach either an hour before you eat or two hours after you eat. In addition, thyroid pills have to be taken either four hours before or after your last calcium pill. This requirement is because the calcium binds to the thyroid pill, rendering it ineffective. For Terry, this lead to a scheduling nightmare. At one point, given real-life events happening at the time, she took the thyroid pill when she woke up, waited an hour before eating, then four hours later started the calcium routine. Life changed (mostly because waiting an hour to eat was becoming impossible since the last meal of the day was usually noon or 1:00 the day before), so she switched to calcium pills in the morning with breakfast, didn't eat for four hours, took the thyroid pill, waited an hour, had lunch, then four hours later, finished the calcium. Life changed again, so she tried taking the thyroid at night. There went those before-bed snacks!

After diagnosis with osteoporosis, Terry talked with the rheumatologist, who said it would be all right for the thyroid medication to be altered to accommodate her lifestyle. (Certainly wish the endocrinologist had suggested that!)

Because of the dry mouth due to the chemo, you may have to brush your teeth with a prescription product called Prevident®. This has to be done usually before bedtime, and you can't eat or drink for half an hour afterward. It is preferable to also brush first thing in the morning, but if you have to take Actonel, that would have to be done a half hour after brushing your teeth, then wait another half hour, take the thyroid medication, this time wait an hour, then eat. The heck with it! (NOT one of her most positive attitudes.) Terry brushes her teeth with the Prevident at night now and has substituted another drug for Actonel.

If you are on medications that require specific timing, talk with your doctor(s) about how to manage all of the scheduling. Your recuperation depends on your making it work. While Terry and Alexis have written about this a bit lightheartedly, it is critical the regimen you establish assures no complications occur with or between any of your medications.

You may also have been on Coumadin during chemo. This was to keep your blood from clotting, especially if you had an infusaport or PICC line implanted. Once you have had those removed, the Coumadin will either be discontinued or reduced, depending on your PT/INR counts. With Coumadin, you have to limit your intake of green leafy vegetables and garlic, all of which contain vitamin K, the blood-clotting agent. However, there is the possibility you can eat these foods/spices, if your dosage is adjusted taking those items into consideration. Check with your doctor first to see if this is a possibility. One doctor told Tom under no circumstances was he to eat green leafy vegetables; another doctor said the Coumadin dosage could be adjusted. Tom limits his green leafy vegetables, but incorporates them into his diet occasionally, because of the vitamins and nutrients in them. Terry also buys multi-vitamin tablets without vitamin K for him. You have to shop around for those, too. Sometimes mass-marketed vitamins without K will also have other significantly reduced ingredients.

If you are a man diagnosed with prostate cancer, you may be on a ton of medicines, which can include Casodex, Cytoxan, DES (*diethyl-stilbestrol*, available only through Professional Arts Pharmacy in Baltimore, MD), Eligarde or Lupron, Prednisone, Simvastatin (if you aren't eating properly and have a cholesterol problem), and/or Uroxatral. If you have back pain caused either by arthritis or bone cancer, you also may be taking Cyclobenzaprine HCL, Hydrocodone BIT, or Lidoderm 5% (patch). If you're having trouble sleeping, you might also be taking a relaxant such as Atavan or Lorazepam. If you decide to become a couch potato despite repeated warnings from the doctor about blood clots forming as a result a number of these medications, you will also likely be put on Coumadin. However, none of these medications will require any substantial alteration in scheduling when you take the meds. With Tom, he has to take some pills first thing in the morning with water and breakfast; some pills are required at dinner with food and some pills are required at bedtime. Some of the medications Tom takes are intra-venous and are done at Dr. Rapson's office once a month, but he can both eat and drink while having them inserted (if he's not sleeping). He will most likely be on these medications for the rest of his life, unless his prostate cancer becomes hormone refractory again, which will necessitate changes in his meds regimen.

Regardless of whether you have cancer or not, please, even if just for yourself, develop a list of all medications and any supplements you take, surgeries and shots, such as flu and pneumonia. (Go to http://www.SoYouveSurvivedCancer.com to download a free wallet-sized sample.) This is helpful when you go to the doctor, dentist, or have to go to Emergency. Terry has made a chart for both Tom and herself; it includes the name of the medication, the dosage, the doctor who prescribed the medication and the purpose. When you have cancer, medications can be discontinued, and then, as your condition changes or is not responding to a current drug, one you have already taken may be re-prescribed. This is also noted on the chart. It helps if you have it on computer, so updates can easily be made, and you can print a copy any time you may need it for yourself, for your caregiver or family member, or for your doctor or the hospital. You should design any kind of a recording form or system you think would be most beneficial for you, as long as it includes all the specific information you anticipate needing for yourself and for your doctors and health care providers; it can be revised at any time as the need arises.

A sample recording form you may consider adapting for your needs follows.

Medication Tracking Journal
John Doe
(Date of birth)
Updated August 16, 2010
John has Stage 4 Prostate Cancer that has metastasized into his bones and lymph nodes.

Name	Dosage	Doctor	Diagnosis/Purpose
Cytoxan	50mg, 2x/day	(Name)	Prostate Cancer
Coumadin	8mg/day	(Name)	To Thin the blood; blood clot in leg
DES	1mg, 1x/day Discontinue— 3/08 Reinstate-6/09 Increase-to3mg	(Name)	Prostate Cancer
Lorazepam	1 mg/day	(Name)	Not sleeping
Lupron IV	Discontinue 2/8/08	(Name)	Prostate Cancer
Etc. ——–	As needed.		

Being what some people think of as anal retentive, Terry color-codes the writing—green to signify "health" for current medications, red for "updates and changes," black for "previous" medications/dosages. You may need more columns on your meds journal, i.e., a date column, one for reactions you experience to each med, or notes you want to be sure to tell the doctor, or annotations regarding any mistakes you made in taking a med as scheduled. If you keep your journal on computer, you can update, print and take it with you to every appointment.

Radiation After-Effects

One of the few things NOT covered while you are undergoing cancer treatment or later, while you are recuperating after having survived it, are warnings about the after-effects you might experience if radiation was part of your treatment. This is true if you've had cancers as varied as neck and throat cancer, or Hodgkin's Lymphoma. As long as ten or twelve or even thirty years after your cancer treatments have been successful, you might wake up one day to discover that your carotid arteries are 60%-100% blocked, or you've had a heart attack and needed a coronary bypass, or your spinal cord is impacted, or you've developed breast cancer. Any or all of these conditions are likely the result of the life-saving radiation you had during your treatment for cancer. If you had radiation ten or twenty years ago, it is likely that neither your oncologist nor the radiation oncologist were aware of any after-effects at all. Other potential side effects you should watch for include: bone problems, fertility issues, hypothyroidism, problems with your intestines, secondary cancer, vascular problems (such as stroke or heart attack), and neuromuscular or musculoskeletal problems. Because non-oncological doctors are largely unaware of the after effects of radiation, they might diagnose your symptoms as fibromyalgia or insist your symptoms are not caused by the radiation you had so many years ago. Not everyone who has received radiation will develop after-effects. As mentioned earlier, each person reacts differently to each of the medications and to the various treatments used in their cancer-fighting regimen. Even if you and your best friend had the same radiation for breast cancer, one of you may have after-effects, the other not. But the bottom line is: you will have a 15% chance of getting a different cancer other than the one for which you were treated initially.

We have been unable to find much information and only a few resources about the after-effects of radiation. Actual data regarding prior cancer patients who are having confirmed late effect disease or high-risk health conditions due to radiation treatment, or the severity levels, or the degree to which those conditions are linked causally to the radiation, are unknown.

Fortunately, in this day and age, the administration of the radiation has gotten much better than it was as recently as the 1980s and 1990s. The technology, the treatment options, even the chemotherapy have improved immensely. If you've had neck and throat cancer or lymphoma, your heart and lungs would be more carefully protected. When Terry had radiation, the measures taken to protect her body were meticulously executed. The majority of radiation oncologists now have a safety plan they put into operation to assure, the best they can, the radiation will NOT trespass into any other areas of the body. Radiation oncologists now have to pass stringent tests to demonstrate their knowledge of the field and how to properly administer radiation, before they can become licensed to perform these procedures.

What you, as the patient, need to do is stay on top of all your medical concerns and symptoms. Document all the treatments you had for destroying your cancer, including your current diagnoses and medications. Also, refer to: http://www.asco.org/treatmentssummary and/or http://www.livestrongcareplan.org for other samples. You may be totally asymptomatic for heart disease or bone problems, but while you are answering your doctor's questions during an annual checkup, symptoms may be revealed unexpectedly. If you haven't been getting an annual physical in the past, make sure you do it in your present and future. Be sure you speak with your oncologist (who you should be seeing once a year after you survive, and probably for the rest of your life), your primary care physician, and each of the other doctors (endocrinologist, rheumatologist, whoever you are seeing), to make sure they know you have had radiation and to keep watch for any medical concerns that might appear. If you've had radiation near your heart, ask for an echocardiogram to establish baseline data. Your job now, will be to also educate your physicians, whether specialists or general practitioners. Doctors can't be expected to know every little detail in areas outside their practice. (There is something like over 280 pieces of research generated EVERY DAY for doctors to read.) Most will be grateful for the knowledge you share with them. For Tom's primary care physician, Dr. Wheeler, he was exploring new territory with all the Provenge and Zytiga issues but as he said, what we were telling him might help another of his patients at some point. Tom was not Dr. Wheeler's only patient with prostate cancer.

For those of you reading this who are about to embark on your journey through cancer, please know that we are NOT advising you to NOT have radiation. If Terry had to do it again, she would do so without a second's hesitation. However, to have or not have radiation is a decision you should make after consulting with your oncologist, radiation oncologist, spiritual advisor, any other trusted health care professional and/or close family member/friend. We are simply saying that you need to educate yourself, and sometimes, your doctors. The good news is that you are a survivor (or about to become one). More good news is that you will live longer and have time to experience these after-effects—if you even have any of them. Most cancers or other problems caught early are very treatable. And since you now know there might be these little problems afterward, you can face them head on, and have them treated as well.

Runny Nose

> If your nose runs, and your feet smell . . . you're built upside down.
>
> *(thanks, Tim, for this saying!)*.

A runny nose after chemo and stem cell transplant is very common, although not usually mentioned by physicians. That nose will run anytime, anywhere. There is also a slight possibility that you are now more allergic to things than before chemo. Check with a dermatologist to see if you have developed any new allergies or whether any of the allergies you had prior to treatment appear to have changed.

Whether you have had chemo or a stem cell transplant, you nose will run continuously for the first year or so, then intermittently, but far more often than normal afterward. It will drip during dinner, while brushing your teeth, changing diapers, watching a sunset, laughing at a joke; it can appear out of nowhere, for no good reason and with absolutely no warning. Take out stock in a tissue company and load up with tissues when you go out, because you might single-handedly help the company earn more profits. Just kidding, except for the loading up part. You will need them!

Sense of Direction

For many people, one of the after-effects of chemo and radiation is the loss of a sense of direction. If you didn't have this sense before chemo, it doesn't work in reverse—you will simply have a worse sense of direction. Terry used to be able to drive into any town on the planet, take a left here, a right there and end up either two blocks from where she wanted to be, or right in front of the place. That gift is totally and completely gone. It could be likened to walking forever in circles; now there are no directions for Terry at all. Fortunately, the ability to read maps is still present. No one knows why this happens. It could be the medications you are taking, fatigue, sleep disturbances, or any number of things. It may be tied to "chemo brain" somehow. There are a few researchers who are currently exploring the causes. In the meantime, you just have to get used to it, cope with it as best you can, and move on with your life. There are worse things than losing your sense of direction (not to be confused with the sense of direction for your life). Whether this is a short-term or permanent condition will vary from person to person; it can be either.

Sex After Cancer

This is another section where we did quite a bit of research, both books and websites. We needed to do this especially for the section on men, since neither one of us happens to be one, although one of us lives with a man and as his caregiver, has vicariously lived through what he has been going through with prostate cancer.

Let's get a few things out of the way first:

- *Sex does not cause cancer.* Sex after treatment for cancer in no way will bring it back. *Viruses* can be passed on through unprotected sexual contact: squamous cell carcinoma of the penis, rectum and vulva to name a few. If you have Hepatitis B and C, you may pass that on and increase the risk of liver cancer. If you have the Epstein-Barr virus (mononucleosis), it may increase your risk of some cancers. If you happen to have any of these viruses, you may never contract cancer or give it to anyone. But *SEX does NOT cause cancer.*

- *Women who smoke tend to have higher rates of cervical cancer.* But sex does not cause cancer; it is the smoking that correlates with the contraction of cancer, not the sex.

- *Cancer is not contagious.* Have as much sex as you are comfortable with (use protection and consideration for your partner, please), but your cancer cells will not enter your partner's body and cause cancer. Cancer cells are actually delicate and need a proper environment in which to grow. In all likelihood, your partner's own immune system would detect it and destroy it.

- *Treatment for cancer does not usually make sex dangerous.* However, it is wise to check with your doctor first about having sex, because of the kinds of drugs you will be taking. Err on the side of caution—always wear a condom while undergoing chemotherapy and radiation, and for about two weeks afterward. The other "however" is that your immune system may be weakened, making risk of infection a possibility. Check with your doctor to see if having intercourse is possible, and if not, ask your doctor how soon after treatment s/he would recommend you wait before resuming your normal sexual activities.

- *Cancer treatments may causes birth defects in fetuses.* Check with your doctor about what types of birth control are best for you to use with the kinds of cancer treatments and medications you are taking.

Sex is an important and integral part of any relationship. This refers not only to the actual sexual act ("sex") but also to the feelings that accompany closeness or intimacy (sorry, guys) in any relationship ("making love"). It is important for us find ways to keep sexual excitement and intimacy alive in the bedroom (or kitchen or by a stream, if you are so inclined). "Sexuality" is defined as how you personally feel about sex, and it is those feelings that are an integral part of sex. We personally don't believe sex is any more—or any less—important to men than it is to women. We are culturally brainwashed that sex is of supreme importance to men (and it probably is, maybe even supplanting cars and tools), and women often get left behind the mainstream because they are the "nurturers," the "caregivers," and the ones who also earn money to support the family, do the housework, do the laundry, fix the meals, take care of the children, etc. Women—it's time to claim our own sexual heritage.

People often feel uncomfortable talking about sex, whether it is with their partner, or with the doctor. We get embarrassed, tongue-tied, feel very vulnerable, and then wonder if someone is going to judge us by what we express: "Ewwwwww, how can they do *that*?" or "They did *what*?!?" Doctors can also be quite uncomfortable discussing sexual issues with their patients.

Men and women quite often lose interest in either sex or their sexuality while undergoing chemotherapy, radiation or a stem cell transplant. Your main focus has become: "How am I going to survive cancer?" In addition, you are faced with depression, worry about your family and finances, and may be coping with nausea, pain and fatigue. Chemotherapy can also alter your natural hormone balances. Even if you do feel like having sex, it may be best to wait a minimum of two to three days after your most recent chemotherapy session. (If you are still nauseous after chemotherapy and vomit during that special moment, wear gloves to clean it up!) Radiation can sometimes cause burns that make it uncomfortable to have sex. If so, wait a few more days until the soreness leaves, and then see what comes up. (No pun intended.)

Your spouse/partner may not feel up to having intercourse or "be able to" after receiving chemotherapy, or because of the other medications s/he is on, so just try to be patient. Let him/her know that when s/he is ready, you will be there. And sometimes, things don't go as they normally did. If that happens, you can still hug, laugh, touch, and most importantly, say "I love you."

Because of the chemotherapy and radiation, people may refrain from having sex, and perhaps even cease being intimate for an extended period of time. Sometimes in women, other factors, such as vaginal dryness, which causes discomfort during intercourse, can make them reluctant to engage in the sexual act. This puts further pressure on a relationship in which cancer has become such a huge part. Often men, as well as women, are afraid to resume their previous sexual activities because it has been so long, and their bodies have changed so significantly while undergoing chemotherapy and radiation. Regardless of how you may have been changed as a result of your cancer, it is critical for two people in a relationship to fight for maintenance of their intimacy. If the two of you can just forge ahead, those special "intimate" moments may become the key to saving your life by supporting and sustaining you throughout your fight for life.

Please keep in mind that "normal" sex can mean a variety of things to different people: three times a day, once a month, once a year ("and tonight's the night, honey!"). Different positions are normal. Normal is whatever feels right for you and your spouse/partner, as long as no one is being hurt in the process, physically, mentally or emotionally. It is also normal to enjoy your sexuality up until you take your last breath. Sexuality isn't just for the young.

It is also important to realize that as we age, the abilities to achieve an erection for men or an orgasm for women can sometimes require a longer period of time. (But hooray for that—it brings an end to the "wham-bam" approach, or, before the kids are out of the house, having to rush through things before they wake up and want a drink of water.) This is especially true because cancer is usually found in people over the age 50. According to the American Cancer Society, if you are a man between the ages of 40–49, about 30% of you will have trouble maintaining an erection. The difficulty goes up to as high as 90% if you are over the age of 70.

It is estimated that over 14 million women have had chemotherapy and radiation. About 12.5 million women have had hysterectomies, with both ovaries removed. This can lead to vaginal dryness, because of decreased levels of estrogen, which leads to discomfort during intercourse.

According to some theorists, there are basically five phases in sexual response:

- Desire (an interest in sex)
- Excitement (being "turned on")
- Orgasm (sexual climax)
- Resolution (body returning to its normal state)
- Refractory period (the time it takes to be able to achieve another orgasm; men usually have to wait for a period of time; women can have multiple orgasms)

Remember, if one of you is experiencing difficulty, this has an impact on your spouse/partner. Both of you need to discuss it and talk with a doctor, who might be able to rule out stress, diabetes, high blood pressure, or urge you to quit smoking. If there is nothing physically causing the problem, or if medicines or surgery can't help, then a qualified sex therapist may be the next step. If either of you has a "problem" with seeing a therapist, ask yourself: what is more important—your ego or your relationship with your spouse/partner?

So, speaking of ego—let's start with the men.

Chemotherapy, radiation and a stem cell transplant will have an impact on your sex life, at least initially. Period. Count on it! (Women, this also applies to you.) Talk with your doctor or another member of your health care team you feel close enough to about what you might expect, depending on the type of cancer and treatment(s) you have had.

Some chemotherapy treatments may lower your sperm cell count, may reduce the motility of the sperm or may cause other abnormalities. You might become temporarily or permanently infertile. Some drugs may damage parts of the nervous system, which may have an impact on your erections. Chemotherapy, in general, should not affect your ability to have intercourse; the major problems that will inhibit your sexual activity might be fatigue and lack of desire. If you are having chemotherapy, be sure to wear a condom, because chemotherapy may damage your chromosomes. You will need to ask your doctor if the chromosomal damage will be a temporary condition, or a permanent one.

Some types of treatment for cancer will prevent a man from achieving an erection. If you have treatment for some forms of brain cancer, or if you have had chemotherapy or radiation on your spinal cord, this may damage some nerves or muscles, making it difficult to even get pleasure from simple touching. Even if you are physically unable to get an erection or have an orgasm, there are other avenues to explore to provide you with some satisfaction. It is important to open your mind to other possibilities, and not keep yourself locked into what had been the "one" or "acceptable" way of doing things. Your "usual" routine may be permanently altered AC, or after chemotherapy. Be inventive, and talk with your spouse/partner about what is pleasurable now for him/her. *In this case, silence is **not** golden.* COMMUNICATION IS CRITICAL. If you are not comfortable talking with your spouse/partner, then ask your doctor or other health care professional to help.

A man's sexual drive can be present, and he may be able to ejaculate, but may not be able to have an erection depending on the type of cancer and the treatment(s) administered. Other men may have an orgasm, but not be able to ejaculate. Premature ejaculation can also be a problem (even in healthy men), so there are exercises that can be done to delay gratification, including the taking of anti-depressants. Talk to your doctor about what helpful options might be available for you.

Some types of cancer treatments will preclude having an erection, but once treatment has ceased, there are surgical procedures or other medications that might restore this function. Thoughts can play an important part, too, and you will already have been through so much. If you, as man, become worried about not being able to have an erection, odds are, you won't. So, even though it may sound too simple, just relax, believe in yourself, and let nature take its course—then, most likely, it will.

If you experience pain during an erection, or if ejaculation is painful, <u>tell your doctor right away</u>, so treatment can be introduced. There is a condition called "Peyronie's disease" in which a "knot" or curve occurs during an erection. This can also be found in men who are not being treated for cancer, and then is often due to scar tissue in the penis. Both of these two conditions are usually treatable.

Other medical conditions or procedures that can interfere with either erection or ejaculation are:

- *Radical Prostatectomy* (prostate cancer; removal of the prostate and seminal vesicles)

- *Radical Cystectomy* (bladder cancer, removal of the bladder, prostate, upper urethra and seminal vesicles outside the body or the construction of a new bladder)

- *Abdominoperineal* *(AP)* resection (colon cancer—removal of the lower colon and rectum)

- *Total Pelvic Exenteration* (large tumor of the Colon, removal of the bladder, prostate, seminal vesicles and rectum; this is a rare procedure)

- *Orchiectomy* (removal of one or both testicles)

There are different ways of doing all of these surgeries, and better methodologies are being found all the time. Each of these surgeries can interfere with having an erection by damaging the nerves that allow blood flow to the penis. Since the nerves "fan out," it is often difficult for the surgeon to see them. Some men are fully able to have erections after these types of surgeries, but a lot is dependent on the type of cancer, the method of surgery used, what other damage has already been done, and your overall health going in to the surgery. If you have a total pelvic exenteration, the ability to have full erections will not be regained. It can take up to two years for you to regain full erections for the other types of surgeries. The younger you are when having one of these procedures, the more likely it will be for you to have full erection restored, once again being able to achieve and sustain an erection. If you had good erections before surgery, you will likely have the same level, or close to it, after surgery. Should you be dissatisfied with your post-surgery performance, there are procedures that can be used a few weeks after surgery to help you achieve better erections. Check with your doctor to see what might be best for you.

If you receive radiation for prostate, bladder or colon cancer, this treatment can also have a negative effect on erections. It depends on the amount of radiation received, and the size of the area that was radiated. Radiation can damage the arteries carrying blood to the penis. As a result of the radiation, scar tissue will form. Other problems include a hardening, blockage or narrowing of the arteries, affecting the nerves that help bring about an erection. It is estimated between 1/4 to 1/3 of men having radiation treatments will develop a lessening of erections for about a year after treatment ceases. In some cases, firm erections are no longer possible. If you had "normal" erections prior to treatment, then by five years after treatment, only about half of the men were reported to have become, what seems to be, permanently impotent. Again, if you are older or are a smoker, your chances of becoming impotent increase substantially. Testosterone levels usually return to pre-radiation levels in about six months after the radiation is ended.

If you are having chemotherapy, most men likely have normal erections for a while, but find them waning the longer they are in treatment. After a week or so of not having chemo, your erections return, but you may also be dealing with fatigue. Chemo slows testosterone production. If you have had a graft stem cell or bone marrow transplant, having a "host" donor, rather than being an "autologous" or self-donor, you will more likely have long-lasting testosterone depletion. You may need to have supplemental testosterone replacement therapy for a period of time. Genital herpes or genital wart infections may increase if you had had them before your chemo or your transplant, and the infections may eventually cause life-long infertility.

As mentioned earlier, treatment for prostate cancer involves the administration of female hormones. Prostate cancer feeds on testosterone, so in order to kill the cancer, the testosterone has to be eliminated from the body. These low levels of testosterone will have to be maintained for the rest of your life. Side effects include hot flashes and growth of breast tissue. There may also be a decrease in the frequency with which you have intercourse. But, fear NOT! Female hormones will NOT make you become a woman. If you were attracted to women before, you will not suddenly find yourself attracted to men. You may simply not be able to achieve an erection or maintain one, but touching, intimacy, tenderness, and consideration for your spouse/partner are always possible for you.

If you have prostate cancer or testicular cancer, as examples, and you still wish to father a child, go to a sperm donor bank BEFORE YOU EMBARK ON ANY CANCER TREATMENTS, and RESERVE YOUR SEMEN. For those interested in sperm donor programs, a study was recently conducted in the United Kingdom (U.K.), and the results were reported (October 2010) in the *Annals of Oncology;* see http://annonc.oxford journals.org, and http://biomedme.com/general/many-male-cancer-patients-are-missing-out-on-spermbanking_18744.html. It was found that about half the oncologists and the hematologists in the U.K. had information available on sperm banking. Unfortunately, many were unaware of the policies surrounding sperm banking. The study suggested that any male, including teenagers, who might wish to start a family someday, should store his semen.

Some chemotherapy can immediately affect your sperm count, which may cause infertility that can either be short-term or lifelong. Some chemotherapy can damage the nerves that control the prostate, seminal vesicles and the opening to the bladder. As a result, you may have what are called "dry" orgasms—no semen is released. If you have had your prostate or seminal vesicles removed, you will most likely also have dry orgasms (if the semen is there but doesn't come out, it has been released back into the bladder; this will NOT harm you. The next time you urinate, your urine may look cloudy.). Another side effect is that your orgasms may not feel as intense as before treatment. It is normal for the intensity of male orgasms to decrease as you age, and chemotherapy may contribute to a further decrease. Talk with your doctor and your spouse/partner about this to see if there are any treatments available.

And now for that all-scary type of cancer: cancer of the penis, or penile cancer. Gentlemen, as delicately as we can put this, if you have cancer of the penis or the bottom end of the urethra, you may have to have all or part of the penis removed. (Whew, there, we've said it.) This happens rarely, but if it happens to you, it doesn't matter whether it's rare or not. If found early, usually chemotherapy and some radiation will take care of the problem and you will have little or no side effects in terms of sexual pleasure and function.

But what if chemo and radiation will not solve the problem? There are two options:

1. a partial penectomy—which removes only the end of the penis. There will still be enough of the shaft remaining to ensure both sexual pleasure and functions are maintained. You will be able to have orgasms and normal ejaculations.

2. a total penectomy—a surgeon will install a new urethra. If this is your condition, you do not need to stop having sexual relations, unless other health concerns preclude such activities.

It will take some effort and experimentation on your part to find what is pleasurable for you. For example, stroking the skin behind the scrotum may be pleasurable. There is also the possibility of rebuilding the penis. It is rare for this to occur; it is a complicated surgery and a skilled surgeon is necessary. If you decide to explore this procedure, be sure to ask about success rates, whether there will be any scarring and how that might impact your sex life, what complications can occur both during surgery and afterward, and most importantly, what experience your surgeon has had with this procedure. You will want to bone up (sorry about the pun) on the research currently available and have a thorough discussion with your medical team before deciding whether this is a viable option for you. You can always seek a second opinion if you feel the surgeon you have contacted doesn't have sufficient experience with this type of surgery. However, please remember, this surgery is still rare, so you may have trouble finding an expert doctor in the field.

There is some discussion now about circumcision and its relationship to penile cancer. Research seems to indicate that circumcision shortly after birth is the best course of action. There are fewer cases of penile cancer and of urinary tract infections in men who were circumcised while still an infant. Research has shown penile cancer is extremely rare among Jewish men, for whom circumcision is a ritual performed shortly after birth. It is more common in Muslim males, believed to be because circumcision is performed after puberty. The studies find penile cancer is most common in men who have never been circumcised.

The website cited below is provided as a courtesy of The American Cancer Society; it documents possible male sexual problems caused by cancer treatments. http://www.cancer.org/Treatment/Treat mentsandSideEffects/PhysicalSideEffects/SexualSideEffectsinMen/ SexualityfortheMan/sexuality-for-men-with-cancer-summary-table-ca-treat-and-sex-and-fertility (accessed on February 2, 2011; no author was cited; last revision was made on 5/17/2010.)

Regardless of what type of cancer and treatments you have had, there may be lifelong changes in how your sexuality is affected. The best time to learn about this is before you start treatment, so you will know beforehand what to expect, and so you can learn about the length of time for recovery, but since the topic of this book is mostly about what happens AC, that piece may be too late. (However, if you or your spouse/partner are reading this and at the beginning stages of treatment, it will be timely for you.) Talk with your doctor and with your spouse/partner if you are concerned about the potential sexual side effects. While statistics exist that might predict you will have a problem, you may be in the fortunate group that doesn't have the problem. Statistics are just numbers—good numbers to have, certainly, but you are still an individual with your own set of concerns, who will respond to treatment with your own distinct physical reactions and outcomes.

The first thing your doctor will do is to determine whether the loss of normal function is due to a medical condition. It is most likely a medical condition (and permanent) if the lack of ejaculation or erection occurs in all situations. A plan will be formulated to help you deal with this. One of the studies that may be done is the number of nighttime erections. Or the doctor may check the blood flow to the penis using several different techniques. If the problem is medical, treatments can range from medicines to vacuum constriction devices, penile implants (which include rods and pumps) or penile injections. If you are considering using herbs, studies indicate they are largely ineffective.

On the other hand, your sexual problems may be sporadic and something that may, or may not, have a medical treatment. If you experience feelings of inadequacy, loss of desire, or have trouble reaching an orgasm, talking with a competent therapist can often help. Yes, men, we realize this would be a difficult concept for you to conceive or accept. After all, culturally we are raised being told men should be men, they have no problems, must be self-sufficient and strong, and they will take care of everything, and be a stud from the first breath to the last. Who in the world ever thought of all these requirements for manhood? What a burden to carry! (You guys certainly have our sincere sympathy.) Did you ever ask yourself upon what your sexual code is based? Did you ever ask yourself if that sexual code is interfering with your leading a satisfying, fulfilling life? Remember, sexuality is forever; it may diminish as we age but there is no reason that it should totally and completely stop. And if your spouse/partner is asking you to get some help, for heaven's sake, get it; do it together!

And, now, ladies, it's your turn . . .

First, a little history to put things in perspective: Women have had to endure centuries, perhaps even millennia, of misunderstanding about sexual pleasure. If you think about it, there is probably a good reason that "hysteria" and "hysterectomy" are etymologically linked. Women are supposed to be hysterical, non-logical, and prone to "attacks" and other stereotypic behaviors. It was originally thought that women became hysterical because of sexual frustration (and who could blame them?!?). Clitoral orgasm was prescribed as a treatment for hysteria. Doctors would manually induce orgasm to reduce the hysteria. However, this could be quite a waste of a doctor's valuable time (especially when it was estimated that 75% of women could be affected with this hysteria), not to mention boring and unfulfilling for the doctor, so this job was turned over to midwives. Vibrators came into fashion to help relieve the perceived hysteria. In the early 1900s, needlework magazines were advertising electrical vibrators so women could try them in the privacy of their homes; in time, this became the fifth electric appliance to make its way into a woman's home—after the sewing machine, fan, coffee or tea maker and the toaster.

Women can find it hard to talk about sex, even with a doctor or their spouse/partner. Perhaps it's because of our cultural conditioning—we are taught from an early age that women are supposed to be the nurturers, take care of the men in our lives, keep a neat and clean house, be a good cook, greet our husband as he comes through the door after a hard day at work in our high heels and our hair freshly styled, with all the laundry done, the clothes ironed, the sewing done, the bills paid, the kids nicely mannered and cleaned-up, so we can now—wait on him—so he can relax. And somehow or another you have to be modest in dress and actions, stay virgins the rest of your life and all children are "magically" created—through even more immaculate conceptions. And for heaven's sake, don't dare to talk about **sex**, or even say you're interested in **sex**. Be there for your husband and ignore your own feelings, which you're not supposed to have anyway because you're a brood mare. *Shhhhhhhh*!

Well. Just in case you did NOT know this—WE'RE GLAD THOSE DAYS ARE GONE! At least, we pray they are gone for our daughters and granddaughters, just as we pray our guys do not any longer have to live up to their MAN-GOD role.

Regardless of our gender, the truth is that when you first heard the diagnosis of cancer, you had many of the same questions men have: how will this affect my sex life? How will it affect my husband/partner? What will be "normal" after cancer? And to whom can I go in order to talk about this?

Even today, many oncologists and oncological nurses feel uncomfortable talking about sex with their patients. For Terry, the one exception to this was Tania at Karmanos. When Terry said part of the book would include a chapter on sex AC, Tania said, "It's about time someone talked about this!"

There was an interesting sexuality workshop done by Christel Wendt (University Hospital, Lund, Sweden) and Corien Eeltink (VU University Medical Center, Amsterdam, The Netherlands), sponsored by the European Group for Bone and Marrow Transplantation. The aims of the workshop were to increase nurses' knowledge of changes in patients' sexuality that could be caused by cancer and/or its treatment, and how to address sexuality on a daily basis. And it may be a two-way street: perhaps oncologists don't know if they should broach the subject, and patients aren't sure if they should, either. The workshop identified sexuality problems and asked the question of when or if patients should ask their doctor(s) about sex. One interesting observation on the PowerPoint was that "Gynecologists are afraid of cancer; Oncologists are afraid of sex." One of the questions asked of health care professionals was: "Do you feel uncomfortable in terms of issues around sexuality?" The overwhelming majority answered either "No" or "Sometimes." When asked "Do you raise questions about sexuality with your patients?" the overwhelming response was "No", "Sometimes" or "Rarely." The same response was given with the question of whether patients raised the issue with the doctors.

What is even scarier is the data documenting that over half of men and 80% of women will have "long-term sexual problems after high-dose treatment and/or hematopoietic cell transplantation for malignancy." For further information about this issue, please contact either C.Eeltink@VUmc.nl or christel.wendt@skane.se.

So—what can be done?

Women can have a variety of orgasms: sometimes nothing happens, sometimes there is one orgasm with a sexual encounter, sometimes the encounter is multi-orgasmic, but as we age, it can take much longer to achieve one. Sometimes women can have orgasms with sexual intercourse, but a lot of women need extra genital stimulation to create complete arousal. Orgasms during intercourse are neither better than, nor worse than, genital stimulation. Orgasms can also occur during sleep, or while fantasizing. And there's still that old bugaboo about both people reaching a climax at the same time as the absolute best thing that could ever happen (next to chocolate, of course). People, it mostly doesn't happen that way, so just relax and enjoy what does happen. That's one myth that needs to become extinct.

As with the men, women should learn as much as possible about what impact cancer and treatments will have on your sexuality. If you're too embarrassed to talk to your doctor or nurse, you will never learn what is possible and what isn't, and, as a result, an important component of your life may disappear. If physical intercourse isn't possible, then touch each other in ways that are pleasing. Keep an open mind about what is pleasurable, and don't be afraid to explore new touches, new comfort levels or new positions. Sometimes cuddling or embracing is more pleasurable than the actual act of sexual intercourse.

There are some cancer treatments that disturb your hormones, leading to vaginal dryness and a very definite lessening of sexual desire. Quite often, pain accompanies sexual intercourse, caused by changes in the vagina's size or lack of moistness. This can occur after pelvic surgery, radiation and the previously mentioned hormone fluctuation. If a woman has *vaginismus* (the muscles around the vagina become tense), sexual intercourse is impossible. Vaginismus is treated through counseling and muscle relaxation exercises. For the most part, once treatments have ended, sexual desire returns in time. Orgasms return unless the genital area has become numb or the spinal cord was damaged through treatment.

Genital and reproductive areas of the female body that may be involved in cancer surgeries of the pelvic area include the uterus, cervix, fallopian tubes, ovaries, vagina, bladder, vulva (which includes the area where the clitoris is) and the rectum. With any of these surgeries, there will undoubtedly be some impact on future sexual activity, even if only temporarily, while recuperation occurs. But obviously, some surgeries will permanently change your sexual options.

A *radical hysterectomy* can be performed as the initial treatment for some cervical cancers. The uterus and the connective tissues that hold it in place are removed (hooray, hooray, no more periods! No more "oops" in the middle of the night that leads to a bundle of joy in nine months). In addition, the cervix and maybe one or two inches of the vagina are removed. If you have uterine or ovarian cancer, less is removed as a part of the radical hysterectomy. The ovaries may or may not be removed. Your age, along with the actual diagnosis, will determine what must be taken. If you are under the age of 40, the surgeon will try to leave at least one ovary to prevent early onset of menopause. If you are between the ages of 40–50, a decision will be made whether or not to keep one or both ovaries, or to remove both of them entirely. The main reason to remove both ovaries is to prevent the possibility of ovarian cancer in the future. However, findings from a recent Canadian study, have determined that having a bilateral oophorectomy (both ovaries removed) increases the risk of lung cancer. See the *International Journal of Cancer,* May 11, 2009, by Koushik A, Parent ME, Siemiatyck J, et. al. There is also a Harvard Nurse's Study indicating higher mortality in other areas, including cancer. An earlier Japanese study found that women who took hormone replacement therapy following a hysterectomy and a bilateral oophorectomy, had an increased risk of lung cancer (*International Journal of Cancer*, 2005, Liu Y, Inoue M, Sobue T, et. al.) However, if you are over the age of 50, the recommendation is likely to be made that you have both ovaries removed.

A hysterectomy does not preclude a woman from experiencing orgasms. Although the vagina has been shortened a bit, the clitoris and vaginal walls are still active and intact, and can provide sexual pleasure. If you encounter a problem, it usually concerns lack of lubrication; some pain may occur as a result, and a feeling that the vagina is "too small." Most of these symptoms disappear after six months or so.

A *radical cystectomy* is performed in an attempt to control bladder cancer. A whole ton of stuff gets removed—uterus, bladder, ovaries, fallopian tubes, cervix, the front wall of the vagina and the urethra. This might result in more difficulty achieving an orgasm, but all is not lost. The vaginal wall can often be rebuilt, and with lubrication, intercourse will not be as painful. A lot depends on how much of the vagina you have left. "Thrusting" during intercourse may be difficult until you find ways to compensate. The good news is that you get to experiment with different positions. Since Terry is a former teacher, she will tell you to do it until you get it right! The one thing you need to talk to your doctor about before your cystectomy, is keeping the nerve bundles in the vagina as much intact as possible. This will help with orgasms. Also talk with your surgeon to try and keep as much of the urethra as possible; the urethra helps to fill the clitoris with blood, aiding in your ability for experiencing sexual arousal.

If you've had a radical cystectomy, you will also need to have an *ostomy*. An ostomy is the surgical construction of an artificial excretory opening in the abdomen, so waste can be eliminated from the body. Since urine is being eliminated, it's called a urostomy. This is a plastic pouch outside the body that fits in a plastic plate around the ostomy and is glued in place. During sex, you will need to take a few precautions: empty the bag first; check to make sure everything is in place before starting. If a leak does occur, both you and your partner will get to jump into the shower together, have fun cleaning yourselves up, and then jump back into bed to try again. It is also wise to try and avoid foods that might cause a strong odor. Asparagus is one of these, so there is a dilemma—asparagus is also good for possibly preventing Bright's disease (a disease of the kidneys), so maybe have asparagus one night and have sex the next night. There are now new techniques where a bag isn't needed; a catheter is inserted and you withdraw the urine a few times a day through a "nipple." Make sure your partner doesn't lie on top of the bag. Figure out different positions so this doesn't happen, or you will find yourselves in the shower once again. Wait! What are we thinking! Showers can make sensual scenes for some great foreplay, and who knows, but what you two may even discover new positions, just right for some successful shower opportunities.

An *abdominoperineal* operation is used in the treatment of colon cancer. Usually only the lower colon and rectum are removed, but in some cases, the uterus, ovaries and rear wall of the vagina are also removed. If you have this procedure, a colostomy is created to help solid waste be excreted. This does not impinge on a woman's ability to have orgasms, but lubricants might have to be used because of vaginal dryness, especially if the ovaries were removed. The rectum helps cushion the vagina and when it is removed, the vagina may "move around" more. Again, you may have to experiment with different positions to find what is comfortable for you. If you've had a colostomy, you will do the same things as for the ostomy. Since the colostomy isn't active all the time, you might be able to plan a time of day to have sexual intercourse. If you clean out your colostomy before sex, you can probably get by with just a patch. The key here is to avoid eating foods that cause gas before you think you might have sex. Have beans the day before, to get in your protein and fiber.

A *vulvectomy* is done when you have cancer of the vulva. Depending on the extent of the cancer in this region, you may have a *partial vulvectomy* (only the affected area and a small portion of tissue for preventive purposes), a *modified radical vulvectomy* (removal of the affected area, some tissue and occasionally some lymph nodes in the groin; if there is cancer in or near the clitoris, it may have to be removed, as well), or a *radical vulvectomy*. The surgeon removes the clitoris, the inner and outer lips and lymph nodes. Usually the vagina, ovaries and uterus are not removed. As a result of the radical vulvectomy, women may find that wearing jeans or tight slacks will be painful, because the "padding" has been removed. In addition, feeling sensations could be radically different. Women may also experience a swelling in their legs and in the groin area; this is called *lymphedema*, which can be a problem during sex. If you've had a vulvectomy, you may experience difficulty in experiencing an orgasm. It depends on how much of the vulva has been removed. If the clitoris has been totally removed, orgasms may be impossible to achieve. If you have had a partial vulvectomy, but still notice a kind of numbness in the clitoral area, this lack of feeling should disappear in about six months. Some women have reported it taking from one to two years to fully recuperate from this surgery. They also said it takes a great deal of persistence and practice to discover what would work in their new body to create pleasurable sexual encounters.

Radiation can also have an impact on your sex life. If you've had radiation that affects your vagina, it may feel tender for several weeks after the last dosage. As the radiation burns heal, scarring may occur. The walls of the vagina may become "tough" and you may find they do not respond in a normal manner during intercourse. The lining of the walls may become thin; then bleeding often occurs. Sores can appear and take months to heal. If you do not have bleeding from tumors in your bladder, uterus, cervix, vagina or rectum, you should be able to begin to experiment with sex. As long as your spouse/partner is gentle, even with pelvic radiation, sex should not be impeded. In general, radiation done outside the body will not come in contact with your spouse/partner. Some women receive an implant into their bladder, vagina or uterus. In that case, sex is prohibited. However, check with your doctor first to make sure sex is possible and permissible during your radiation treatments.

If you think you still want children, talk with your doctor before chemo starts. Some chemos can damage the ovaries and reduce fertility. Be sure to use birth control during chemo, because these chemo drugs may harm the fetus. Alexis and Andrea would like to have more children, but the oncologist has told Alexis to wait five years before getting pregnant because of her breast cancer. The length of times may be shorter for different types of cancer. Remember that even if you are still menstruating while receiving chemo, you can still get pregnant. Don't forget—use birth control!

Chemo can also cause yeast infections. If you notice a whitish discharge that looks a little like cottage cheese, get to the doctor right away. Chemo can also aggravate genital herpes or genital warts, if you have had them before. Any infections you may contract need to be treated right away, because your immune system is being compromised and can no longer protect you from unforeseen infections. To reduce your risk of infection, don't wear pantyhose, nylon panties, tight jeans or slacks. Wear loose-fitting clothing, and as much cotton as possible so moisture isn't maintained in the vaginal area. Wipe front to back after urination. Do not douche. If you're having sex, practice safe sex from start to finish. You do NOT want to get any kind of sexually transmitted disease while undergoing your treatment.

Women (and men, as well) can sometimes feel unattractive while undergoing treatment for cancer. The two "biggies" are probably hair loss and weight gain or loss. You might also have catheters inserted for the administration of the chemo. Now this can really get in the way of feeling particularly sultry and seductive, or of having a pleasurable sex life. This is especially true if your treatments go on for months. If you have a PICC line, you have to be so careful not to get an infection, and in the heat of the moment, always have to keep one eye open for pulling on the tube. Not exactly music, candlelight and roses. But these are things that with some care and consideration can be worked around. As Andrea said to Alexis, she didn't care if Alexis was bald, had no arms and no boobs, as long as Alexis was alive. Your spouse/partner can have a lot to do with how you feel sexually while going through cancer treatment and afterward. You might have to wait months for your hair to grow back, so you can finally, once again, feel like a woman.

In our culture, breasts play a major role, both for men and women. Breasts pretty much define who and what a woman is, in terms of her attractiveness level and measure of her womanhood. Men and women alike buy into this farce. Even though we can logically say a mastectomy, a double mastectomy or a lumpectomy is medically necessary to save our lives, there is still the emotional impact of losing your breast(s). The nipples and breast caressing can play a large part in sexual stimulation. When they are gone, that stimulation portion of lovemaking is also gone. Sometimes women feel uncomfortable having their husbands/partners on top during sex. They fear it would be quite noticeable that one or both breasts is/are missing. Even with a breast prosthesis, it can be awkward and uncomfortable. Some women experience long-term pain in their chests and shoulders. If a lumpectomy was performed and radiation was administered, the breast may become somewhat scarred, and feel misshapen, or become a different size (and NO, that size is NOT usually larger).

In the long run, there should be no adverse affects sexually if you have had one or more breasts removed. It in no way interferes with the ability to have an orgasm. If it bothers you to not see your breast, if you feel like you're not much of a woman without breasts, usually reconstructive surgery can be done, but the feeling there once was will no longer exist. It will simply be for aesthetic purposes, or a morale booster. One of the things Alexis noted after her double mastectomy is how much insulation her breasts had provided for her. Now she not only didn't have boobs, but also was colder in the winter, and in spring and fall.

If you have been through menopause, whether naturally or induced through hysterectomy, hot flashes will likely return. In Terry's case, they returned after a week in chemo and continued throughout chemo and the stem cell transplant. Then they went away. They came back about 17 months after her last chemo, and she still gets them for about one minute every hour. The website below is provided, courtesy of The American Cancer Society; it summarizes some of the possible sexual problems and conditions women may experience during the course of their cancer treatment and after: http://www.cancer.org/ Treatment/TreatmentsandSideEffects/PhysicalSideEffects/SexualSide EffectsinWomen/SexualityfortheWoman/sexuality-for-women-with-cancer-summary-table-ca-treat-and-sex-and-fertility (accessed 2/4/2011; no author cited; last revision 3/3/2010).

Sometimes women with cancer, and older women in general, appear to lose the ability to achieve sexual satisfaction. The desire is there, but the intensity of previous experiences simply doesn't appear to exist anymore, or at least cannot be aroused anymore. Thus, the vicious cycle has begun. The inability to reach satisfaction will negatively impact not only your relationship with your spouse/partner, but can also lead to severe depression and other psychological disorders for you. You then begin to feel even stronger feelings of inadequacy that often accompany the lack of sexual satisfaction. This can also be the case if you have had a hysterectomy or encounter the vaginal dryness that occurs in women as they age. (Incidentally, childbirth can also cause a loosening of the vaginal wall, which impacts sexual pleasure in much the same way, causing similar bouts with depression and failure to achieve the sexual satisfaction so desired.) A Truism:

> *"The cycle that repeats itself is the one most traveled—*
> *the one that goes to nowhere; break ranks—get off the*
> *track, and make a new path for your own new journey*
> *to ecstasy, then jump off, and make another."*

The lack of sexual intimacy may also rest with the spouse/partner; s/he may be going through some kind of mental or physical turmoil (psychological, depression, medicines that are being taken, their own expectations of prior sexual intimacy not achieved, lack of caring or a growing distance between the two of you that was actually present before cancer entered the scene, but had gone unresolved, i.e., poor physical condition, some stressors at work, trouble with your communication, fear the relationship was failing, concern about where your lives together are going, just to name a few).

For women there can also be another cause. As we age, have had children or fail to exercise properly, there is a weakening of what is called the *pubococcygeal* muscle or (as it is more commonly abbreviated) the PC muscle, which is located about two inches inside the vagina. For a more in-depth discussion of these effects, check the website http://www.VeryPrivate.com.

So—what can women do? Men, pay attention, because this can also help you. There is an exercise, quite a simple, unobtrusive exercise, which can be done even while you urinate. The exercise is called "Kegels," named after Dr. Arnold Kegel, who accidentally discovered it. The exercise is simply contracting and then relaxing the PC muscle. As an example, while you are urinating, stop the flow of the urine. Hold it for a few seconds, then urinate some more. Repeat the process until your bladder is emptied. Then repeat and repeat and repeat *every time* you go to the bathroom for the rest of your life. Pretty soon it becomes habit, and you won't even consciously realize you are doing it. It is simple and non-invasive (some women after childbirth often resort to surgery to shorten the muscle). If you are incontinent, you might also want to try this. There is a device available known as the KegelPro. Neither of us has tried it, so we can't attest to its effectiveness, or lack thereof.

If you've tried the Kegels, or are experiencing pain or discomfort during intercourse, and still are reluctant to resume previous sexual relations, women can do some or all of the following: in a private part of the house and day, put some lubricant on your clean fingers and explore what is pleasurable to you and what isn't. If that feels good, insert a finger to reopen the tightness of the vaginal wall. You may need to do this for several days, increasing the numbers of fingers that are inserted. Share what feels good with your spouse/partner, and allow him/her to touch you, always communicating what feels good, what doesn't and what you fear. As your confidence levels build and you aren't in as much discomfort (both psychologically and physically), then explore full penetration. Both of you need to remember that "normal" reactions may take some time and some practice; you might not hit a home run the first time at bat.

Sex after 50 doesn't have to diminish. Sex AC doesn't have to diminish. Sex after 50 <u>and</u> AC can be the most liberating, most satisfying, most intense part of your life. Yes, there can be vaginal dryness as our estrogen level decreases (or if you've had chemotherapy), but there are wonderful lubricants available to help you reach all the summits of which you have dreamed. And now, considering all you have been through together, we suggest you have no fear. A Truism:

> *"Your love is deeper and more intense than ever before in your lives—your expression of that depth and intensity can register with no less magnitude; let it be —give it wings."*

Other cancers and their possible impact on sexuality:

A *laryngectomy* removes the larynx, commonly referred to as the "voice box," a part of the respiratory tract that contains the vocal chords. Following this surgery, you will breathe through a hole in your throat. At first, you may be startled by the air coming through the hole in your throat, particularly while making love. This can be especially noticeable if you've eaten garlic for dinner. Sometimes communication can be hindered because it takes a lot of effort to "talk" through this hole. While you are learning how to use it, it can be exhausting. Usually there's not a whole lot of talking that goes on during lovemaking, so this shouldn't be a problem. However, if you wanted to whisper sweet nothings into his or her ear, the whispering part will be O.K., just not into the ear unless that person spends a lot of time near your throat area (maybe they're shorter than you are . . . .). In general, most patients who have had a laryngectomy do not report many sexual difficulties. The biggest concerns are related to depression and a reduced libido. These issues are not caused by the chemo or radiation you might have had, but are more likely related to having had cancer in the first place.

Cancers of the *head and neck* can be devastating, simply because they are so evident—parts of the bone structures of the face will have been removed. If you've had surgery on your jaw, tongue or palate, it can affect the way you talk forever. Even with advances in restorative surgery, the "you" you once looked like and talked like will never be the same. As mentioned earlier, a lot of sexuality is in our minds. If you feel unattractive, if you feel no one could ever love you again because of the way you look and sound, or how you talk, these feelings from the place of a diminished self-esteem will have a negative impact on your sex life, if you let it. In saying this, there is no intent to deny the significance of what these issues might be like to live with, but we know without doubt, your mind and your attitude can lift you out of that place, to where you recognize and love who you are again. Sometimes distance from the surgery and a growing acceptance of the new you will resolve your concerns. Other times, therapy and an understanding partner will be needed to help you feel whole again.

If you have had bone cancer, sometimes the *amputation* of a limb has become necessary. In many cases an artificial limb is used to replace what was lost. Then the questions arise: Do I use the limb during lovemaking? What happens if I do and it's painful to wear? The answers are simple; it depends on how you and your partner feel about it. Sometimes a prosthesis can get in the way. Sometimes prostheses are painful to wear, especially in the beginning stages of learning how to use and deal with them. You will definitely have to explore alternatives in lovemaking, depending on which limb or limbs have been removed. Sometimes prostheses can help you maintain your balance during lovemaking. Other times, straps can get in the way and become a distraction, obviously ruining "the moment." If these side effects become too much of a distraction or you find it too difficult to allow you to physically manipulate your body for successful sexual encounters, talk with your doctor about other possible alternatives.

In summary, people do change after cancer. That's a fact. Cancer changes how you see yourself, especially sexually. Grief is a natural part of surviving cancer. You have to say good-bye to the old you and learn how to welcome and accept the new you. Grieving may recur long after you think you are finished. Cancer carries with it great costs— financially, in time lost with friends and family, your career and sometimes your faith. There is this struggle to balance the need to protect your friends and family by not telling them what's bothering you—you don't want to "burden" them. Most often, what happens when you do that is an insurmountable wall of silence appears and grows; over time, it festers, until a massive chasm or break occurs, that crushes all the structures that bound and held your lives together. A Truism:

"Burdens shared decrease the loads all of us carry."

Friends and family can sometimes withdraw. Anger, resentment, depression and other emotions both on the survivor's part and on the part of friends and family can rise to the surface. If you have had the type of cancer that requires a prosthesis of some sort (a voice box, a penile implant, a colostomy bag), the anger or depression can occur because the actual piece can be a reminder of how close to death you came. Your brush with death also reminds others how close they have come to their own mortality. Chemotherapy can also change the way you look, which is not only difficult for you, but also your friends and family. Don't give up on each other; friends and family members— don't give up on the survivor. Be patient. The person they are deep inside is still there, but there will be some changes. For every negative thought, give six positives. Friends and family members of survivors need that just as much as the survivor does. No "pity parties," No "poor me" or No "poor you," please.

And if all the information above isn't enough, there is always the World Wide Web. As a *CAUTION,* though, when you do a search, please enter something like **"sexual health"** (including the quotation marks). If you simply enter "sex," your computer will download about a bazillion entries, and you could possibly be inundated forever with pornographic spam.

Shingles

If you ever had chicken pox in your life (and about 90% of us have), you carry the virus with you forever, putting you at risk of contracting Shingles later in your life. The virus is alive but usually remains inactive. It finds a home in nerve roots in your body and can lay dormant for years. There is no way to determine who will get Shingles or when it may occur. About one million people will be diagnosed with Shingles in a year, usually starting at around age 60; if you live to be 85, one out of two of you will develop Shingles. Apart from advancing age, the other risk factor for Shingles is an immune system that has been compromised by a disease such as cancer, but could also be because of other medications you have taken.

Shingles may initially be felt, but not seen. Symptoms include burning, itching and/or tingling. Once those symptoms manifest themselves visually, a rash containing fluid-filled blisters will appear, usually on one side of the body or face (Terry's mother-in-law had them all over her back). The blisters may take up to four weeks to heal. Even after the rash heals, pain may last for months or years. If there is long-term nerve pain, it is because Shingles damages the nerves. You have to watch for possible decrease or loss of vision or hearing, muscle weakness, paralysis on one side of the face, scarring and skin infection. An excellent resource for more information is http://www.shinglesinfo.com.

What was a surprise to Terry was that she could not receive the Shingles shot to prevent an outbreak because it is composed of live virus, which would have given her Shingles. As alluded to earlier, she can't be around people who have an active case of Shingles (good luck avoiding that in crowds), or who have recently had a case of Shingles. Terry recently flew for the first time in March of 2010, and forgot to ask the ticketing agent about NOT sitting next to a person on the plane if s/he has/had an active case of Shingles. So far, nothing has appeared on her skin, but it is a precaution she probably should NOT have forgotten. It would be helpful for us to hear from people in the airline industry about the best way to handle this. What is the protocol? With whom do we need to speak? What documentation do we need? Is screening even possible? You can e-mail us at: Theresa@SoYouveSurvivedCancer.com and/or Alexis@SoYouveSurvivedCancer.com.

Skin—Side Effects, Over-the-Counter Stem Cell Treatments

We are only going to mention this in passing since neither of us has experienced it. That is, we experienced it during treatment, but not after. You might experience dry skin or other skin irritations after chemotherapy. What happens is that chemotherapy cannot distinguish between the healthy and the cancerous cells. Your skin is comprised of cells that rapidly divide, in a constant state of renewal, sloughing throughout normal day-to-day activities, even while you sleep. Chemotherapy may disrupt this process. If you develop dry skin or other skin irritations, check with your oncologist who might refer you to a dermatologist. If there is no particular medication that can help, try taking short baths or lukewarm showers and then putting a moisturizer on your skin. Once again, be careful that what you are putting on your skin does not contain carcinogenic chemicals. One company particularly well known for non-carcinogenic skin products is TilVee Eco Ethical Skincare, http://www.tilvee.com. There are probably others, but this is a company whose products we have both used and like. Burt's Bees also makes some nice products (http://www.burtsbees.com).

While in the doctor's office one day, Terry picked up one of the gossip magazines to peruse (to keep up with the great-nieces and their interest areas). She discovered an ad for "Stem Cell Therapy—Young Again Program." Out of curiosity, she called to try and talk with a real person about the stem cell process used in the product. No such luck. The ad had said "100% free," but the recording said that for $49.95 (plus shipping and handling), they would send a 30-day supply and a free 30-day supply. She hung up before the recording even finished. It didn't sound "100% free" to her and she's not that vain. To her, A Truism:

"Every wrinkle is a badge of honor for a life well-lived."

After sleeping on it, she decided to give it a whirl, purely in the interest of you dear readers (and so she could deduct it from her income taxes as research for the book. Be grateful: she was on the phone for over 15 minutes wading through all the special offers; she stopped counting after 6 and put the phone down until the voice stopped. There was no short cut to get to the finish; then it was wait for "10–14 business days" to get the product. Then it was even more special offers on the phone. She hung up.).

Anyway, she finally did try the product, but in the meantime, she had sent several e-mails to the company ("BioLogics") to try to get some information. There were responses the first few times, but when she asked "Why do you call it 'stem cell' therapy when there aren't any stem cells in it?" the only response was to send the same blurb that came with the product. She used it twice a day for almost two months, including a sample on her arm for comparison purposes. Then she asked for some opinions with regard to which arm appeared to show fewer wrinkles. Over 80%, an admittedly small sample, guessed the wrong arm. While she can make no recommendation either way based upon her 'little' study, she found further reinforcement on the side of caution whenever making any kind of purchase. "Don't believe what you read, believe only half of what you see, and nothing of what you're told." Isn't that what THEY say?

Sleep Cycle

The good news is that once you stop chemo, your sleep cycle will readjust itself over time. The bad news is that sleeplessness may recur again and again. After her stem cell transplant, Terry was getting pretty good sleep, but around the 18-month marker, she was back to getting from one to three hours of sleep a night. What is not known is whether the decrease in the numbers of hours of sleep and the concomitant stress of not getting sleep was merely a factor or a large causal factor. Her brain simply wouldn't rest, wouldn't "shut off" at night. Naps in the afternoon sometimes did—and sometimes didn't—affect her sleep at night. During chemo she had taken a prescription drug to help her sleep that mostly didn't work, but after chemo, was afraid she would form a dependence on pills. She had quit the pills "cold turkey" and suffered no greater loss of sleep than with the pills. Neither walking, nor other forms of exercise seemed to help her get to or stay asleep. At this stage, she has asked for a prescription for sleeping pills, but will eventually begin to taper off slowly, and hope her body readjusts to the point where, once again, she can begin to experience a natural, good night's sleep.

Spirituality

"I said to myself: 'Why is it that all men fail to adhere to truth instead of believing falsehoods?' It seemed to be in the nature of man, which is weak and sluggish, even though man aspires to know the truth and the hidden things of nature, this endeavor is difficult and can only be attained with great labor and patience . . . Hence people hastily accept whatever they have heard from their fathers and shy away from critical examination. But God created man to be the master of his own actions, so that he can be what he wills to be . . . "

—*Hateta Zera Yaekob, The Essay of Zera Yaekob, the Ethiopian Philosopher (1592–1692)*

"All the cosmos is a single substance of which we are a part. God is not an external manifestation, but everything that is."

—*Baruch Spinoza, Ethics (1632–1677)*

"Take the first step in faith. You don't have to see the whole staircase, just take the first step."

—*Dr. Martin Luther King, Jr.*

Once you have been diagnosed with cancer, you may find your spiritual or religious beliefs will change. Once you have survived cancer, you may find your beliefs will have changed again. For some, their faith or belief systems will have been strengthened; for others, questions may arise regarding the reason or purpose for having gotten cancer and what it should or will mean to them. Family and friends of someone who has been diagnosed with cancer may also find themselves questioning their own beliefs. It's different for everyone and please believe, it IS normal, or at the very least, common, not only to question what has happened, but also...to question all things you have believed BC.

We have both struggled with this area, not only before we had cancer, but during and after. Now as we begin to write this section of our book, we are struggling even more. What on earth could we possibly write that would be meaningful to, or helpful for, anyone else, especially a cancer survivor? We have even considered NOT doing so, of eliminating the section altogether, given that spirituality is so very personal, and so widely examined by writers from all realms of life since the beginning of time. But as we endeavor to isolate and discuss those issues most critical AC, few other topics have emerged with such clarity as an inescapable priority for inclusion, if we are to be at all helpful to you, our readers. Spirituality is a must for the book, for us, and we believe, for you. So bear with us, as we enter the *infinite* realm of the "unanswered," or perhaps, "answerless" questions—those that evoke our greatest thinking and the most challenging introspection into our own lives.

In her formative years, Alexis attended a Russian Orthodox Church; shortly after, she attended every other denominational church you can imagine, winding up in a strict southern Baptist church in her teenhood. In her youth, Terry attended a sort of a Baptist-Evangelical-Holy Roller-Pentecostal kind of church. Religion was poured down the throats of all the children. On Sundays, there was Sunday School in the morning, church service after that; Sunday evenings were another sort of Sunday school and another church service; Wednesdays were prayer meetings and choir practices; Saturdays were the youth groups. Terry spent one week each summer at Bible camp, where they were encouraged to be "saved." Terry has been "saved" about 100 times and spent a lot of time "witnessing" to people. She spent many evenings at the local mission playing her violin or viola for all of the inebriated, who were looking for a free meal. (It's amazing that her playing didn't drive them to drink even more, or to leave town on a permanent basis.)

As kids and young adults, we were both curious. We wondered about the six big questions—the who, what, when, where, how and why of things, not only "why are we here?" but also, why is there so much hatred in the world when all these religions are supposed to be about love? Why are there different brands or denominations of religions (and even multiple sects within these religions), when it's all the same God? Why is it people cannot get along and learn tolerance of others and their differences? And these are only a few of the many, many questions we had about our religion and our beliefs. (In the original draft of this book, the questions go on for four pages, and even those 100-plus questions had not begun to scratch the surface of all the issues about which we sought answers.)

When we asked our religious leaders why something was the way it was or why something had happened, quite often the response was

"Because God wants it that way." But if that were the case, then why bother getting an education, or learning how to read, write and compute? Why try to find a cure for cancer or other diseases? Why bother to learn how to balance your checking account or pay your bills? (Terry once heard of a pastor of a church who refused to pay his mortgage because Jesus was coming any day now.) Why bother with earning a living to support our families? Our priests and pastors had no answers, at least not any which made sense. Like the doctors mentioned earlier, when you asked them a direct question, they mumbled a lot and changed the topic or rushed off to greet another parishioner. But that's not the worst part. Today we have first century beliefs dictating our political strategies, scientific research and the K-12 education system.

Both of us independently began on paths to try to get some answers to our endless questions. Church for us became increasingly uncomfortable, and as we learned and lived more, it became increasingly irrelevant. The racism, sexism, homophobia and exclusivity that were extant in these churches became increasingly intolerable in our eyes. Even early on, the God we believed in was one of unconditional love, and we couldn't find that love within the churches we had searched, nor were we able to find that sense of a loving God within the majority of the people who attended those churches. As we read, studied and learned, we realized we really didn't have (to borrow Lawrence Gardner's phrase) Christ-ianity, as much as we had Peter-ianity or Paul-ianity, both very much human, and NOT divine at all. To quote Ashleigh Brilliant, "The purpose of an institution is to perpetuate the institution."

We also realized that nearly all of these religions were "*fear-based*," mostly to help members cope with this horrible fear of death that human beings seem to possess. Fear, as an emotion, is one which envelops us all with the avoidance reaction. This avoidance aspect of fear is the enabler of all those who would take power and control over us. If you are afraid or are made afraid, it is much easier for anyone, or for any organization, to shape and determine your beliefs and behaviors, seducing you to act in accordance with their wishes, fulfilling their purposes, which most frequently are NOT necessarily those of God (or the God we believe in). For us, the primary objectives of organized religion appear to be self-serving, designed purposefully to ensure institutional propagation through the maintenance of power and control over members through the invocation of *fear*. Ultimately, we have both decided that the life review, if one is conducted upon the occasion of our passing, will be done with compassion and unconditional love by a merciful and just God.

St. Augustine, in the fourth century, reportedly made two arguable proclamations:

1. that it was O.K. to lie in order to protect the church, and

2. that curiosity was a "<u>disease</u>," and leads people to discover what they "<u>should not wish to learn</u>."

Both contentions are not only problematic, but contradict biblical teachings. Consider curiosity for a moment; it has been curiosity that has stimulated exploration, discovery and learning. As a result, curiosity has enabled us to understand more and more about how the human body works to help people live and grow in this environment, send people to the moon, discover more about the universe in which we live, create the Internet, develop differing art forms, create music that speaks to the souls of people from all over the world, manufacture vehicles and mass transportation systems, find ways to make life safer and easier to do productive work, and find medicines to treat cancer and other deadly diseases. Ask yourself this question: Would you really want to go back and live in the first century?

And yet there was that yearning for something deeper, that feeling there was Something or Someone, a Source or Power, out 'there' Somewhere, that was a necessary and integral part of our lives. This became increasingly important as we were diagnosed and treated for cancer. The questions weren't so much why we had cancer; we never asked, "Why did God give us cancer?" Rather, our questions were: How is this journey with cancer we are on going to help us, and could it help us help others? What lessons can we learn from this? Is this journey going to help us become closer to God (or the Great Spirit or Jehovah or Yahweh or Allah or whatever name you choose to use; for us, it's all the same omnipotent Entity), or will the experience drive us away from that Entity? Cancer had realistically given us a second chance at life—it was not only a "wake-up call," but a motivation to reassess our lives as well, providing us the opportunity to redefine our lives, and to reach out to others we encounter in life, to recognize how much we are all interconnected, and to redefine how our lives could be fulfilled, whether personally or professionally.

And there was another important question that for us, had to, or at least needed to, be resolved, one for which we are still searching for resolution. What is the difference between "religion" and "spirituality"? Can it be that the two are elements of a "faith" continuum, falling at different points across the spectrum of believers? Where do we fall on that continuum? How does it apply to us? And will it help us with cancer? Do we come back to the "church" and the institutions of organized religion, or do we seek community and knowledge in other places and from a wide variety of sources? (For Terry's atheist friends, she has read some of the books by Sam Harris, Richard Dawkins and Christopher Hitchens, thoroughly enjoyed them, and understands completely why this portion and others of our book may be anathemas to you.) We have no intention of evoking denunciation of our book because of our questioning minds, but we do intend to inspire your thoughts and your questioning to help resolve what we have found to be very profound, complex, contradictory and confusing issues. If nothing else, moving from an unsure state of mind regarding your spirituality to one that offers you a sense of resolution and surety, may free your mind and body to focus your energies upon your healing, which is critical now that you have survived cancer.

In the July/August 2009 issue of Spirituality & Health, an article appeared entitled "The Difference Between Spirituality and Religion?" written by Rabbi Rami Shapiro. He defines religion as being . . .

> ". . . *about belonging, community, shared values, shared rituals, and mutual support. Spirituality is about living your life without a net, forever surrendered to reality and meeting each moment with curiosity, wonder, gratitude, justice, humility and love. The two are not antithetical. Religion is often a container within which spiritual practices are preserved and passed on. Some find the container as helpful as what it contains, and choose to belong to a specific religion. Others simply take what they need from the containers and fashion their own way. I do (Rabbi Shapiro does) a bit of both."*

And for some of you who are going through cancer treatments and have survived cancer, you may find your beliefs (not your faith; we make a distinction between the two) either challenged or strengthened. We don't have all the answers for you. In fact, we may not have any. We can only relate what we have discovered which may—or may not—have relevance for you.

There are passages in the Bible which we have interpreted in vastly different ways than you will find in most institutionalized religions. There are countless references in both the Old Testament and the New Testament that allude to "Ye are gods." The Hindus have a custom of greeting everyone they meet with hands in the "prayer" position, which is to acknowledge the God that is inside each person. For us, Spirituality (or God) isn't "out there"—it is an intrinsic part of our very inner souls. From the book of Revelations, we don't interpret the prophecies as hellfire and damnation; rather, we interpret them as the unveiling or "revelation" of truth, of enlightenment and of wisdom. "Apocalypse" means to unveil, or to reveal. (And for those of you who are thinking we are heretics, the etymology of "heretic" is "seeker of knowledge," which both of us unabashedly acknowledge and embrace.) There are some cultures that believe the Apocalypse, or what to them means the end of the world, *is* coming; that in fact in 2012, the world, as we know it, will disappear. What we believe is if something does happen in 2012, it will be what Albert Einstein alludes to—the God we have worshipped in the past will now be devoid of dogma and theology. The time will come that the dogma of original sin, which is a man-made concept, will be replaced by the notion that God is inside us. The new interpretation will be that the "Temple" of God is the temple of the mind, at which point we hope there will be a way for religions and science to be united. The *Gospel of Mary* says that the treasure we seek (dare we say the Holy Grail, the eternal quest) is the "Mind."

For both of us, ridding ourselves of religion was a must—the fear-based life, the guilt, the shame and the humiliation and condemnation that accompanied it—in order to find God. We had to reach those depths inside us that we felt certain were a part of a larger Whole, which was comprised of unconditional love. *We had to get rid of out-dated first century beliefs, the man-made rules and regulations, the dogma in order to find God.* It was wearisome to go to church every Sunday and have fear, guilt, shame, humiliation or condemnation be a part of every sermon. Author Gershen Kaufman has said that shame is a "kind of soul murder." We became convinced that to find unconditional love, we had to chart our own course in search of the God who bestows upon us unconditional love.

This search for unconditional love connects with the unquestionable need to fully embrace and sustain a positive attitude throughout the time you are undergoing chemotherapy, radiation and a stem cell transplant. If you are wallowing in guilt, shame and accepting that you are a sinful creature, that somehow God did this to you, that somehow you have been "bad," and this is your punishment, those thoughts and feelings could be detrimental to your ability to regain your health, or to succeed in your battle with this pernicious disease. If you believe you are doomed, you probably will be. A Truism:

> *"When you allow negative beliefs to grow within you, they are what you will harvest."*

In these times, it appears that others, whether facing a life-threatening disease or not, are also seeking meaning in their lives outside the institutions of religion. A 2008 survey by the Pew Forum has shown that the number of "nonbelievers" in America has doubled since 1990; by non-believer, the surveyors were referencing those who do not now belong to, or do not plan to become a member of, an organized religion in the near future. Thirty percent of Americans now refer to themselves as "spiritual" but NOT "religious." According to another 2008 poll conducted by Harris, nearly one-quarter (24%) of Americans now believe in reincarnation, up from only 6% a few years ago. As we read and study more, we have found ourselves asking, "What is it about religion and/or people today that is bringing about such a shift in people's lives, and in their thinking and belief systems?" For what are they searching?

Psychologists originally thought we humans were somehow "wired" in the parietal lobe to believe in God, and that it is inevitable, at some point in all of our lives, we will believe in Him. As it turns out, that might not be the case. Gregory Paul, writing in the online journal, *Evolutionary Psychology*, finds there might just have to be an environmental cause to trigger neurological connections to belief in God, and that social progress can serve to decrease religious belief. It may be then, that religion or faith in God may not only be a way to cope with death, but also the means to cope with the stressors of a diseased, dysfunctional environment.

The other side of the dilemma, though, is that both of us have friends who have cancer and are "religious." They absolutely, firmly, unequivocally, undeniably, totally, completely, you betcha, uh huh, believe in and practice the rituals, rules and regulations of their respective institutions, whether Christian, Islamic, Jewish or whatever their affiliation. And they have done quite well in their recovery and are among those who have survived cancer. For them, the "community" Rabbi Shapiro talks about is very important, and has helped them cope with their medical conditions, and to fight their disease successfully. Acknowledging the reality of these instances further confounds the dilemma with which we are struggling, and makes finding the "answers" even more elusive.

According to the February 23, 2009, issue of *Time* magazine, you might just gain an extra two to three years of life if you go to church (or, we're assuming, synagogue, mosque or other place of worship) regularly. This is based on research conducted by Dr. Daniel Hall, an Episcopal priest and surgeon in Pittsburg, PA. It is in religious communities where people go for friendship, support, and help in times of crisis. This is that sense of community Rabbi Shapiro feels is so important—the "net" that embraces us all about which he speaks. There appears to be evidence that faith just might bring us health. "People who attend religious services do have a lower risk of dying in any one year than people who don't attend. However, people who believe in a loving God fare better after a diagnosis of a serious illness than those people who believe in a punitive God."

Neil Krause, at the University of Michigan, has found regular churchgoers (and we are assuming a synagogue or mosque) cope better with economic crises (cancer can bring about economic crises of gigantic proportions), and that people who receive support from their religious institution do quite well health-wise—but, <u>do even better *if they are doing the giving,* rather than the receiving</u>. His research also has found a feeling of gratitude reduces depression; another piece of research shows people live longer who believe their life has meaning and purpose.

African-American churches have also played a vital role within their communities. For many African-Americans, church is the very center of life as it affects community, religion or spirituality, and politics. Many African-American churches are joining forces with scientists in the health care arena to get their members to eat healthier, learn how to exercise more and how to improve their fitness. Many churches are now serving healthier foods during their events. A program in North Carolina was so successful they ultimately named their project "Body and Soul," and have produced reading materials, DVDs and cookbooks to spread the work of the program into the broader community. The initiative was developed in collaboration with the National Cancer Institute and the American Cancer Society.

In the Islamic faith, the concept of original sin is not acknowledged within the writings or teachings. An illness or suffering in life (such as poverty or disease) may be a function of God testing you in this life, in order to make your next life in Paradise better. But for them, the bottom line is that God is Love, and love can be seen as a form of reformation.

Doctors are often at a loss regarding whether to talk about any spiritual or religious concerns with their patients. And yet, most people, some studies have shown as high as about 90%, would welcome such a discussion. There is a program in the New York City area called HealthCare Chaplaincy. Religious leaders of the Christian, Jewish, Muslim and Zen Buddhist faiths are now part of more than a dozen hospitals. They work hand-in-hand with hospitals and doctors to assure that spiritual/religious care is coordinated with medical care. This has eventuated into an effective partnership; people can discuss life and death matters that concern them, and receive not only excellent medical advice, but spiritual counseling as well, including referrals to other health care providers, psychological help, and in some cases, the services of a social worker to assist the families in crisis when life-threatening illnesses occur.

Studies have shown that faith and prayer have a positive impact on health. To get technical here, for a minute, the frontal lobes of your brain are engaged during prayer; they are the ones that rule focus and concentration. According to Dr. Andrew Newberg at the University of Pennsylvania, if your frontal lobes are functioning well, it can also boost memory. In the book *Train Your Mind, Change Your Brain,* by Sharon Begley, the author documents that Buddhist monks, who have meditated for years, have actually changed the function and structure of the brain, which leads to changes in how they think and feel. This is accomplished through a process called *neuroplasticity.* The brain is not fixed. Even as we age, our brains are capable of adapting, healing and renewing the neurons. We aren't stuck with the number of neurons we had at birth. We cannot only improve the depression that often accompanies ill health and/or aging through meditation and prayer, but we can also teach, and most importantly learn, compassion through these same avenues. From existing evidence, the world today is certainly suffering from a short supply of genuine compassion, with rare, but compelling exceptions in those situations of mass disaster. We base this observation upon the frequency in everyday life in which people are moved to take action on behalf of their fellow human beings living in deplorable circumstances, whether fault can be discerned or not.

In addition, there appears to be some kind of link between prayer and good health. Even the progression of AIDS seems to regress a bit if a person believes in God and prays. However, since a researcher can't accurately measure how much, how often and for what duration of time prayer occurs for a person in ill health, *actual data cannot be generated that could be used to conclusively determine the extent of its effectiveness.* Studies have shown that people who prayed for another person with heart disease, for example, *appeared to have generated no measurable effect*, despite the prayers they offered. There were still very high rates of complications. What does seem to matter, though, is *whether the subjects in the research study know or don't know* they are the subject of another person's prayers. In a few studies, it was demonstrated that if a person was prayed for "in secret," there was a slight elevation in the extent to which complications arose. If the subjects are told they are being prayed for, they believe it and, like a sugar pill, a placebo effect takes place. (The same thing can happen to a patient who receives medicine for cancer; believing the medicine attacked the tumor, it went away. When the patient was later informed the medication held no therapeutic value, the tumor actually grew back.)

And yet, both of us do very much believe in the power of prayer. At one point, Terry had people praying for her who were Anglican, Animist, Baptist, Buddhist, Catholic, Coptic Christian, Episcopalian, Orthodox Jews, Reformed Jews, Lutheran, Methodist, Muslim, Native American medicine women, and by people with no particular set of rules or affiliations, but who simply possess a faith in God. And her atheist friends were playing their parts by doing medical research or sending funny e-mails, which Terry considered a form of prayer (they probably wouldn't be happy with that). She is immensely grateful to each and every one of them. Even before delving into some of the research on prayer and faith, and its impact on health, we always told people we were praying for them, even people in chance meetings in grocery stores, restaurants or wherever we happened to be. Alexis also had her prayer warriors doing what they do best around the clock. The denomination was not an issue; what did matter, however, was the truth, honesty and love that lifted her in their prayers of healing. She had people who were not exactly "spiritual" offer worry stones and books and food. All were blessings, regardless of the form in which they came.

There is an organization in the Denver, Colorado, area called Common Tables. They use mealtimes to bring people of different religions together. Basically, up to eight people from differing belief systems get together four times a year to have dinner and learn about each other's beliefs. Questions can be raised in a "safe" environment about faith, family and rituals. The one cardinal rule—there shall be NO proselytizing. (For further information, call Dave Corby, at 303-690-3900, or log onto http://www.commontables.org). Wouldn't it be a great idea to form something like this for those who are going through cancer or who have survived it? We not only need to expand the "circle of understanding" about differing beliefs, but we all need to be united in the fight against this disease.

Somehow we find it ironic that in our book the discussions on Sexuality and Spirituality are two of the longest sections of the "Now What?" chapter. Yet each, in its own way, plays a major role in our lives in surviving cancer or other health concerns. We believe some form of spiritual, or religious, beliefs, in conjunction with other life factors, but definitely including clearly successful sexual-life experiences, are key components to great health, both physical and mental. But we both like the Buddhist concept that states: *"There are many paths to the same place"* (thanks to Joseph Campbell for this insight; pick up his *Masks of God* series; his books are worth every minute of your time). Not everyone will agree with the concept that many paths could take you to the same place, of course, and each of you will have to search and find those beliefs that work for you within your life situations. A Truism:

> *"Be aware—over time, even those beliefs you hold most firmly today may change tomorrow."*

Stem Cell Recuperation

Stem cells can be found in bone marrow, in your blood, in the umbilical cord and in embryos. (There are also cancer stem cells, but those are a whole different subject, one that neither of us feels adequate to discuss.) Embryonic stem cells can grow into any type of cell in your body, but bone marrow stems cells cannot. Stem cells from bone marrow can grow into white blood cells (fight infection), red blood cells (carry oxygen to the body) and platelets (helps the blood to clot). At this point in time, the only cancers that stem cell transplants readily help are leukemia and lymphoma. The other areas currently under exploration are for breast cancer, for sickle cell anemia, aplastic anemia, and a few immunodeficiency diseases. Stem cells can be used to treat myelomas, but ordinarily chemo will still have to be administered for the rest of the person's life. There are two types of stem cell transplants: autologous—you can be your own donor; and allogenic—you have to find a donor, which may be a family member, or be acquired through the marrow donor bank. Stem cells may also be gleaned from the umbilical cord of an unrelated donor. Donors are matched as closely as possible to the recipient's own tissue to avoid the risk of rejection. This is called an HLA (Human Leukocyte Antigens) procedure. The procedure to remove the blood to obtain the stem cells is called "apheresis." Bone marrow from the pelvis bone is not used as much today, because the donor has to go to the hospital to have it removed. Once the stem cells have been collected, they are frozen until they are needed. The time limit before expiration of the frozen stem cells is three years.

Stem cell recuperation will take some time; by some estimates, it will require as much as three to five years to be fully restored. You will have to be patient with yourself, as will all those who will be around you. You will initially make several trips to the transplant unit or a clinic, where your blood will be repeatedly monitored to make sure your body is producing enough healthy red and white blood cells and platelets. They will check to make sure you aren't running a fever, whether you have any nausea, if you have any mouth sores, or are having diarrhea, and whether you are regaining your appetite. Your PICC line may have to be in place for up to six months, depending on how well you are progressing toward recovery. Extended time with your

PICC line is more likely if you have used a donor. The risk of graft-vs-host disease (GVHD)—or transplant rejection, infections and graft failure—are quite real and the health care staff will want to make sure you are truly recovering. It might take from six to twelve months before you feel any real energy, because your blood cells and immune system require a great deal of time to recuperate and become fully operational again.

Graft-vs-host disease usually occurs within 90–100 days of transplant, because the stem cells slowly attack your body. Acute GVHD usually occurs more than 100 days after the transplant, and can last for the rest of a person's life. Symptoms of this condition are itching or a rash that starts on your palms or feet and gradually spreads over your entire body, nausea, loss of appetite, vomiting, cramping and diarrhea. Doctors determine how severe the rejection is by how severe your diarrhea is. If you have jaundice (yellowing of the skin), this is a signal of potential liver damage. If you have acute GVHD, you will be treated with glucocorticoids. If you have chronic GVHD, you will be treated with steroids, from which you will gradually be weaned (<u>never, ever, unless the doctor tells you, quit steroids "cold turkey"</u>). If you are older when you get your transplant, you are more likely to develop GVHD. In order to try to prevent GVHD, regardless of your age, doctors will prescribe medications to suppress your immune system. Also, to the extent possible, doctors will try to use umbilical cord stem cells to reduce the risk of rejection. Until more umbilical cords are donated, and umbilical cord stem cell transplants become the standard of treatment, benevolent donors will have to be relied upon heavily to increase the rates of successful stem cell transplantation.

Possible side effects from stem cell transplants vary greatly dependent upon the donor source used for the transplant. If you use an allogenic donor, the side effects may include: cataracts, new cancers, infertility, and damage to the lungs, heart, liver or kidneys. People who use their own stem cells—an autologous donor, for transplant in treating leukemia will more often get the disease back than if they had used an allogenic donor or umbilical cord stem cells. Allogenic or donor stem cells recognize the new cancer cells as a foreign body and attack them. The return of the disease occurs with an autologous donor because stem cells from one's own body don't recognize the new cancer as foreign, and allow it to grow and multiply. Does this mean that every person who had an autologous stem cell transplant will have a relapse? No, but the odds are increased. In these cases, immunotherapy will be used to stimulate the immune system to counteract a relapse of the leukemia. There is, however, one fact to keep in mind as you make decisions about the method(s) you want your doctors to use to treat your cancer; *stem cell transplants are frequently the only treatment option currently available that can save, or even prolong, a person's life if s/he has been diagnosed with leukemia or lymphoma.*

Once you get home, your life will involve many significant changes. First, you have to get used to living in a germ-ridden environment all over again, no matter how clean you keep your home. You are no longer in a safe, sterile environment, but the health care staff will monitor your blood counts to make sure your immune system has recuperated enough so this does not become a factor slowing your recovery. You must protect yourself from every kind of infection. The really good news is that this means you should NOT do any housecleaning for a month or so after you get home. Someone ELSE will have to clean the toilets, sterilize kitchen countertops, scour the stove, dust and polish everything, and take out the trash (Oh—How awful! No housework to do!)

You will now be showering or bathing at least once every day, with towels and washcloths dedicated for your use only. Find a soap that is gentle and non-drying. Use lotions two or three times a day to keep your skin moisturized; avoid any lotions that have alcohol in them. You and your caregivers will have to remember to wash your and their hands constantly, especially in the preparation of food and after going to the bathroom. It is preferable to wear glasses, but if you do need to wear contact lenses, make sure they are cleaned thoroughly. Eye makeup used before your transplant should be discarded, and new makeup should be purchased. If you simply have to take out the trash, wear a protective glove and wash your hands thoroughly afterward. Sexual intercourse may be resumed when the doctor reports that your platelet count is over 50,000 **and** your neutrophil (a type of white blood cell) count is above 1,000. If you are experiencing vaginal dryness, use a water-based lubricant.

Dental hygiene is also critical when you go home because of your heightened risks of infection, and the fact that your mouth has more germs than any other part of your body. Check your mouth every day for emerging sores. Check your tongue to see if there is any bleeding, cracks or white patches. Brush your teeth with a soft bristle brush, and brush gently. You want to avoid having your gums bleed, which can lead to infection. Use a fluoride-based toothpaste such as Biotene or Sensodyne. It is better to wait to floss until your platelet count reaches 50,000 or more. Again, you want to reduce the risk of bleeding and subsequent infection. However, your oral oncologist may have a different recommendation; in that case, follow whatever advice s/he offers. If you feel a "bad taste" is in your mouth or you worry about bad breath, use a non-alcohol-based mouthwash such as Biotene, or make a mixture of baking soda and water (see the "Dental Concerns" section). If you do not have access to an oral oncologist, ask your regular dentist to speak with your transplant doctor before having any dental work done. You may need to be on antibiotics to prevent infection anytime you go to the dentist for at least one to two years following your transplant.

If you are at some distance from the hospital where you received your transplant and you will need frequent additional blood transfusions or blood work, arrangements can be made with the local Visiting Nurses Association (VNA). You will also be seeing your transplant health care team quite regularly for at least the first six to twelve months, depending on how well your recuperation is progressing. Blood tests will be given every time you visit your doctor to make sure your immune system is improving. At each visit you will be asked numerous health status questions, such as how your appetite is, whether you have been nauseous, whether you have had diarrhea or constipation, whether your eyesight has changed, if you have any numbness or tingling in your fingers or toes, and a whole lot more.

If you go home with a PICC line or other catheter, be sure to keep it clean and sterilized. When you go out to public water play places, avoid getting into any lakes, oceans, hot tubs or swimming pools because of the high presence of bacteria; even at your own home, do not get into the hot tub or swimming pool. It is always better to take a shower than soaking in a bath. Do not let the PICC line or catheter get into a tub of water.

To avoid infectious complications from bleeding, do NOT play contact sports, don't do heavy exercising, use only an electric razor, blow your nose gently, use a digital mouth thermometer to take your temperature (sterilize it after each use), and avoid taking aspirin unless directed by your physician. Call your physician right away if you notice bleeding in your stool or urine, if you see bleeding in or around your gums that is hard to get stopped, or if you see a rash of little pur-plish spots in your skin (petechiae).

Your children will also have to be medicated differently, especially when it comes to vaccines. They should not receive a live virus vaccine for at least one year after your transplant. If they have to have vac-cines, ask the pediatrician to inoculate them with inactivated vaccines. If you have a baby, or your friends have babies and children who have been immunized for polio or chicken pox, you cannot, under any cir-cumstances, be around them for a minimum of eight weeks after your transplant. Avoid people who have contracted measles, pink eye, or colds. If someone has something as simple as a stuffy nose, avoid him/her as well, until it is gone. If you are inadvertently exposed to any contagious diseases, you must contact your doctor immediately.

If the adults in your life have been inoculated with inactivated or killed flu vaccine, it is fine for you to spend time with them. However, if any of them have been inoculated with the flu vaccine that contains a live virus, you cannot be around them at all. Check with your trans-plant doctor to see how long it must be before you can personally interact with them again.

Initially, you will have to restrict going to any places where large numbers of people may gather—the grocery store, malls, movie the-aters, ball games, parks, restaurants, and even the schools your kids attend. If you have to or want to go to these places, wear a mask. Take alcohol swabs to wipe the handles of shopping carts, and around the rims, in case you accidentally touch the rims. You will also have to avoid flying, taking the train or bus for probably a year, unless your doctor feels your body can withstand the potential for contracting a disease. If you go out, avoid the sun as much as possible. Wear a sun-screen protection factor (SPF) of 15 or more, and apply it frequently. Do NOT lie in the sun. Wear a wide-brimmed hat and wear clothing that covers most of your body.

Eat healthy foods. Nutrition is a key component for your recov-ery. Avoid foods with bacteria in them, such as blue cheese. As always, you or your caregivers should wash hands thoroughly before, during and after fixing food. Use one cutting board for meats and one for other fruits and vegetables. (To really clean the meat from a cutting board, take a handful of salt and rub vigorously over the surface; rinse thoroughly.) Leave eggs in the carton in which you purchased them; do not put them in the refrigerator door or the plastic container that comes with your appliance or any other kind of container. Keep your refrigerator at or below 40 degrees F. (4 degrees C.) and your freezer at 0 degrees F. (-18 degrees C.) Use a refrigerator/freezer thermometer to make sure these temperatures are accurate. If you want fruit, cut off the bruised sections. Do not eat fruits that come from vines (strawberries, grapes), as they contain a fungus. Avoid anything with raw eggs (eggnog) or shellfish (crab legs, shrimp, etc.) for at least six months.

You may find your taste buds have changed. What you used to like you no longer do. You may also discover you need to continue eating smaller portions of food many times a day because it is better for your digestion. This is the time to really load up on milkshakes. They will be easy to swallow, contain calcium, and will not cause blisters or sores in your mouth. It might make food taste better if you clean your mouth before eating. You may find eating tart candies such as lemon drops, or even sucking on a lemon, will bring your taste buds back to at least a semi-normal level of flavor intensity. Eating high protein foods is also helpful.

If you have mouth sores, avoid spicy foods for awhile. If you have diarrhea, drink clear fluids for 24 hours or so, then begin to add foods into your diet one at a time to try to determine which ones are causing the problem. Cook or eat food within two days of purchase, or put it in the freezer. Once you have finished eating, refrigerate any leftovers immediately. Throw out any food that has been left in the refrigerator for two or more days. The Food and Drug Administration (FDA) has more tips on the safe handling of food, as well as a chart you can download to help you track freshness dates. Go to http://www. fsis.usda.gov/Fact_Sheets, or call the FDA at 1-800-535-4555.

If you want to go out to eat, avoid salad bars and buffets. Do not share your drinking or eating utensils with anyone, whether you initiate the gesture or your companion does. At home, wash all eating or drinking utensils thoroughly with hot water and detergent; since you will need to avoid the chemicals that can be in dishwashing soaps, always rinse thoroughly as well. But, remember to let someone else do the dishes, at least for the first few months—or years if you can get away with it. Avoid alcohol until your platelets are over the 50,000 mark, and wait until your doctor says it is safe for you to begin to drink—in moderation, of course.

Avoid, totally and completely, any cigarette smoke, pipes, cigars and marijuana. Your respiratory system is also compromised, and you must use extreme caution to take care of it. For at least a year after your stem cell transplant, go only to those restaurants and other places that are totally, completely, you betcha, smoke-free. There are a few enlightened states that now have by law non-smoking restaurants, university campuses and other public facilities. Remember, it can take up to a year for the carcinogens in these places to be completely gone once smoking has stopped.

If you have started construction in your home, see if it can't be postponed until you have recuperated more. If the construction has to go ahead, then avoid those areas and get someone else to thoroughly clean that space for you. Try to avoid chemicals and fumes found in gasoline, fertilizers, cleaning supplies, paints and pesticides. People may want to bring flowers and plants to help you recuperate, but they will have to wait until the doctor gives you his O.K., which may take up to a year. Do not put your hands in soil; do not mow your grass, or pull your weeds. This may also require a year or so before you can do these things again. Do not empty water that has been sitting around outside. Someone else will have to do all these things for you.

Continue your exercise program once you get home and settled. Start slowly, gradually building up both stamina and strength. Don't feel like you have to train for the decathlon or a marathon. Take a year to build up to those kinds of strenuous efforts and even then, only with your doctor's permission. It is better to do short periods of exercise, followed by rest. For most of us, a car is not only a symbol of freedom and a means of independence; it is as necessary as breathing. However, once you are at home, the doctor will want you to wait a bit before you start driving. The reason is that your energy level is low and your reflex time could also be slow. There is even the possibility that some of the medications you are taking could cause drowsiness.

Check with your doctor about when you can safely return to work, and what your schedule should look like. Work with your office and colleagues to let them know what you can and can't do. If you are teaching (done well, teaching is strenuous), you may be able to go back only for half-days for the first few months and then only with a mask (remember, kids are walking germ factories). You may find your stamina, plus your "chemo brain," impacts your memory and ability to put things together in whatever work you do. Take your time and as we said earlier, "**Be patient with yourself.**"

After your stem cell transplant, your doctor will most likely have prescribed a number of medications, such as Acyclovir, which will help prevent infections. Another drug might be Bactrim, which helps prevent a fungal infection in your lungs. Take all medications as prescribed by the doctor, and don't quit until instructed to do so. Avoid aspirin and other over-the-counter pills such as Motrin and Advil; they can irritate the lining in your stomach and decrease the ability of your platelets to recover. Also avoid laxatives, unless prescribed by your doctor. If you are of the Islamic faith, check to see which medications you can and cannot take (some medications use meat products to coat the pills). Do not take vitamin supplements, especially Vitamin A, until you talk with your doctor first. As for flu and pneumonia shots, it is usually better to wait a year after your stem cell transplant before getting them. And remember, your childhood vaccinations will have to be renewed. This will probably be done over a two-year period; the first year after transplant you will get the first round of the vaccinations, and after the second year, you will complete the cycle.

If you have pets who are an important part of your life, for the first month or two, it is better for you to find a safe place for them to stay. You have to be so very careful around pets. You should have them checked for parasites before you arrive home and begin to live in the environment where they were. After the first 60 days or so, you may be able to allow them to come home, with your doctor's approval. Then, wash your hands every time you pet your animals. Avoid mopping their urine or feces. If they lick you, wash wherever they licked right away. <u>Do not clean aquariums, cages or litter boxes; ask someone else to do all pet care cleaning activities for you</u>. This also includes most of the pet grooming activities. Do not get a new pet without checking with your transplant doctor prior to making the investment.

Your emotional recovery from a stem cell transplant is just as important as the physical recovery. For most people, the reason they had to have the stem cell transplant was the very real possibility of dying without one. Facing your mortality, regardless of your age, is a daunting prospect. Beyond that, there is the fear your body will reject the transplant, and the fears of potentially life-threatening infections, osteoporosis, problems with your lungs, being a burden to your family and friends, and not being able to work. These emotions impact not only you, but those around you, as well. Recovery will take time, but it will happen. In a study conducted by lead researcher Karen Syrjala, Ph.D., Fred Hutchinson Cancer Research Hospital in Seattle, Washington, and printed in the *Journal of the American Medical Association*, it was found at about a year after transplant, the physical aspects of the stem cell transplant were easier to overcome than the emotional aspects. A year after transplant, 79% of people were still fearful of rejection (if they had a donor), or a relapse back into cancer. Three years post-transplant, 42% of the study group said they still worried about rejection, relapsing, being a burden, etc. However, by the fifth year post-transplant, only 13% of the study group reported any significant worries. If you feel depressed, it will likely take longer for you to physically, let alone emotionally, recover. Please give yourself the time to recover—it may take as long as five years, or with some people, depending on their age and general physical condition, may be longer. This is normal. If you are really feeling distressed, talk to your doctor about being referred to someone for help. There is no shame in asking for help, in fact, it will be quite brave of you to realize you need emotional support. It may even be helpful to invite your family and friends to participate. Remember—you are not the only one who has cancer; your friends and family are also struggling.

Stress Management

In our fast-paced lives, with all of the pressures to multi-task and be all things to all people at all times, it is no wonder people often feel at loose ends. People who are facing, or who have faced, cancer are also coping with wondering if they will be cured, or if they will go into remission or if the cancer will recur. Even with all the miracles of modern medicine, the diagnosis of cancer can raise anyone's anxiety level to alarming proportions. After all, cancer is still perceived by many people as a death-sentence, and it sometimes is. Negative emotions, or what you may refer to as worries, also contribute to increased stress levels, run rampant during the course of treatment and sometimes, long after. If you experience a recurrence of cancer, those increased stress levels return, even higher this time, and neither subside as quickly, nor as completely, after a second survival.

What is stress? It can be physical, mental or emotional, and is a reaction to the tensions in everyday life. Stress occurs when the demands on our life are greater than the resources we have at hand to meet them. Stress is perceived as challenging, demanding, threatening and exhausting. Stress can also be defined as "responsibility with a lack of control." (Thanks, Mims!) It is frequently characterized physically by an increased heart rate, a rise in blood pressure, muscular tension, irritability, and even depression. Stress can contribute to a greater vulnerability to colds (something cancer and stem cell transplant survivors must avoid until their immune systems are fully functioning), wounds healing more slowly, high cholesterol, heart disease, weight gain, and an increased risk of diabetes due to the lack of sugar control. Clearly, these conditions constitute a state in which no one would choose to remain for any length of time!

Three steps you can take to reduce stress are as follows.

1. Determine why you are stressed. What is there in your environment (perhaps toxins in the workplace) or in your life (arguments? finances? your child going through "the terrible twos" or becoming a teenager)? Are your medications making you "jittery"? Are you feeling angry, resentful, developing ulcers, having difficulty sleeping, have increased your drug, including alcohol, usage, are fearful, or withdrawing from others with whom you would normally enjoy spending your time? These are questions that may help guide you to identify your stressors, if you are able. Sometimes there is more than one factor involved and it will be hard to separate one from the other. Remember, if you cannot identify the stressor, you cannot move on toward alleviating the problem.

2. Try to change your negative attitudes or responses and your automatic skeptical assumptions into positive feelings, thoughts and reactions. Your ideas and thoughts, especially negative ones, often trigger feelings of stress within you that only grow out of control over time.

3. Find a way that works for you to cope with the stress. Do you need more information about the situation? Should you make an appointment with a therapist? Should you talk with your best friend, spiritual advisor or doctor? Can you identify physical activities, such as deep breathing exercises, stretches, etc.,

that assist you in releasing your stress? Whatever your approach, <u>you must find something that allows you to cope with or manage your stressors and your reactions to them</u>.

These stressors cannot be allowed to dictate the aura or life force you exude, because it has been proven there is a positive correlation and strong link between a positive outlook and positive attitudes to sustained cancer recovery.

Caregivers are especially vulnerable to stress. For some, caregiving is a positive, life-changing experience, one they would not trade for anything in the world. For others, it is a burden; they feel trapped by the situation, one that is driven by the alternative of guilt and sense of failure to fulfill expected responsibilities. Caregivers can become exhausted, angry, and fearful, feel that their relationship with the person who has cancer has changed (and not for the better), can worry about the financial aspects of cancer and worry about dealing with the health care system. Caregivers, especially partners/spouses/significant others of the one who has cancer, also tend to suffer more from depression, and an increase in health problems, such as high blood pressure, arthritis and muscle pain. For both the caregiver and the survivor, there is also the decrease in the frequency of contacts with the medical staff members with whom you have become so close while going through cancer treatment. These people, who have been such an important part of your life, who have provided such life-saving care, support and comfort and upon whom you may have begun to depend, are now having to turn their attention to others who are in crisis—just as they had to do with other survivors in order to take care of you. You may find yourself feeling as though you have been abandoned, which will only add to the stress you are already carrying.

For both the cancer survivor and the caregiver, it is essential you take time for yourself, reach out to others now for assistance, search for and find the meaning and purpose in what you have gone through, and keep appointments with doctors, especially for your annual physical. Other strategies for managing stress (or perhaps "coping" is a better word) are yoga, regular exercise, a balanced diet, and, with your physician's approval, taking vitamin B-complex and vitamin C, both of which may be helpful.

Stress and its causes are areas that are currently being studied. There is no question that cancer patients, survivors and caregivers are certainly stressed. In the case of people who need additional help coping with stress, there are a couple of questions that need to be addressed: What form should stress management take and for how long? One-on-one therapy with a licensed practitioner is expensive, and surprisingly, not as effective as something that is self-administered, which can be less than 2/3 of the average cost of a professional. The self-administered types of programs include audio/video tapes and books available from bookstores and libraries, and self-help booklets patients/survivors/caregivers could take home from the offices of their health care provider or social worker. You should be aware there are a few therapists out there who specialize in stress management for people dealing with cancer; your oncologist or his/her office staff people should be able to make appropriate referrals for you.

Sunburn

One of the cancers that is most rapidly increasing is melanoma, or skin cancer. Melanoma has been classified as the most deadly form of skin cancer. It has been reported that if a person has had five or more sunburns in their lifetime, the risk of getting melanoma doubles. If your child or adolescent gets one sunburn, the risk of contracting melanoma later in life is doubled. There are two types of non-melanoma skin cancers: basal cell carcinoma and squamous cell carcinoma. These two are directly correlated with years of sun exposure. These carcinomas usually begin on the face, ears and hands, although they can appear on other parts of the body that are not usually (hopefully) directly exposed to the sun's rays. What normally triggers the melanoma is an intense exposure to the sun that has resulted in a sunburn, accompanied with blisters on the epidermis, followed by peeling of multiple layers of skin.

Teenagers, especially girls, are more prone to use tanning beds without sunscreen in order to "look good." There is some concern now being expressed about tanning booths being "addictive," regardless of the age. Adolescents tend to believe that getting burned in a tanning booth or bed makes it not only better for you when you go out in the sun, but also safer. And where do adolescents get their role models? No surprise here—it is usually from their parents or other important adults in their lives. If the parents model sun bathing or use of a tanning sunlamp, bed or booth, the odds are high their kids will, too. However, data show there is a 74% or 75% greater risk of developing melanoma (the most deadly form of skin cancer) if you started using tanning booths or beds before the age of 30, and if the tanning bed emitted UVA radiation—and most do. Another study demonstrated the use of a tanning bed quadruples your risk of getting melanoma. **Tanning booths and beds are not safe at any age. Period!** There is such a long history of research with documented evidence against the use of tanning beds, sunlamps, and even sun tanning itself, that there are no more questions left as to the link with melanoma—the relationship is causal! So why, then, is melanoma the most rapidly growing form of cancer when we know what causes it? No one believes it will happen to her or him, just to somebody else.

Australia has the highest rate of skin cancers in the world. It is estimated two of every three Australians will develop some form of skin cancer in their lifetimes. Approximately 1,000 Australians die from it every year. (Those from the southern United States and people from Europe who migrate to Israel are also at high risk.) The Australians are embarking on a long-range campaign to cut the use of tanning salons by adolescents. Among the strategies being proposed is to limit the age of people who can use them. Other strategies are to require parental consent for their kids to use the tanning salons, to work with the educational system to promote skin safety, explore other approaches to address attitudes and behaviors, and to even develop codes to specify the amount of shade that must be provided in public parking lots. They are also developing an extensive research base on cancers, particularly skin cancers. Two programs, "Timebomb" and "SunSmart" have been put in place to help address these issues. SunSmart is a program in elementary schools in Victoria where 80% of the children wear hats and must play in the shade. Another program has been adapted for use in the United States by the American Cancer Society. It is called "Slip! Slop! Slap!"—Slip on a shirt, Slop on some sunscreen and Slap a hat on your head to protect your face and skin.

Once you have had treatments that included either chemotherapy, radiation, a stem cell transplant or a combination of these three, you will always and forever have to be careful about how much exposure to the sun you get. This is especially true if you live in or visit the southern half of the United States or other countries where sunshine is the norm. Simply put, you are at an even greater increased risk of myeloma or skin cancers. After Terry's stem cell transplant, when she was finally given the green light to begin mowing again, she had to wear a broad-brimmed hat and long-sleeved shirts. Sunglasses with UV protection are also necessary because of the increased likelihood of cataracts developing more quickly. She wears slacks, not shorts (that was probably the decent thing to do anyhow), and socks and shoes, not sandals. It normally takes three and a half hours to mow the lawn at one sitting. If she was going to only mow half the lawn, then occasionally, she would wear a sleeveless top and remove the hat (the rest of the *haute couture* ensemble remained constant). Sunshine does give us Vitamin D, of which some of us living in the northern climes don't get nearly enough.

Exposure to the sun not only increases the risk of skin cancers, but can also cause cancerous growths, which are usually located in and around the eyes. These tumors are invasive and malignant; they usually attack the thin, membranous skin tissues that protect the eyes. Granted, these are rare occurrences, but carcinoma or melanoma can cause disfigured eyelids, vision loss and, if left untreated, can result in death.

Another condition where cancer cells form in eye tissue is called *intraocular melanoma*. This is the most prevalent form of cancer in the eyes of adults; this cancer attacks the eyeball itself. Intraocular melanoma can be detected during a thorough eye exam, so be sure to visit an optometrist or ophthalmologist every year so that, should any of these conditions be developing, they can be caught as early as possible. Conditions the doctor will look for include a dark spot on the iris (the colored part of your eye), blurred vision, changes in the shape of your pupil and/or any other changes in your vision. If caught early enough, the condition is very treatable. Be sure to wear sunglasses that block 100% of ultraviolet A rays. This is the best way to prevent or delay the onset of any of these cancers involving the eyes. Left untreated, intraocular melanoma can cause glaucoma or blindness.

What follows are some tips that should help you avoid too much exposure to the sun, whether you've had chemo or radiation or not. Seek shade between 10:00 A.M. and 4:00 P.M. every day. Do NOT allow yourself to get sunburned. Use a sunscreen (non-carcinogenic) with an SPF factor of 15 or greater—apply it two hours before going out in the sun, and then every two hours after the first application. Always wear a broad-brimmed hat and sunglasses that block the UV rays. Newborns should be kept *__totally__* out of the sun at all times; babies should also use sunscreen even though they should only be in the shade when they are outside. Below are 2 websites to check out: http://www. skincancer.org/Facts-about-Sunburn-and-Skin-Cancer.html, and for our children: http://www.kidzworld.com/article/1014-too-hot-to-handle-the-sunburn-reality.

Taste

There are four basic types of flavors: sweet, sour, bitter and salty. A receptor for each of the flavor-types is contained in every taste bud in your mouth. About 50% of people who have received chemo say the tastes of foods have changed. It is not known why this happens. The technical name for this is "dysgeusia." Some examples of how your tastes may change include: an intense dislike or a craving for sweet foods; having foods such as Brussels sprouts no longer be palatable; the acid in tomatoes and tomato products producing an awful taste in your mouth; you may lose your appetite for meats altogether, or your mouth may register foods as "metallic" in taste. These changes occur because chemo changes the taste receptors in your mouth. Also, some people lose a lot of weight during and after chemo. This could be the result of simply not feeling like eating, but if it lasts longer than a month after chemo has stopped, go to a dietician or ask your oncologist to see if you have any nutritional deficits. These deficits could also impact your sense of taste. Over time, most people regain their previous sense of taste (and smell), but sometimes, the losses become permanent.

Linda and Terry experienced more of a metallic taste in their mouths all the time. It was hard to cook and season food properly, because it was hard to judge what tasted good and what didn't. For them, sugar and salt lost their taste, or, rather, changed tastes. They weren't sure what the new flavors were, but salt was definitely not salt, and sugar was definitely not sugar. Over time some taste has started to come back, but the taste buds are still impacted. For example, Terry doesn't like the taste of jalapeños (or salsa with jalapeños; salsa without jalapeños is fine) in Mexican food, but now orders Thai food that is medium hot; none of these changes make any sense. She now uses Cayenne pepper or cayenne pepper flakes instead of black pepper whenever possible, which had never been a part of her diet. Previously, she enjoyed a variety of flavored waters, but now only one or two flavors taste good to her, and sometimes not even then. The flavors "catch," as she describes it, in the back of her mouth, making it difficult to swallow sometimes. Thankfully, chocolate still has its flavor—WONDERFUL—Scrumptious—Better than Sex (well, at least close)!

There are only a few ideas we have to offer when food does not taste good to you; feel free to try any of the following ideas, until you find some that work for you. First, we once again strongly suggest: *STOP SMOKING!* Being able to taste your food is just one more reason to do so. Rinse your mouth with a mixture of 1 teaspoon baking soda mixed into 1 quart of room-temperature water before every meal. If food tastes "metallic" to you, use plastic instead of metal cutlery. Try bland foods with little smell that take a short time to fix such as omelets, pancakes, oatmeal, and smoothies. Use tart flavors (lemons, pickles) unless you have sores in your mouth; then use different spices you don't normally use—oregano, rosemary, tarragon—and increase the catsup or mustard you use on food. Marinate fish and poultry in lime or lemon, and other meats in a vinegar-based salad dressing. Check with your doctor to see if you have deficiencies in zinc, copper, nickel, niacin or Vitamin A; if yes, ask which supplements s/he would recommend. You may also find cold or frozen foods taste better than warm or hot foods, since hot foods can have an aroma that smells unpleasant to you; the senses of taste and smell are linked. Brush your teeth often, and use dental floss to prevent bacteria formation, and chew sugar-free gum. Drink decaffeinated tea and ginger ale. Go outside your "comfort zone" in terms of food and try new ethnic dishes. Oh, and, did we say, *STOP SMOKING!*

Thyroid

It is amazing how much the thyroid controls in your body. The thyroid is probably the most important single gland in your whole body. It is the biggest gland in your neck and is shaped sort of like a butterfly. It is located below the Adam's apple in your throat and wrapped around the trachea, sort of where a bow tie would be located. Its primary responsibility is to regulate your body's metabolism (converting oxygen and calories into usable energy) by taking in the iodine found in many foods and then producing thyroid hormones. The thyroid is regulated by the pituitary gland, which in turn is regulated by the hypothalamus, both of which are deep inside the brain. The endocrineweb.com website likens the thyroid to a furnace, the pituitary gland as the thermostat and the hypothalamus as the entity that regulates the thermostat. The thyroid also controls your normal body temperature, heart rate, blood pressure, appetite and digestive system. It is important for muscle and bone development, as well as the functioning of the brain and nervous system, especially in young children. Quite often, thyroid problems are genetic, so know your family medical history. Every cell throughout your body is dependent on your thyroid. For further information, go to: http://www.endocrineweb.com.

If you had either a hypoactive (underactive) or hyperactive (overactive) thyroid before cancer treatment, your thyroid will likely change during chemotherapy and will need some time to get readjusted. You will have to be patient and allow the thyroid to become adjusted at its own pace. If your thyroid was "normal" before cancer, it is likely that tests were given in the course of your normal blood work; these tests were for the purpose of keeping track of your thyroid function. The doctor would be looking for signs of thyroid conditions such as hypothyroidism or hyperthyroidism. It is possible you will be required to have yearly thyroid checks after your cancer treatments end, simply because of the importance of this gland to your bodily functions, as well as to find any growths on the thyroid as quickly as possible before they become malignant. Thyroid nodules and cancer may not show up for years after chemo or radiation has ended. If you have had radiation anywhere near your throat, are female or were treated for cancer at a young age, you are especially at risk for developing thyroid nodules. Having your thyroid tested is critical if you have had Hodgkin's disease. One estimate indicates that 75% of patients diagnosed with Hodgkin's disease and treated with chemotherapy and/or radiation will survive, but are at risk for long-term development of thyroid problems, as well as other serious conditions (cardiovascular disease, scoliosis, and secondary malignancies). If you are a young female and want to have children, check with your primary care physician *before getting pregnant*, because your baby could be born with developmental problems. It is also critical to have thyroid tests during pregnancy, so problems can be detected and treated early. If you do happen to contract thyroid cancer, the good news is that it responds very well to treatment and has about a five-year survival rate of 97%. There are several different types of thyroid cancer, some of which can be treated with surgery, while with others may require more extensive protocols such as radiation and chemotherapy.

Tinnitus (Ringing in the Ears)

After having received chemotherapy, some people experience tinnitus, or what is commonly referred to as ringing in the ears. (For further information, please see the American Tinnitus Association, http://www.ata.org.) The other possible noises you could hear are buzzing, chirping, hissing, humming, tinkling (not when you go to the bathroom!) or roaring. Tinnitus caused by chemo may be ototoxic (damages the inner ear), or it could be a temporary condition. The amount of damage seems to be related to the type of chemotherapy drug(s) administered (such as Arimidex, Cisplatin or Tamoxifen).

Tinnitus is generally caused when the acoustic nerve sends a message to the brain for noises that are not produced by sound waves. What you are hearing is something inside your head or your ears. If the cilia have been damaged, they don't "flow" normally; they are erratic and constantly irritated. Tinnitus is not just one disease, but rather symptoms of underlying conditions. Tinnitus may be found in the outer ear, middle ear, inner ear, or may be because of a brain abnormality. Some tinnitus is normal—at night when it's really quiet (if you live in the country) you might hear some light buzzing in your ear (not related to mosquitoes). If you played in a rock band, shot firearms, used a power saw or a jackhammer without adequate ear protection, you may already have tinnitus. We are surrounded by constant noise in our daily lives—vacuum cleaners running, TVs going, radios blaring, sirens screaming their way to the hospital, iPods plugged into our ears at full blast; over time, this takes its toll on our ears. If you are highly stressed, the tinnitus may be exacerbated. Chemotherapy may aggravate the tinnitus. For example, in addition to the ringing in your ears (or swooshing or other noise), you may be able to hear some frequencies better than others (lower frequencies may be the most difficult to hear; higher pitches may drive you to the edge). Tinnitus can last for as short as two weeks or a month, or may go on for nine months or longer. Your particular personality may determine how well you tolerate tinnitus.

Before you go to an audiologist to evaluate you for tinnitus, ask either your oncologist or regular doctor to check whether you have any wax buildup in your ears. If you don't, and if the tinnitus persists for an exorbitant amount of time, schedule a complete evaluation with an audiologist (be sure to take a list of all medications you have taken before, during and after chemotherapy, including over-the-counter medications and any herbal supplements you may have taken during the same time period). The evaluation may include an auditory brain-stem response, checking if your Eustachian tubes are blocked or staying open too long, if you have mucus in your ears, whether the cilia (hairs inside your ears) have been damaged, or if you have otosclerosis (bone growth in the middle ear). It will also include checking to see whether you have high blood pressure or migraines, whether there is any hearing loss on one side or both, whether that loss is greater in one ear than the other, or if your eardrum has been perforated, all to determine the amount and type of damage that has occurred.

Your treatment will depend entirely on the cause of your tinnitus. It could be as simple as removing wax from your ears, to reducing your sodium intake (salt builds up fluid in your ears), to changing your medications, to eliminating caffeine, alcohol, and nicotine, to using hearing aids. Some research studies have shown, *taken as directed*, gingko bilboa, B vitamins, magnesium, melatonin, and zinc may reduce some tinnitus symptoms. Do NOT self-medicate with these items. Please—check with your doctor first to make sure there is no conflict with the medications you are taking. If the tinnitus has become so severe it impedes your daily life, you may need to learn sign language or how to lip-read. You may also need to ask people to speak slowly and more clearly, but not to shout. Gestures may also help you understand. In the long run, tinnitus may simply be an exercise in patience, because not all treatments work all the time with every person. In the end, you may need to just learn to live with it.

Travel Tips

When you have cancer, and even after you have survived it, you need to carefully consider what you need to do when you travel. If you either have or have had a chronic or acute illness, you need to think ahead before going on a trip to make sure your health will not be jeopardized. The July 10, 2010, *Health Alerts* from Johns Hopkins has some nice tips:

- *Check with your physician(s) first* to make sure you are physically able to make the trip you have planned. If you are planning a long flight, this may increase the risk of blood clots, depending on the medicine(s) you are taking, so make sure you get up frequently and walk. If you are planning on travelling to a different country, make sure there aren't any pre-existing health factors that would put you at additional risk.

- *Develop a "health profile" with your physician(s).* This should include what you are currently being treated for, medications (both generic and brand names) and dosages, the names and phone/fax numbers for your physicians, emergency contact persons and their relationship to you, and photocopies of your identification (passport, insurance card, driver's license, other). If you will be travelling to a country that does not speak your language, try to have this information translated into that country's language. If you are located near a university or there are ethnic organizations in or near your community, there may be people who are capable to help you with the translations. Alternatively, there are two websites where you might find other assistance: Microsoft HealthVault (http://www.health-vault.com) or Google Health (http://www.google.com/health). These two sites have a variety of options (keeping track of your medications, you can put all your medical records at one site, find tools and other devices to allow you to find other medical information) and could come in handy when you are travelling.

- *Include a letter from your physician(s)* detailing your medical condition and your medications, especially if you are taking a prescription that includes usage of a syringe and needle. Also, if you have had any kind of metal implant, a letter from your doctor regarding the implant is a good idea. (Although these letters may seem redundant, they could come in handy when you go through security checkpoints at an airport or other entry locations, such as cruise line ports of call.) Keep all medications in their original labeled bottles or containers. Place all medications, along with the letter, in a clear plastic bag. This should be placed in your carry-on luggage. Make sure you have enough to last the entire trip. Some insurance companies are reluctant to give you a refill on your prescription earlier than would be normal, so be sure to work with them prior to your scheduled leaving date. If some of your medications should be kept cool, travel freezer packs are available. Check with your pharmacy or do an online search (we tried "medical travel freezer packs" and over 300,000 listings came up).

- *If you need to use oxygen, be sure to work with the airline or other carrier before booking your travel destination.* Some carriers prefer you rent their equipment rather than take your own. Even if you bring along empty equipment (such as an oxygen pack or tank), you may be charged an additional fee in order to carry it on board. Also work with the carrier if you need a service dog, walker or wheelchair.

- *Be aware that Medicare will not provide coverage outside the United States.* Partial coverage may be offered by Medigap. Regardless of what type of insurance you carry, check with a representative of that company before booking your trip. Remember to get the person's name you talk to, their telephone number, a fax number if possible, and detailed notes of what you discussed. Even though it's a pain, be sure to read your insurance policy to determine what might be covered should you need medical care and/or hospitalization in another country.

- *If you feel your health insurance is inadequate for travel outside your own country, short-term health insurance is available.* Your travel agent, doctor or pharmacy may be able to help. In the United States, check the Department of State website: http://travel.state.gov/travel/cis_pa_tw/cis/cis_1470html. For traveling anywhere in Europe, check http://goeurope.about.com/od/insurance/Health_and_Travel_Insurance_Companies.htm, and/or http://nriol.net/europe-travel-insurance. Should you want to travel in Asia, check the info at: http://www.travelmedicalinsurance.asia. For any other countries, use a search engine and enter "short-term health insurance" and the name of the country you will be visiting.

- Once you have resolved all the issues listed above, it's time to *research where the hospitals are located for the county/shire, state, city or country you are visiting.* Your physician, friends, travel agent or carrier might also be of help in this area. Make a list of the name(s) of the hospital(s), address(es) and phone number(s) and keep it in the same bag as your medications or other safe, secure location. For international travel, a good resource is the website for the International Association for Medical Assistance to Travelers, http://www.iamat.org.

Thrive, published by the University of Michigan Comprehensive Cancer Center, offers these additional tips:

- *Consider taking along a binder that has all or most of your medical records, especially the most recent or most pertinent.* If you are traveling with someone, let them know where the binder is and what it contains. It may also be a good idea to work with the airline, cruise line or other carrier to let an appropriate person know it is available and where it is kept.

- If you are thinking of traveling to a country that requires shots, *check with your physician to see if any of the required injections conflict with the medications you are taking.* If so, you might have to postpone that trip until you are no longer on those medications.

- *Request a wheelchair if you are flying into a large airport.* Even with moving stairs, it can be exhausting to get from one section of the airport to another, or even getting to the luggage claim area. And remember—at airports, the gates often change, and they are either back at the first place you walked past, or are now at the very end of the airport corridor. You want to save your energy for the place(s) you want to visit. Standing in line is also exhausting.

- Airplanes can also carry some other risks for your health. *Be sure and drink plenty of liquids to stay hydrated while airborne but stay away from anything with caffeine or alcohol.* If your lymph nodes are still swollen, get a compression _garment_ (it's like a stocking) to help prevent/reduce the risk of causing and/or complicating lymphedema. Wearing a compression garment is also easier when going through security. Compression _wrap-_

pings (essentially bandages) make the security people understandably very nervous.

- While you are recuperating is not the time to go on adventures, whether white water rafting or just sampling that roadside food vendor. Almost all people who travel to a different country suffer from some kind of intestinal ailment when they drink foreign water (yes, even people who come to America). *Stick with bottled water* (at home it's a waste of money). *Always carry a hand sanitizer*—either a plastic bottle or the tissue wipes, and *be sure to wash your hands frequently.* The exposure you encounter to bacterial and viral infections in all travel centers poses high risks for you during your recovery when you are so vulnerable.

- *Allow yourself extra time to get to your destination,* whether flying or driving. First, it reduces the stress of the trip. Secondly, if something unforeseen arises (you missed your connecting flight, you have a flat tire, or road construction), you won't have an additional worry. Keep in mind, while you are recovering, you will simply need more time to get from one location to another. Remember, this is still the time to pamper yourself. You don't have to do it all.

Vitamin and Mineral Supplements

Cancer survivors often take vitamins and supplements to try and strengthen their immune system, but, for most, their actual health benefits have not been determined, even for multi-vitamins. A couple websites on this topic come from Science Daily: http://www.sciencedaily .com/releases/2008/02/080201090851.htm, and from the *Bangkok Post*: http://www.bangkokpost.com/news/health/35100/the-pros-and-cons-of-multi-vitamin-supplements.

According to a Science Daily article, 61% to 81% of those surviving cancer take supplements, compared to 50% in the general population. In a study conducted by a cancer institute in the United States, it was found that men who mega-dosed on multivitamins and other supplements increased their risk of getting prostate cancer. Vitamin and supplement usage is generally higher with breast cancer survivors, and lowest with prostate cancer survivors. Increased usage of vitamins and supplements are common with females and those who report a higher level of education. Most doctors are unaware of any vitamins or supplements being used. BIG mistake! Whether you have cancer or not, you should disclose any vitamins and supplements you are taking. Folic acid, beneficial to pregnant women, may actually cause cancer in some people. Beta-carotene (usually found in carrots and other vegetables) has been found to cause lung cancer, particularly in heavy smokers. However, physicians, nurse practitioners, physician assistants and nurses also have the responsibility to ask and to make sure they write it down.

The Mayo Clinic advises that exercising regularly, eating a balanced, nutritious diet, maintaining a healthy weight, and using alcohol in moderation probably help more than the additional supplements. Exercise can be as simple as parking further away from your office or the grocery store, and taking the stairs rather than the elevator, but these efforts are no substitute for a regular exercise routine. Fatigue, a big factor after all treatment has stopped, may mean there will be some days when you can't exercise. That's fine, and you should not feel guilty, but don't make taking breaks from regular exercise a lifestyle pattern, either.

There is increasing evidence indicating exercise can prevent cancer from recurring. In one Finnish study, men who exercised more than 30 minutes a day had a significantly reduced risk of dying from cancer. Another study conducted by the American Cancer Society found that those who report sitting more than others in the study may be at increased risk of death. And as strange as it sounds, the more exercise you do, the less fatigued you will be. Even if further research doesn't bear this out, it is still important for your cardiovascular system. Why add any other problem to all you have been dealing with all ready?

As for a balanced diet, there is no research to indicate that Diet A or Diet B (except a vegetarian diet; see references to the Campbell book, The *China Study*, in the Diet and Nutrition section) will prevent a recurrence of cancer. As a part of your diet, however, it is generally best to eat fruits, vegetables and grains (alcohol does not count as a fruit, vegetable or grain), eliminate the caffeine, and reduce your intake of animal products. Vegans need to be aware they may be failing to get their minimum daily requirements of vitamin B-12, iron, zinc and calcium. In general, people in higher socioeconomic countries are not vitamin or mineral deficient—just look at a side panel of a cereal box to see all the additives, which also includes humungous amounts of sugar or high fructose corn syrup. Always remember and remind others that—CANCER FEEDS ON SUGAR AND HIGH FRUCTOSE CORN SYRUP. There is no difference in the death rate between those who take supplements and those who don't. If you and your doctor decide to add a multi-vitamin or another vitamin, follow the directions carefully. More doesn't mean better and, in some cases, can be detrimental while you are recovering from cancer. If you have questions about what it is that comprises a truly balanced and healthy diet, log onto the national website at: http://www.health.gov/dietaryguidelines.

As mentioned earlier, there are all kinds of products that say they are "all natural," or have "no side effects" or "supports the immune system" or promise the most miraculous results. (Some of the supplements that claim to promote strengthening the immune system actually weaken it.) You also have to be wary of pills that are reported to be the equivalent of real fruits and vegetables. They simply are NOT, regardless of the manufacturers' claims. Our favorite words for these types of supplements are "quack medicines." There is even a website on this: http://www.quackwatch.com. Watch out for the buzzwords like "organic," "stress-reducing," "oxygenation,", or "boosts the immune system." Be especially cautious if you have to buy something in order to find out about the product. Quack medicines account for over $1 billion a year in sales. Notice ads for diet pills—they always recommend you follow a low calorie diet and get lots of exercise. Pills for boosting the immune system almost always say, "Eat a balanced or nutritious diet and get lots of exercise." So why waste your money on diet supplements? The phrase "money back guarantee" is also a frequently used buzzword. If you try to return the product, assuming you even make the effort to do so, then you must follow through with the process, even though it is often lengthy and cumbersome. These places are counting on you NOT to return the product or even make the effort.

The Food and Drug Administration (FDA) does not consider vitamins and supplements as a food or drug, so there are no regulations. The only way the FDA can get involved is if a track record emerges to indicate a product is dangerous. Notice that there is always a disclaimer saying that such-and-such has not been proven to cure, or treat or diagnose an illness. Saying that something is "natural" is not a guarantee, either. After all, there are many "natural" things that are not good for us (ingesting poison ivy is one example). After you survive cancer, you will still most likely be on one or more medications. Some vitamins and supplements will prevent your medications from working properly. For example, if you are taking Coumadin (a blood thinner), you will want to reduce your intake of green and leafy vegetables, which contain vitamin K, a blood-clotting agent. If you are able to take a multi-vitamin, you would need to buy one without Vitamin K.

Weight Gain (Fat Is Where It's At)

Whether we like it or not, being excessively thin (which we don't believe should be a goal, and not just because we can't achieve this!) is promoted many times a day. If you are a tabloid reader, while they decry actresses or models who are wasting away, they also promote it by showing them. Girls, especially, are mentally and psychologically assaulted from an early age to be thin. New cases of bulimia and anorexia are on the rise. And yet ironically, it is highly likely magazine and tabloid publishers have the photographs of the most emaciated celebrities airbrushed to make them appear healthier than they are.

The type of cancer you had and the treatment you received may determine whether you gain or lose weight, and has an impact on the diet you will need to follow once treatment has stopped, in order to either prevent or delay recurrence. For example, prostate cancer survivors run a greater risk of recurrence if they eat foods with high saturated fat content. In addition, since metabolic rates vary from one individual to another, and yours may have changed as a result of your fight with cancer and the medications you were or are still taking, you may have to experiment with different diets to determine which one allows you to meet and sustain your weight goal.

Both of us have had to fight the "Battle of the Bulge" since chemo ended. It is a constant battle. We wage war at breakfast, lunch and dinner. Both of us have gained over twenty pounds since chemo was finished, and we struggle to take off even one pound. We both exercise and watch what we eat, but it's frustrating to not lose the weight. Since both of us have been very, very heavy earlier in our lives, we are not willing to go back to those bodies. At best, we are both healthier. An improved diet and exercise will certainly help so we don't have other health concerns, such as high cholesterol and triglycerides, and so our glucose stays normal . . . but, we don't like the weight, or its distribution. Breast cancer survivors who received chemotherapy are more likely to gain weight in different ways—muscle is lost and fat replaces it; they will normally gain between five to eight pounds over the course of treatment; once again, we are ahead of the curve—"over-achievers" that we are. Melissa, the nurse at the radiation oncologist's office, has become a breast cancer survivor since Terry had her radiation. She is also fighting weight gain and has learned that breast cancer survivors have to decrease their caloric intake by 300 calories a day in order to either take weight off or maintain what you have, especially if you have taken Tamoxifen or have gone/are going through menopause. Yikes! That's one meal! We (Alexis and Terry) are concerned that gaining the weight and not taking it off will increase our risk of developing other cancers as we age, or may even cause our cancers to recur. On the other hand, we must recognize our bodies are still adjusting to the drugs we took in order to save our lives. It can take up to three years (or more for some people) for the chemotherapy to leave your body after it is stopped. So—after the three years, we will have to come up with a whole new set of excuses for not losing the weight . . .

We both do strength-building exercises in the form of hand-held weights. Alexis has to be more cautious because of the risk of developing lymphedema (arm swelling), due to the removal of lymph nodes during her surgery. This helps improve muscle tone, and replaces fat with muscle. It's not helping much on the scales, but is helping in the wardrobe department. What we also have to remember is: we are survivors, we have been through a lot, and until the weight becomes a serious health issue, we should focus on eating properly and getting enough exercise.

Weight gain is common in breast, prostate and ovarian cancer, largely due to the medications taken during and after treatment. Some medications will cause you to retain fluid in your body. If you are experiencing weight gain, try to reduce your intake of salt, and ask your doctor to prescribe a diuretic, if compatible with the medication(s) you are taking during your recovery. If you are interested in referencing some websites that offer more information on weight control issues log onto: http://www.cancer.gov/cancertopics/life-after-treatment/allpages, http://www.acsevents.org/docroot/NWS/content/NWS_2_1x_Breast_Cancer_Weight_Gain.asp, http://caonline.

amcancersoc.org/cgi/content/full/51/3/153, or you can also check out the medical website at: http://www.medicinenet.com/script/main/art. asp?articlekey=18684.

Weight Loss (Thin is *NOT* In)

We recognize there are others who fall at the opposite end of the spectrum, and who have lost too much weight. Men will often say that weight loss and the loss of muscle tone is worse than weight gain. For those who have this problem, we suggest you start with smaller meals several times a day, and focus on foods you really enjoy. If you have lost your taste for your formerly favorite foods, use this as an opportune time to go exploring. What might also help is to go for a walk before eating, to increase your appetite.

Childhood and Cancer

Childhood Cancer and Its Ramifications

One of the most traumatic events in life is to either have a child, or know a child, who has been diagnosed with cancer. For a parent or other relative, and family friends, their whole worlds can cave in, and no option or choice of treatment will go unsought or untried. Somehow, it seems just outrageously unfair that this young, innocent person has this horrid disease invade his/her body. There simply is no rationale or belief system that can be used to ever make childhood cancer seem fair. There is an impotent rage felt by everyone, that this young person may not have the chance to grow up, have children of his/her own or live a "normal" life, that for this child, life's full potential may never be realized. For us, neither is it fair, nor could any reason be offered that would make it right. (And, please, don't even remind us that "Life isn't fair.")

At the outset, let us reinforce that neither of us is an expert in, or had any personal experience with, childhood cancers. What follows should be considered as very basic information, a starting point for you on the subject. We are including the topic to provide you with information we have acquired through our journey, and to offer guidelines for how to formulate questions you may have for doctors, should you ever have the need. And please know, we pray you never do.

A recent study by Weaver, Rowland and Alfano, published in the online journal *Cancer*, June 28, 2010, estimated that in the last two years, 18% of people diagnosed with cancer and 14% of cancer survivors are parents with one or more children living at home under the age of 18. The authors estimate during the past two years, there were in excess of 500,000 children who had a parent beginning cancer treatment for the first time. This is an astounding figure! It becomes even more alarming when the rates are applied to our entire population, yielding approximately 1.5 million cancer survivors and 2.8 million children. This is one huge group of children who are in need of support and financial services. But there is yet another set of children who need even more; these are the children who are diagnosed with cancer themselves.

In "The Childhood Cancer Survivor Study," it states, ". . . more than ten million cancer survivors are alive in the United States (and Canada), at least 270,000 of whom were originally diagnosed when they were under the age of 21." Health defects that arise many years later in life AC, known as "late effects," are the subjects of research by Les Robison, Ph.D., at the St. Jude Children's Research Hospital in Memphis, Tennessee, and funded by the Childhood Cancer Survival Study through the National Cancer Institute.

According to the St. Jude Children's Research Hospital, it is estimated that one of every 350 people in the U.S. develops one form of cancer or another by the time they are 20 years old. Well into the 1950s, few children survived cancer, but in the early 1960s, approaches had been discovered, tested and approved to combine chemotherapy, radiation and surgery for improving the chances of youth survival. These new combinations of treatments increased the survival and remission rates for children, and provided actual cures for some.

Today, more than 80% of children diagnosed with cancer will become long-term survivors, which means having survived five years or longer after treatment, and may be considered "cured" of cancer. That's the good news. That's also the bad news because, as a result of these miraculous treatments, survivors run risks to their health, which must be dealt with for the rest of their lives. This is both an opportunity or challenge and an obligation. The opportunity or challenge lies in acquiring new knowledge to further improve treatment, and to develop strategies to increase survival, improve the quality of life in future decades, and to learn how to minimize harmful side-effects. It's an obligation because survivors, and their parents, siblings, other family members, friends and teachers, need to be educated about the possible risks after having the chemotherapy, radiation and surgery, as well as be provided with the necessary programs needed by survivors. This education must include the prevention and detection of effects that might occur in the future.

It is estimated that today one in 500 young adults who had cancer as child is a survivor of pediatric cancer. This is certainly good news, and is a tribute to the researchers, doctors and other medical staff. As with adults, there are many long-term side effects which can last decades after treatment has ended. Some of these side effects include other secondary cancers. In a study done by researchers in Scandinavia, it has been reported that survivors of childhood cancers have a tendency to develop unrelated second primary cancers *throughout their lives*; this risk increases with age. They also frequently experience problems with fertility, learning difficulties, psychological and/or social and emotional problems, premature menopause in women, stroke and organ dysfunctions related to the types of cancer therapy and treatments administered in childhood. See http://www.cancer.gov/cancertopics/coping/ccss.

The Childhood Cancer Survivor Study found that 13.8% of the five-year survivors who were diagnosed between January 1, 1979 and December 31, 1986, had died by December 31, 2002. The cause of death for 57.5% of these deaths was attributed to cancer that had recurred. Other causes of death were from cardiac, pulmonary or other medical causes. It was estimated the probability of survival for 30 years after diagnosis of cancer was 82%. After 20 years of survival, the death rate caused by a recurrence of cancer exceeded that of all other causes.

In addition, more than 200 chronic health conditions were reported, which included cataracts, hearing loss, and heart and lung conditions. The good news is that these conditions were reported in less than 3% of the survivors. More good news is that "a very small percentage" of survivors were impacted by any one severe or life-threatening condition. Women were at much greater risk than men of having a chronic or life-threatening condition. (See Childhood Cancer Survivor Study, lead author: Kevin C. Oeffinger, MD, Memorial Sloan-Kettering Cancer Center, New York; the *New England Journal of Medicine*, October 12, 2006, and the Massachusetts Medical Society.)

As a result of this study, other data were extracted. A few, very few, other studies are listed below. Many of these articles may be found in either the *Journal of the National Cancer Institute* or the *Journal of Clinical Oncology*. In these journals, other articles related to late-term cancers may also be found. (Since most of us do not readily have access to these journals, the authors are cited below for your reference, should you want to contact them for further information.)

For example, in a study conducted by Paul Nathan, et.al., at the

Hospital for Sick Children in Toronto, Ontario, Canada (see the *Journal of Clinical Oncology*, September 20, 2008), it was found that survivors who were black, older at the re-interview or who were uninsured, were not as likely to have received risk-based or survivor-focused care. However, from the *Journal of Clinical Oncology*, September 20, 2005, those claims had not been found to be entirely accurate, as reported in the study: "Minority adult survivors of childhood cancer: a comparison of long-term outcomes, health care utilization, and health-related behaviors from the childhood cancer survivor study," SM Castellino, et. al., Department of Pediatrics, East Tennessee State University Quillen College of Medicine, St. Jude Children's Research Hospital, Memphis, TN.

Children who develop cancer at a very early age (as early as nine months) may be at special risk. It is estimated that as many as 40% or 50% of children who have been treated for cancer can have negative long-term cognitive effects that impact thinking and learning. They may have very subtle learning difficulties, which may not show up until as late as sixth grade, by which time kids have become experts at hiding, coping with, or compensating for their learning difficulties. This means that tests schools may use for assessment might not be discriminating enough to pick up on problems related to memory, the ability to problem-solve, the ability to focus and pay attention, the processing of visual and/or verbal abilities, or how to put all these functions together in a coherent way. It is likely some form of neuropsychological testing will need to be performed to determine actual skill levels. This assessment would be especially helpful if the child has to have an IEP ("Individualized Education Plan") developed at his/her school. Neuropsychological testing should be conducted (depending on the age at the time of diagnosis) at 18 months to 2 years, at the beginning of Kindergarten, third grade, at the start of middle or junior high school, at the start of high school and after graduation. For further information, you may check the Disabilities Education Act (http://www.idea.ed.gov, and http://www.ada.gov/cguide.htm); you may also refer to the Rehabilitation Act of 1973, Section 504 (http://www.hhs.gov.ocr/504.html, and the federal site, http://www.ed.gov/about/offices/list/ocr/504faq.html) to learn more about your child's rights in school.

In comparison with their siblings, teen survivors of cancer are at greater risk to have symptoms of anxiety or depression, and are more likely to have anti-social behaviors, especially if they previously had leukemia, neuroblastoma or CNS tumors. This age group, in the best of situations, is already a difficult time in the social and emotional realm, but is complicated ten-fold by the disease. Refer to the *Journal of Clinical Oncology*, August 20, 2007, "Behavioral and social outcomes in adolescent survivors of childhood cancer: a report from the childhood cancer survivor study," by KA Schultz, et. al., Department of Pediatrics, University of Minnesota.

Children who are five-year survivors of leukemia and brain tumors, especially if the brain tumors were treated with cranial radiation therapy with doses greater than 30 Gy, are at an increased risk of stroke. See the *Journal of Clinical Oncology*, November 20, 2006, "Late-occurring stroke among long-term survivors of childhood leukemia and brain tumors: a report from the Childhood Cancer Survivor Study," written by DC Bowers, et. al., Department of Pediatrics, from the University of Texas Southwestern Medical School.

In another study, "Survivors of Childhood Brain Tumors: the Potential for Late Effects," conducted by Sara Bottonley at the Texas Children's Cancer Center, children who have survived specifically brain cancer are at high risk for "physical, medical, cognitive and or psychosocial late effects," depending on the age of the child, the type of cancer, location and extent of the brain tumor, or the treatment (surgery, chemotherapy and/or radiation). If the child was an infant or very young when diagnosed and treated, there are higher risks of side effects. What was also interesting was that a very small number of children had inherited rare conditions that predisposed them to potential side effects. Possible (and possibly not) additional long-range effects are: learning disabilities; changes in thyroid, growth and reproductive hormones; fertility (especially brain tumors during puberty); hearing loss; speech delays; tinnitus; altered emotional responses; loss of vision and/or development of cataracts; stroke; and dental concerns such as increased cavities, missing or small teeth, and abnormal growth of the jaw.

The development of other cancers into adulthood has also been noted. These were cancers primarily in the genitourinary system, gastrointestinal tract and head and neck areas. (See *Journal of Clinical Oncology*, January 20, 2006, "Risk of selected subsequent carcinomas in survivors of childhood cancer: a report from the Childhood Cancer Survivor Study," M. Bassal, et. al., Division of Pediatric Hematology/

Oncology/BMT [Bone Marrow Transplant], University of Colorado Health Sciences Center, Denver, CO.) In addition, young women, especially those who have been diagnosed and treated for Hodgkin's disease or lymphoma, and who have had radiation in the chest area, are at increased risk of developing breast cancer 10–20 years later.

A study was also conducted to determine whether race or ethnicity has had any negative impact on long-term childhood cancer survivors. In this report, there were no adverse outcomes for Black or Hispanic childhood cancer survivors compared to whites. The study also reported that Black survivors appeared to have less risky behaviors and practiced better preventive care measures. Hispanic childhood cancer survivors had the same access to cancer-related health care. See the *Journal of Clinical Oncology*, September 20, 2005, "Minority adult survivors of childhood cancer: a comparison of long-term outcomes, health care utilization, and health-related behaviors from the childhood cancer survivor study," SM Castellino, et. al., Department of Pediatrics, East Tennessee State University Quillen College of Medicine, St. Jude Children's Research Hospital, Memphis, TN. For another viewpoint, refer to Paul Nathan, et.al., at the Hospital for Sick Children in Toronto, Ontario, Canada in the *Journal of Clinical Oncology*, September 20, 2008.

One of the concerns for female survivors of childhood cancers is the potential for long-term negative health effects as it relates to reproduction. One study found that among some female survivors, there was an elevated risk for the fetus in that s/he does not grow as well as it should *in utero*, and that there was a higher proportion of premature births. This was especially true for women who had received radiation in their pelvic area. (See "Female survivors of childhood cancer: preterm birth and low birth weight among their children," by Lisa Signorello, et. al., International Epidemiology Institute, Rockville, MD.) Women also face the likelihood of early onset menopause before the age of 40, compared to the average at age 51, especially if they had radiation on the abdominal or pelvic areas, or received chemotherapy treatment with alkylating agents. (See the *Journal of the National Cancer Institute*, October 18, 2006, Charles A. Sklar, MD, et. al., Memorial Sloan-Kettering Cancer Center, New York or the *Journal of the National Cancer Institute,* July 5, 2006.)

While cancer in teens is rare, certain kinds are especially likely to develop. For example, teen-aged girls rarely get breast cancer, but today, boys tend to get more testicular cancer than older men. For your teenage son who contracts the disease (may God protect him from all disease), and who might wish to have children in the future, it is worth exploring how to store his semen **BEFORE** treatments start.

Leukemia is one of the most prevalent of childhood cancers. Leukemia enters the bone marrow and can travel to the bloodstream. Leukemia can cause bleeding, anemia, bone pain and infections. If it metastasizes, it can impact the lymph nodes, liver, spleen, brain and testicles. Treatments usually include chemotherapy, radiation and stem cell transplants.

Osteosarcoma, or bone cancer, sometimes appears during the growth stages that occur during the teenage years. It affects twice as many girls as it does boys, and seems to be in people who are taller than average. The most common symptoms are pain and swelling in a limb, an arm or leg, and may be accompanied by a lump. Treatment ranges from chemotherapy to surgical amputation, which is only performed to prevent further spread of the cancer. Sometimes treatment involves removing only the portion of the bone that is affected, accompanied by the insertion of a metal rod to take the place of that bone.

Ewing's Sarcoma primarily affects teens and young adults; it is usually found in the leg or hip, in the pelvic area. This type of malignancy generally responds well to chemotherapy and radiation. Both Ewing's Sarcoma and osteosarcoma normally respond well to treatment, and are usually curable.

Brain cancer is not frequently found in teens, but there are two types that occur most often. The first is called *astrocytomas,* which originates from cells in the brain; it usually does not spread outside the brain or spinal column, and usually doesn't affect other organs. The second type of brain cancer is called *ependymomas,* which usually begins in the lining of the four brain ventricles or cavities; these ventricles are the pathways for the fluid that cushions the brain and spine to protect them from trauma. There is no known cause for this type of cancer; treatment for ependymomas may include surgery to remove the tumor, if possible, which will be followed by chemotherapy and radiation. Depending on the size and location of the tumor, there is also a high likelihood of being cured.

Lymphoma develops within the lymph system, which includes lymph nodes, thymus, spleen, adenoids, tonsils and bone marrow. There are two types: *Hodgkin's* and *non-Hodgkin's*. Hodgkin's can appear in adolescents and young adults. Chemotherapy and radiation are used to treat Hodgkin's. Non-Hodgkin's lymphoma, which is similar to leukemia, is usually treated just using chemotherapy; radiation is not generally needed. Again, the chances for being cured are excellent.

Other cancers teens can get are *testicular cancer,* which *only occurs very rarely*, or *rhabdomyosarcomas*. Testicular cancer is most common in men ages 15–35. It is almost always completely curable, **when caught early.** Rhabdomyosarcomas are soft tissue cancers that are rare, and primarily occur in infants, young children and teenagers. The malignancies usually develop in the skeletal muscles of the trunk, arms or legs. Types of treatments and cure-rates depend on where the tumors are, and whether they have metastasized or not.

As noted by Philip M. Rosoff, MD, Duke University School of Medicine, long-term follow-up health care is not usually the norm for childhood survivors of cancer. After cancer, children (if they have health insurance) are mostly referred back to their pediatricians, their family doctor or another type of physician who has not had training in post-oncological issues. This means that while these other doctors have great knowledge and experience, great compassion, concern and empathy for their patients, they have simply not had any training in what these kids have gone through and what it might mean for their future health concerns. The other problem is that for the lay person, whether parent, grandparent, aunt, uncle, friend or next-door neighbor, the medical field changes daily (hooray), and it's difficult to stay current in terms of "right now" treatment, and what has to occur in the future. Many of the research articles are not "user friendly" for the typical parent to pick up and read—simply because they are overwhelmed with facing what their child is going through, and not because of any intellectual constraint.

A new Childhood Cancer Survival Study, covering the years from 1987–1999, is being conducted to determine whether the advances in diagnosis and treatment, as well as life-style choices (such as smoking and obesity), have had any affect in survival statistics. The previous group (1979–1986) will also continue to be monitored, to see what impact aging has on their future health concerns.

If your child has cancer, ask for a child life specialist, even after the cancer has been brought into remission. For example, the Child Life Program at the University of Michigan offers help to work first of all, with the family, especially siblings, once your child has been diagnosed. The staff will also work with the school to help with the transition back into academics. Two people who work with the Child Life Program are Sheila Morris and Jenni Gretzema (Ms. Gretzema also uses Art Therapy).

The first hurdle comes with the siblings of the child who has cancer. Often the sibling becomes angry and confused, and perhaps somewhat frightened, about all the attention and time being given to your "sick" child. Then the sibling's emotions may begin to be expressed through a behavioral transformation from his/her normal appropriate actions, into a prevalence of inappropriate acting-out types of actions, both at school and at home. The sibling may further exhibit the troubled emotions through the failure on his/her part to perform at his/her normal academic levels in school. The Child Life staff will work with the whole family during this phase, not only at home, but also at school, and will work with the teachers and administrator.

When it's time for your child to go back to school, the Child Life staff helps to make the transition from being a cancer patient, back into being a student in the classroom. The staff at the Child Life Program will work with teachers and students to help them understand what your child has been experiencing while undergoing treatment for cancer, and to learn how the school can assist in the transition.

Another hurdle children who have had cancer face is the extended absence from peers and homework. While school districts may provide homebound services, it's often difficult for students who are ill to focus and keep up with the schoolwork. Coming back to school, with its schedule, academic pressures, fast pace and the important social task of rebuilding friendships, can be overwhelming for any child. If the child survivor has experienced disfigurement in any way, such as an inordinate weight gain or loss, or hair loss, even if both are temporary, or perhaps a missing body part, from a surgery, chemo and other drugs used in treatment, s/he may have developed a heightened sensitivity about his/her self-image. The condition may also lead to a depressed level of self-esteem. Additional concerns are related to the factors around "chemo brain." For an unknown period of time, the child will have great difficulty in remembering even the simplest of things. The ability to concentrate may also be problematic. The school mates will have so much energy, particularly in high school or middle school in going from class to class, and the survivor will struggle, just managing to get from place to place in his/her own time. The child should be afforded great patience and understanding, and allowed to work at his/her own pace and level for an indefinite number of weeks. Another option is to let the child leave his/her class a couple of minutes early in order to not have to deal with the crush of students in the halls.

Often several meetings take place between school staff, the student and his/her peers, the parent(s) and the Child Life staff. These meetings may include any one or all of the parties with Child Life staff. Information disseminated might include: the type of cancer, the treatment received, current side effects and limitations, how to control for infection, what to do if the student isn't feeling well, realistic expectations for academics, and any accommodations the child might need, such as extra time on tests and adjusting teaching styles. This is especially critical for high school or middle school students. Both the student and parents are encouraged to be advocates for themselves, and to be part of a real team effort to help the student be as successful as possible. In elementary schools, hands-on materials, such as dolls and vinyl bones, are often used to explain what has happened. For further information, contact the Cancer Center Child Life Program at the University of Michigan Cancer Center: http://www.mcancer.org.

How to Talk With Children About Cancer

First of all, Terry wishes she had known some of this information before meeting with Tom's adult children, in order to help them help the grandchildren. Alexis, being in the medical field, had more knowledge beforehand, and could help Calen. Secondly, every child is different; their levels of understanding will vary by age and perceptiveness. Calen (a.k.a. "Pea") was only six when Alexis was diagnosed with cancer, but you could talk with her like a young adult because of her perceptiveness (and, let's face it, innate intelligence). Niece/sister-in-law Monica, in her 30s, had a much more difficult time handling our diagnoses. She was older, she had had more life experiences than a child, and because of her intelligence, knew what a lot of the ramifications could be, and therefore could ask many more questions immediately. (Sorry, Monica, we know you aren't a child, but it was a good example to try to explain about differences when it comes to the age of the person to whom you are talking.) And being an adult, Monica would rebound much more quickly, and knew when and how to help. As mentioned earlier, Calen also stepped up to the plate in short order, and almost mothered her mother. What follows below are some general guidelines, which should be tailored to your individual child or children. If any of the suggestions feel strange, fearful or uncomfortable for you, there are many qualified therapists and social workers who can help you find more appropriate approaches for your particular situations. We urge you to reach out for any kind of help you may need.

It is natural for adults to want to protect children from all the pains and woes of the world; this is especially true when you have to tell your child that someone they love and are close to has a serious illness. But kids have built-in radar that can discern lies, sense subterfuge, and know when you are trying to hide something or keep a secret. Kids can quickly feel the change in the atmosphere in your home; they will notice things that are out of their normal routines— excess doctors' appointments, "tests," adults whispering or shutting off conversations as soon as the child walks into the room. Kids will pick up on bits and pieces of information, which are sometimes misinterpreted. Or they will hear things "in the street" or see and hear things on TV, which can also convey false information. Kids have vivid imaginations and will fill in the "gaps" with scenarios that may not reflect the reality at all. Kids worry. A Truism:

> *"The Fear of what may be, or of what can be imagined,*
> *is far worse than knowing what is; fear is debilitating*
> *. . . truth is freeing and motivating."*

First and foremost—be as open and honest as you can, or should be. This does not mean you proclaim, "I HAVE CANCER AND I'M GOING TO DIE!" or "YOUR SISTER HAS CANCER AND IS GOING TO DIE!" or "YOU HAVE CANCER AND YOU'RE GOING TO DIE!" Depending on the child, you may need to break the news gradually, a little at a time, and as they begin to show understanding of what you are telling them, bring in more details. Uncertainty is harder for children to deal with, as it is for adults, and makes it harder for anyone to cope with any situation. As a part of that honesty, if you don't know something, say you don't know, but that you will try to find the answer for them. Not telling your children the truth about your illness (or theirs or their sibling's) could erode their trust in you far into the future.

Children feel the whole world revolves around them. If you are the one who has cancer, it may be that your children will feel it is their fault you are sick, thinking something they said or did made you get sick. They can keep this guilt and fear a secret for a long time before they will talk to you about it. You should reassure them in your initial honest talk that this is just something that has happened, that NO ONE is to blame (unless you were/are a smoker, or are obese and have had a poor diet all your life; then you could say some of the choices you made in your life helped to create this illness within you; if they ask what choices, tell them—you have a real opportunity to teach and to help them NOT to "do as you did").

Step 1: You know your child better than anyone. You are their parent, teacher, guidance counselor, spiritual adviser, occasional friend, and occasional disciplinarian; you are everything to your kids. You know their capabilities and their limits. You have given your love, your time, your total effort and energy into and for these children. When getting ready to talk to them about either your cancer, their cancer, or someone else's cancer, think through and rehearse what you are going to say and when you are going to say it. For example, during the time your child is getting to do something special, or when s/he is deep into a video game, or when s/he is tired, are probably not good times to talk about it. If necessary, rehearse with a close friend or talk with a member of your health care team. It is not only the words that are important, it is also the feelings with which you say them and what your body language is telescoping. Remember, kids have built-in radar, and it can zoom in like a laser beam to pick up all of your unspoken words and feelings.

Step 2: Take your time. Go through things step by step. Monitor for understanding and ask periodically if s/he has any questions. Keep track of your child's emotions and his/her body language. They will signal you when they have had enough, and don't want to talk about it anymore. You can resume either the next day, or the next time s/he asks a question about the subject. Let them take the lead on further conversations, unless the timing for activities related to the disease is eminent, and you need to explain something more quickly than comes naturally. Try NOT to let critical issues become last minute discussions.

Step 3: No matter how difficult it is, be as calm and optimistic as you possibly can. Your calmness will help children not be as frightened as they would be if you somehow let it show that you are upset or worried. Remember, your attitude will tell them, without words, what attitude they should adopt about the whole thing. Be the model of how they should be, NOT of what you are feeling inside. This may seem as though you are acting, or not really being honest. But this is an honorable and purposeful honesty that will serve both of you; as you help your child, you will also be helping yourself develop the "survivor's attitude." Be prepared for your kids to be hugely shocked no matter how calmly you tell them. Tears and fears may still be present, regardless of the age(s). And be very careful NOT to over-promise. Both you and your children, and your families and your friends, will all share many challenges and surprises during the course of the cancer treatments and ultimate **RECOVERY**. Can you see it? The power of positive thinking is working again to bring forth yet another survivor. A Truism:

> *"Imagine your child as you want him or her to be in five years; let that vision focus your every step, until it becomes reality."*

Step 4: Regardless of how strongly you believe you are the supermom or superdad or supergrandma or superfriend, LET OTHERS actively help you, including your children, grandchildren, friends and neighbors. People, especially your kids and grandkids, even your friends' kids and neighborhood kids, want to be of help in some way. Learn to say, "Yes, thank you." You don't have to, nor should you, do everything. On the other hand, try not to feel upset if your kids or grandkids don't want to help on a particular day. They are also going through this transitional phase. You may (will) see an increase in "naughty" behavior as they work their way through their own feelings, including fear.

Step 5: Keep the channels of communication open regardless of the age of your children, whether they are 6 or 60. You must make your own health a priority (or the health of your child), but your children and your grandchildren, your nieces, nephews, and children of close friends, all still need you. Being able to talk with you may be the only time they can feel comfortable enough to say what they really think and feel. It is a difficult role for you to assume at best, but you will be afforded the opportunity to <u>empower them to feel heard, understood and reassured that they matter</u> in this whole scary situation.

Step 6: Notify the school your child attends about the situation at home. Tell them what you have told your child and what other information you want anyone else to have. Also ask the teacher to let you know if s/he sees any behavior changes in your child. Sometimes children withdraw when they're upset, and sometimes they "act out" to relieve their own tension and fears.

Children under the age of three or four really don't understand "cancer" or any illness, but you can and should use the word. They simply need to know what is going on at any particular moment in time, and in simple words they can understand. Explain that you (or your child) might be away in the hospital for a few days, but that an aunt, uncle, grandparent or other known, trusted person will be there to take care of them. Parents need to ask if there was a word their child didn't understand, or a word that made them feel fearful. It may take a lot of children, regardless of age, time to think through what they have been told. Most children of this age won't remember, and will need repeated explanations. This is especially true if you will be visiting someone who has had, for example, a mastectomy, and who won't be able to hold the child as closely to him/her as they usually do. You may need to explain to them that in order for you (or your child) to get all better, you will have to take a lot of medications, like when s/he has a cold. Be sure you forewarn them of the times when you (or their sibling) may not feel like playing with them as you normally do; then assure them you will be playing again just as soon as you can. Another issue to consider is that, although you are the parent, you may not feel comfortable talking with your child about this. Should that be the case for you, ask yourself who the adult is in your child's life to whom s/he is the closest, who is trusted and with whom s/he already has established a good relationship? An aunt? An uncle? A grandparent? A neighbor? A teacher? Be sure to first check with the person you choose, to make sure s/he feels equipped to take on this role and is comfortable talking with your child about this subject. And then, go through steps 1 and 2 with them.

As children get older, you can give them more details, even showing them pictures of what your cancer looks like, but again, use the KISS method: Keep It Short and Simple. One of the most important things is to keep the channels of communication open. Listen to their concerns. If they are struggling to find words to express their feelings, give them some words that might help: scared, angry, sad, unsure. Assure them no matter what, the love between you and them will always be there, and that you are willing to listen to them at any time and talk about things that may be bothering them, or just anything else they may want to talk about. Sometimes children find it easier to express themselves through drawing or puppets; older children might prefer to write poetry (don't be concerned if the lines don't rhyme). For this age of child, you can explain that cancer is not contagious. You can still hug and kiss, and they will be safe and will not get cancer.

Explain that their routines may change, but that you will try to make any changes be as little as possible. The next door neighbor may take them to school. Dad may be the one taking them to their games. You can also tell them in simple terms that you might be sick in certain ways—you might be too tired to play. Your hair may fall out, but it will grow back—and maybe even in a cooler color with lots of curls. If your kids are embarrassed about your loss of hair and they don't want their friends to see you like that, you can promise them you will either wear a wig or a stylish hat. It is especially important for children of all ages to have their teachers told what is happening. Behavioral problems may crop up both at home and at school. Kids may have greater difficulty doing what is expected of them, like their homework or their chores, while they are adjusting to this change in their lives. Patience is the key for them, and for you!

Teenagers may have the hardest time coping with this type of news. First of all, they are going through their own set of body and emotional changes—and their hormones are raging. They are also going through the normal peer pressures, the need to spend more time with their peers, more time listening to their peers than their parents, asserting their independence, withdrawing from the family in order to be "grown up"—and along comes this disease from out of nowhere, upsetting their relationships with their friends. All of a sudden, they don't have a life of their own; they face having to think of someone other than themselves. They might feel they have to stay home and take care of you. They might create a distance between you while they are sorting out their feelings. They might feel guilty about their anger and build up even more resentment toward you. And they might have tons of questions. And thanks to the Internet, they may even do some research at school or on the computer at home. If they do, make sure you ask about it, so you can try to make sure they aren't getting false information. There is a ton of garbage and sites with misinformation on the web; you may want to help them learn how to identify valid, responsible sites. Yes, sometimes your teenagers do need to stay at home and help. That won't hurt them at all in the long run, although in the short run, some kids may really develop an "attitude" about it. What usually turns that around is how much support their peers will give your child for being so much help. Once the peers tell your child how great s/he is for taking on so much responsibility, your teen will start to feel important and then might actually start to help with minimal resentment. And it is NOT altogether unrealistic that this could become a truly life-changing, life-inspiring time for your teenager. Some teens have gone through this and decided to become doctors or researchers or other health care professionals just to be able to help others. Compassion is one trait that can be developed out of this experience, one that may be internalized, and carried with them into their adult lives. A Truism:

> *"It happens sometimes that, from out of the darkness,*
> *a ray of light emerges to light our passage onward."*

Another positive outcome that could possibly come from this experience is that, if a particular form of cancer, such as breast cancer, for example, runs in your family, you will have been given the opportunity to talk with your daughter about it (and also your son; males also get breast cancer), and perhaps, have some testing done to see if she carries a genetic marker for the disease. This information could prove to bring about one of the most positive outcomes possible. After all, **early detection does save lives!** You will have played a life-saving role for your daughter and/or a niece and/or someone else, who may just have heard of your case. Now, can you see how your having had cancer can contribute to fulfilling the greatest of purposes, and turn out to be a gift in disguise? A Truism:

> *"This gift of my life is not intended to be squandered upon me alone."*

Once again, from darkness to the light . . . the good that may come from your walk with cancer is boundless.

It bears repeating that helping children (and you) talk about their feelings is of the utmost importance. Cancer*care* for Kids® recommends you help your children learn that there are no wrong feelings. Emphasize that what they are feeling is normal, and is **okay**. Tell them they might feel one way today and one way tomorrow, and that you, too, are experiencing your own feelings, and a wide range of emotions that are continually changing. Knowing you share these feelings can bring you even closer together.

You may have a child of any age for whom talking about the issues involved with cancer are just not within his/her realm of understanding. You may need to seek the assistance of your physician, spiritual advisor, or even school staff to help you find new and different approaches to make the connections you need. If your child has a learning disability with which you may need special help, you might want to check: http://www.cancercare.org/get_help/special_progs/advanced_cancer.php. There is also a book entitled *Getting on with Cancer*, by Veronica Donaghey, Jane Bernal, Irene Tuffney-Wijne and Sheila Hollins.

To the extent possible, keep your children's lives as close to normal and as routine as you can. This is especially true if you will be experiencing any physical changes (loss of hair, weight gain) or having additional people in your home to help care for you. And yet, they also need to be included in the cancer treatment. Depending on the age of the child(ren), they may want to go to the location where you receive treatment and ask questions of the doctors and nurses. They may feel more comfortable talking with a stranger about their fears and feelings than talking to you about them, simply because you are too close. This way, if there has to be a change in their routine or normal life, it won't be as big a shock as it might have been. While kids complain about rules and question what is being asked of them ("Why do I have to make my bed?" "Why do I have to take my dinner plate to the sink?"), and question regular routines, since nothing else is as it was before ("Why do I have to go to bed at 9:00?" "Why do I have to do my homework before watching TV?"), they actually need those rules and routines to feel safe and secure, more now than other times in their lives. These expectations help to maintain a sense of normalcy during the chaos and emotional upheaval that can accompany cancer. And it's also O.K. to ask your children to be on their best behavior, and to take on more responsibility by helping with the house and each other.

One of the biggest fears people have when they have had cancer is: Will it return? And sometimes it does. That is termed "advanced" or "recurrent" cancer. The most notable example of someone with recurrent breast cancer was Elizabeth Edwards, who has since passed away. What an inspiration she was for many people, as well as for her children. Initially, she was an example of "'incurable' isn't necessarily 'untreatable'" (Tom is also an inspiration in this regard). There are treatments that can slow cancer's advance, and still let you have a fairly decent quality of life.

If your cancer recurs, you will have to have a different kind of conversation with your children. Again, the age and perceptiveness of the child will have a great bearing on what you say and do. And of course, honesty is the best way to approach it, but this time you may need to focus on feelings, theirs, as well as yours. Depending on whether you have weeks or months or years as a prognosis, this can give you and your children a chance to make financial and future care decisions. It may also give all of you a chance to decide how you want to spend your time. In the case of a great-grandfather, he may want to spend that time doing more fishing with his great-grandchildren. A grandfather may want to take his grandchildren hunting or hiking. A grandmother may want to talk about her youth and heritage, or spend more time reading to her younger grandkids. A father or mother may want to pass down more family history or a shared craft or hobby, or even do the travelling they thought they would always do—tomorrow, next summer. If you are the caregiver of a person with more advanced cancer, you will have to become a master at juggling even more responsibilities, while at the same time making sure the children don't get lost in the process.

A few resources that might help include the following:

- http://www.cancercare.org/get_help/
- http://www.community.cancercare.org/Page.aspx?pid=647
- http: www.kidscancercare.ab.ca/
- *When a Parent Has Cancer: A Guide to Caring for Your Children*, Wendy Harpham, Harper Collins.
- *The Paper Chain*, Claire Blake, Eliza Blanchard, Kathy Parkinson; Health Press.

With the recurrence of your cancer, it may have become more advanced. When you talk with your child(ren), your conversations will need to focus on these changes to help them understand what is happening and to help them deal with their feelings. This may also signal a time when professional help is sought to help the family through the next phases. Somehow you have to find what "hope" means to you, and what it might be for your kids. Hope will now have to be redefined. Your medical treatment will definitely change; one of the major decisions you will face is: do I continue receiving treatment or is this the time to let go? The situation may even require a discussion of the big "D": the dreaded death discussion will obligate you to be at your very, very best, at a time when you may not have come to terms with the reality yourself. Embrace your strength and hold it steadfast, while keeping your wits about you in the realization that the well-chosen words you select this day will resound in your child's mind for the rest of his/her life (not to put any pressure on you—just had to lighten the moment a bit).

Depending on the age of your child(ren), they may want to have input into your decisions. They will have to mature quickly and develop coping mechanisms. The replacement of the focus on them is equally true if you are the caregiver. Given that the caregiver now has more and more responsibilities, the care of the child(ren) will take on greater meaning and emphasis. Talking with them, helping the communication stay open and making that communication a priority will be the hardest thing you will ever have to do. You will have to develop the ability to skillfully hide your own emotions and struggles with the loss of one you love, all for the greater good in assuring that these young lives come through this experience as "whole" and with as few scars as possible. You will need to reassure the child(ren) many times that **they will be taken care of,** they are **NOT** going to be abandoned, and their needs and feelings are vitally important. The following section offers more specific ideas for effectively carrying out these discussions. A few resources that may help you and your child are:

- http://www.cancerhelp.org.uk
- http://www.breastcancercare.org.uk
- http://www.macmillan.org.uk
- http://www.winstonswish.org.uk
- http://www.mariecurie.org.uk
- National Cancer Institute—*When Someone in Your Family Has Cancer*, http://www.cancer.gov/
- http://www.askkids.com/resource/Talking-about-Cancer-with-Children.html
- Kimmie Cares dolls: these dolls show actual ways for children to see how cancer treatment can affect a person and a person's appearance. They come in several ethnicities and come with an illustrated book. http://www.kimmiecares.com

Talking With Children About Death

Death is the BIG unmentionable, even among adults. And yet, it is inescapably the only way we will end our lives. In some cultures, discussing death is even a bigger taboo than discussing **sex**. Death can be (is) devastating, even after a long, painful battle with cancer. Even with the sense of relief a person may feel when someone they love is no longer suffering, death can still come as a surprise, a horrible shock. It leaves you with a numbness, a sense of unreality, a horrible sense of loss, an empty, gaping chasm in your life, like a part of you is missing and gone forever. If this was a particularly important person in your life, you may now feel directionless and lost in your own sorrow. While you are trying to deal with your own grief, your own mourning, you may also have children to take care of, and help through their grieving processes, and none of you will be doing so in the same manner.

This is a field in which we both felt we needed more guidance. We are both fortunate to not yet have had this experience personally, but for purposes of writing this book, death clearly had a big hole in our knowledge base. A website we found helpful was one for an organization named SheKnows; it is at: http://www.sheknows.com/articles/

804653/how-to-talk-to-your-kids-about-death. Dr. Mia Gregor is a clinical psychologist with The Center for Personal Development in Chicago, Illinois. Some of her insights and recommendations are included in the following discussion. There are also other websites on the Internet, which could be equally helpful. As with other pieces of this book, we encourage you to talk with your oncologist, pediatrician or spiritual advisor, either instead of, or along with, using the Internet. We also found "How to Talk to Your Kids about Death," by Rabbi Earl Grollman, helpful. While this website may seem to have a Jewish focus, there are several pieces applicable to people of any other ethnic or religious group: http://www.interfaithfamily.com/life_cycle/death _and_mourning/How_to_Talk_to_Your_Kids_about_Death.shtml.

If a death is approaching, hopefully there will be time to talk to the children before the person actually passes away. Time will give the child an opportunity to prepare for the impending death. As Rabbi Grollman suggests, it is not necessary to refer directly to the person at first, but rather to approach it as a change and growth. Depending on what the child is familiar with, you may want to draw correlations with: tadpole to frog, leaves in the spring replacing the ones that left in the fall. When things are alive, they have movement. After they die, there is stillness and quiet. The death of a pet can also be used to open up a discussion about the circle of life, and how much joy and sorrow are a part of life. Rabbi Grollman cites a Yiddish proverb: "Not to have had pain is not to have been human." In addition, children are surrounded by death every day, whether on TV or in music. These remote experiences could also be used as springboards into a discussion about death.

As Dr. Gregor points out, children will grieve very differently than adults. As kids grow and develop, their emotions will also develop and expand. This means they may go back to previous feelings and emotions they had felt with the death of someone else they loved. Most children will not have had enough experience in their lives to fully comprehend death or its finality. What they are feeling and their emotions may not be mirrored in the adults surrounding them, and they may wonder why and become disturbed, thinking they are not feeling as expected by the adults in their lives. Children may then exhibit inappropriate behaviors, because they believe acting out to be their only means of expressing the frustration they feel for what they do not and cannot fully understand. Depending on their ages, kids may either still talk about the person in the present tense as if s/he is still alive, and/or still hold hope the person will somehow return. Even so, please address these issues very carefully, with professional help, if needed. Depending on the age of the child, you may want to play with your child, or do art or music together in order to help them deal with their emotions. You might also need to give your child permission to be happy; let them know it's okay to laugh and play and have fun.

In American culture, for the most part, death is an unmentionable. It is hard for most of us to understand or accept that death is a natural, normal process—that it is an inevitable part of the life cycle. In seeking to understand in their two-dimensional, cause-and-effect world, children may internalize the death, and determine the death obviously must have been their fault. This guilt can have its roots in something as simple as not having done what they were told to do when something bad happened. This kind of thinking adds guilt to an already over-whelmed child, who does not understand the feelings s/he has, and does not have enough life experiences to know that over time, these feelings will get better. Coping skills will be learned, along with the growing up process. Most children will not understand death as "final" until they reach between seven to ten years of age. As mentioned earlier, children need stability in their lives; they need routines in order to feel safe and secure. With a death, parents and other adults that surround the child are now dealing with emotional responses that are strange to the child. And if the adults in a child's life, as a function of coping with their own grief, begin to isolate, to withdraw, or to build—what to the child may appear as—a wall, a child's sense of security will be torn apart. Reversion to inappropriate, infantile behaviors from early childhood may be manifested as a means of coping and expressing their lost state; such behaviors as thumbsucking, bedwetting, or needing a parent or other trusted adult or sibling to sleep with them might be manifested. Older children attempt to cope and express themselves by being angry, acting out, or deliberately causing problems at school and at home. If these behaviors are exhibited frequently, tell your child such behaviors are totally unacceptable, and then either refer him/her to a grief counselor, or help him/her develop more effective coping skills. Be sure to include asking if there is something bothering the child s/he would like to talk with you about.

What about funerals? Should children go or not? There is research to suggest that funerals can actually help a child cope with the loss of someone they love. The rituals and ceremonies that accompany death and dying, whether through organized religion or something you create yourself to celebrate the life of the person who died, can help children with their grieving. If s/he is going to attend any of the services, and you may be required to be a particular place away from your child, be sure to make certain someone very close to your child will be beside him/her throughout the occasion. If the child is old enough, allow him/her to decide whether s/he wants to attend the funeral, view the body, only attend the gravesite ceremony, or not go at all. On your child's behalf, it is important for you to assure there will be neither exclusion from, nor pressured inclusion in, any of the memorial activities.

Parents or another trusted adult need to prepare the child for what is going to happen at the funeral. In *Dead by Sunset*, by Ann Rule, the mother of three little boys, all under the age of six, is murdered. The father in the story takes the three little boys to the cemetery where their mother has been buried. He gives them no preparation, only explaining that their mother has died. When the little boys get to the cemetery and see where their mother is buried, the oldest child wonders how she will breathe. As part of the preparation for a funeral, children should be told there will be many sad people at the service, probably some crying, and that there will be a body viewing (if that is to happen). If your child does not want to see the body, don't force him/her to do so. If your child asks questions, once again, answer them as honestly as possible and do so in a clear, calm, age-appropriate way. The younger the child, the simpler the explanations have to be. If you don't know the answer to his/her question, tell him/her you don't know, but will try to find someone who can answer that question. In order to help your child deal with his or her emotions, you also have to be honest about yours. "I am sad today because my weekly breakfasts with (mom, dad, friend) will no longer take place." You are, just like for all of life's experiences, the role model for your children. How you handle the death will either help or harm your child in how s/he is able to cope with the experience and the grief to follow. A Truism:

> *"Challenging responsibilities make of us more than we ever thought we could be."*

It is almost always better to tell the truth—mom/dad/grandpa has died; do not say that he or she is "sleeping" or "has gone away for a rest." Very young children will take this literally, and wonder why the person hasn't gotten up yet or had enough rest. If you tell them that Grandpa is on a long journey, they will wonder when he is coming back. To say that God took someone young because He needed good people is to deny that young, as well as old, die, and that good people, as well as evil people, die. Once the child who has been lied to, however well intentioned, is old enough to understand that death had occurred, there may be emotional and behavioral repercussions later between the two of you, along with the emergence of trust issues.

The following is a brief list of potential symptoms that may indicate your child is having a difficult time coping with a death, especially if any of the symptoms have been present for an extended period of time.

- Inability to relax; having to be constantly busy
- Not caring how she or he dresses or looks
- Indifference to hobbies or school activities that were once enjoyed
- Looking sad all the time
- Having difficulty sleeping, leading to a decline in overall health conditions
- Wishing to be constantly alone and not interacting with the same friends as before the death
- Expressing feelings of worthlessness
- Getting into drugs, including alcohol

These symptoms, if present for an unreasonable length of time, may indicate a need to seek a qualified, competent therapist or counselor. Ask your pediatrician for a referral. In conjunction with the referral, you may want to try working with your child in art and/or music. Studies have reported findings indicating that the arts can help children find and express their emotions, which can finally allow them a release for what they have been holding, locked deep inside their minds. Arts activities can be accomplished with just the two of you, as a family with siblings, by the child alone, or with friends.

And, if your child is happy, that's O.K., too. There can be laughter after a death, and at a funeral, when someone recalls a particularly light or funny moment in the person's life that brought others joy. One of the nice things that happen at funerals today involves the tributes given when people stand and talk about the deceased, what that person said and did that made a difference in another person's life. It brings out aspects of the deceased that may have been unknown by others in attendance; the stories help to sort of "round out" the person by allowing everyone to know other sides of the one they have lost. So often we know only one aspect of someone, and it's nice to learn about and see the person from others' perspectives, to gain a more complete portrait of the person we knew and loved. This can also help older children appreciate the life that has just passed. A particular kindness or a particular skill can help show how much the person was appreciated and loved by others, and can help a child realize that great-grandma was someone other than a person with aches and pains, that she was young once, alive and vital, with hopes and dreams that may have been similar to those the great-grandchild now has today.

After a death and funeral, older children may begin to express a fear of death and tell you they don't want to die. Death is no longer a "concept"—it is now a "reality." If your child is healthy, remind him/her that s/he is healthy, and that you, as a parent, are helping to maintain that state of health by ensuring s/he is eating a proper diet, by getting enough exercise, by seeing the doctor regularly for checkups, and that you are reasonably confident s/he won't die any time soon. Tell him/her you, too, have hopes and dreams for the future and how glad you are that s/he is such an important part of your life. If your child still seems preoccupied with death, it may be time to try a new approach, reinforce the prior one and/or seek professional help. Check with your pediatrician for a referral to a child psychologist or social worker who can help.

On the other hand, if it is your child who has the terminal illness, work closely with the oncologist and pediatrician to find someone with whom your child can talk. Your minister, priest, rabbi, imam or other spiritual advisor can also help, but you want to make sure the person you select is someone with whom your child can effectively connect. This might also be the time for family counseling, because the siblings of your stricken child will also be having their own fears, and dealing with emotions they either can't handle, or at best, are having a difficult time handling. The website for SheKnows has some books listed that may be helpful for you.

Without intending this to be "last, but not least," we offer some words of wisdom from Rabbi Grollman that are applicable to other ethnic and religious groups. Judaism has a sacred commandment to comfort both young and old mourners. Centuries of tradition (one could also apply that to Catholicism) have gone into the rituals that are practiced; these practices are renowned for bringing great comfort, especially to children. Jewish mourning rites are *Kevod ho-met*, respecting the person who just died, and *Kevod ho-chai*, respecting those who still survive. However, in Judaism, there is an attempt to limit the mourning. Rabbi Grollman points out a specific passage in Psalms 23 in the Old Testament, which Alexis and Terry, as Protestants, now see in a new light: "Yea, though I walk through the valley of the shadow of death . . . " The key here is the "walk through." It is unhealthy to remain in perpetual grief and mourning. You have to find some reason for living, some purpose for your life, some purpose in the particular area of the world you inhabit, and move forward. That is why it is critical for you, as an adult, to be in touch with your own feelings and emotions, so that when your child(ren) comes to you, you can help him/her make peace with death, and move relatively quickly back into the land of the living. Treasure your memories of the person you have lost, talk about him/her, but do it in the context of all that remains: family, friends and the love you had shared for one another before the loss, the love you all share now and the love you will all share into the future.

CANCER—
Quick, Down and Dirty

This section is being offered for those of you who are just beginning your journey with cancer. It is being written so that if you have been recently diagnosed, know someone who has been diagnosed, or are engaged in risky behavior (smoking, excessive drinking, poor diet, for example), you will be prepared with information from this brief overview for what is coming in the future.

Everyone knows what cancer is. It's a bunch of cells that run rampant, and that grow uncontrollably. Really, that is it, in a nutshell. However, a deeper analysis shows cancer is actually a cluster of diseases. There are more than 100 different types or kinds of cancer. Each of these types of cancer is a disease of the cells within certain parts of the body.

Normally, cells are constantly dividing and replacing themselves. There is an order to this process, and that order helps keep us healthy. However, when the cells run amok, as in cancer, they divide too rapidly and grow without any order; then, too much tissue is produced. Tumors are formed. *Benign tumors* are generally not dangerous, won't spread and can often be removed surgically; usually they don't return. *Malignant tumors* are dangerous. The malignant tumors are cancer. They become very invasive and can spread without notice. They can also metastasize and form new tumors.

Are you aware of the potential symptoms that might indicate you could have cancer? The symptoms listed below are _not always_ a sign of cancer, and could be indicative of another illness. If any of these symptoms last longer than two weeks, you should make an appointment with your doctor right away. Remember, even if these symptoms are painful, pain is **_not_** necessarily an early sign of cancer.

- A sore that doesn't heal
- Bleeding and discharge that is unusual
- Thickening or lump in the breast or elsewhere
- Indigestion and/or difficulty swallowing
- Change in a wart or mole
- Change in bowel or urinary habits (especially blood in the excrement or in the urine)
- Nagging cough or hoarseness

The earlier your cancer is diagnosed, the earlier you can receive treatment, and the better your chances are for survival. That's one reason why it's critically important to have annual physicals. Often a doctor can spot a potential illness before symptoms appear, and can then prescribe appropriate tests. This is especially true for cancers of the breast, cervix, colon, mouth, prostate, rectum, skin and testicles.

Diagnosis of cancer is accomplished in a number of ways: X-rays, angiograms, radioactive isotopes, ultrasounds and biopsies. Once your cancer has been diagnosed, the oncologist will order more tests to determine the type and staging of the cancer. He or she will formulate a plan of attack to give you the best options available for ensuring the greatest chances of survival. If you wish to ask for a second opinion, your doctor may have a recommendation, or you can contact the Cancer Information Service—1-800-4Cancer.

Biopsies deserve a little bit of explanation. In a biopsy (which means "view of the living"), a small sample of tissue is extracted. Sometimes this is done through surgery (both of us had this procedure), and sometimes through a fine needle aspiration (Terry had this when her cancer metastasized). Once the tissue sample has been obtained, it is sent to a pathologist, who examines it and reports his/her findings to your doctor. The seven types of biopsies are as follows:

- *Excisional*—a whole lump or organ is removed (rarely done now, because of medical advances).

- *Incisional*—a small portion of a lump is removed; this piece is used to distinguish between a benign and a malignant tumor.

- *Endoscopic*—a fiberoptic endoscope ("to see inside") is inserted through a body orifice, the naval or rectum, or through a small incision, such as in gall bladder surgery.

- *Colposcopic*—used if you have had an abnormal PAP smear.

- *Fine needle aspiration*—a needle is inserted into the tumor and thousands of cells are withdrawn for analysis (this is the one Terry had when she was told to holditholditholdit).

- *Punch biopsy*—is usually used by dermatologists to "punch out" a small sample of a rash.

- *Bone marrow biopsy*—is usually taken from the pelvic bone. <u>Regardless of what the doctor tells you—it HURTS! Remember— they have probably never had one.</u> Ask to be totally and completely anesthetized for this type of biopsy. Terry and Pat (who left "claw" marks in Ricardo's arms) had the first one done with a local anesthetic, but for the other two, Terry was "out like a light." They have some really great anesthetics for this. Recovery involves minimal pain, and a "normal" life may be resumed within 24–48 hours.

After the samples have been taken, they are processed in a variety of ways to determine what kind of cancer you have and its developmental stage. Once your diagnosis has been confirmed, in all likelihood, you will be asked to sign an "informed consent" form. This form indicates what approaches/procedure(s) for treatment are recommended, along with the purpose(s), risks, possible side effects and consequences, should you decide to agree to have the treatment as designated. The form will also include information regarding other treatments that may be available to you, should you not agree to the recommended treatment, along with the advantages/disadvantages for each of those options.

When you are first diagnosed with cancer, you are told the medical name of your cancer; you learn the stage of the cancer, which is usually rated between I-IV, the grade of the tumor(s) and whether or not there are other health factors in your profile that may impact the kind of cancer you have. The implications for how this type of cancer will affect your body and your lifestyle are discussed with you, as are those affects most likely to arise from the treatment options you are considering. Finally, the expected prognosis from the use of the various treatment plans is offered to assist you in making your final decision as to how you wish to proceed. In some instances, there is only a single course of treatment possible, with the exception, of course, of doing nothing at all. In the worst of all scenarios, no treatment can be offered, and the prognosis is terminal, which we pray is not your plight. A Truism:

> *"Until such time as your journey reaches its conclusion, no person can determine your destiny—not its direction, nor its end."*

You always have your faith, your hope and the power of your mind to carry you through to the pinnacle of unforeseen outcomes.

Cancer, and the subsequent treatment plan, is determined by where in your body the cancer **begins**. Cancer is diagnosed by the "primary" tumor—where the visible formation or mass is located. When cells break off from the primary tumor and travel to another location, this is called "metastasis." When cancer has spread to another location, it is called "metastatic" cancer. In Terry's case, her cancer "metastasized" to other parts of her body and then became "metastatic" cancer. The interesting part is that if the cancer had metastasized to her brain, she would not have had "brain cancer," but metastatic lymphoma. Linda's cancer started in her lungs, giving her "lung cancer," but after her metastasis, she still had "lung cancer" in her brain. Tom's cancer originated in the prostate and migrated to his bones and lymph nodes. He doesn't have "bone" cancer, but rather prostate cancer in his bones. If several kinds of cancer originate in one location, let's say three kinds of cancer, each will receive its own type of treatment.

Often when the name(s) of your cancer(s) is/are related to you by the doctor, s/he represents them as a broad range of cancers: "carcinoma," or "sarcoma." To do any kind of adequate research into your cancer, you need to know the precise medical terminology for what you have, which your doctor can give you. Be prepared; you may need him/her to write it down for you because there is no way you could spell the name.

Cancer staging tells you how far the cancer has spread. In Alexis's case, she was at Stage 1 A, or maybe B. Terry was at Stage 2 B. Staging is not really applicable to leukemias, which are diseases of the blood. Staging is important, but what is even more important is your general health, your preferences, and what your treatment will entail. Also remember that stages are not the whole story, and a lot depends on your individual diagnosis and treatment, including your overall attitude going into treatment.

Staging is often represented through the use of Roman numerals, which indicate the various levels of cancer encroachment. Stage I cancers are normally curable, and are generally small and localized. Stage II cancers are locally advanced. Stage III cancers usually have some involvement with the lymph nodes or lymphatic system. Stage IV cancer is usually inoperable or metastatic. Additionally, each type of cancer has a different "within-type" rating system, so that Stage II breast cancer will be different from Stage II liver cancer, and each type will most likely receive vastly different treatments.

Cancer can recur months or even years after the initial treatment of cancer, because cancer cells have broken off and found a new home in another location. If all of your cancer has been treated with no signs of the initial tumors remaining, and at some point in time, new tumors become visible, it's called "recurrent" cancer. If the cancer returns to roughly the same area as the original diagnosis, it's called "locally recurrent." If it has migrated to another location, it's called "distant recurrent." If your tumor is a solid mass, there is a more detailed staging called the "TNM" system.

TNM stands for **T**umor, **N**odes and **M**etastases. The definitions of each of these are specific to each cancer. *T* demonstrates the extent of the primary tumor. Zero means the cancer hasn't started to invade other tissues. Four means there is a probable invasion into other tissues or organs, and is usually inoperable. **N** tells how much your lymph nodes are impacted. Only lymph nodes around the primary tumor are considered. If distant lymph nodes are impacted, then it's considered metastatic disease. Zero means no lymph nodes are involved; four means there is extensive lymph node involvement. **M** is for the extent of metastasis and is either a 0 or a 1. Zero means no metastasis; 1 means metastasis has occurred. A person with a *T0 N0 M0* staging means there is no invasion of tissues, no lymph node involvement and no metastasis. Someone with *T4 N4 M1* likely has invasion of other tissues, distant lymph node involvement, and the cancer has metastasized.

Earlier it was mentioned that stages were also broken down into letters—A and B. Alexis was at stage 1A and Terry was at stage 2B. Not all cancers are easily broken down into these groups, and stage IIIa in non-small lung cancer has a greater chance of being cured, even possibly through surgery. People with stage IIIb in non-small cell lung cancer have a worse prognosis. For cancers with no discernable tumors, the staging is again different and the TNM doesn't apply. Since the field of medicine is constantly changing, it's important to keep up to date with as many of the changes as you can. Your staging may change over time, given new research. The National Cancer Institute is very helpful in this area. Log onto http://www.nci.com.

Tumor grading is basically how your cells look under the microscope. The higher the grade, the more aggressive the cancer. If you will recall, Tom's original Gleason Score was given as a 7 of 10, but Memorial Sloan-Kettering ranked it as a 9 of 10. Tumor grading is extremely important for prostate cancer, some brain tumors and some lymphomas. Your pathology report will indicate the grade of your tumor.

Other tests will be conducted before your receive your final "grade." As an example, Alexis's breast cancer cells were found to be Estrogen Receptor Positive (ER+). That means that the cancer cells have markers or "receptors" for estrogen on their surface. The growth of Alexis's breast cancer cells required estrogen. ER+ tumors can be less aggressive and more responsive to treatment. The opposite of ER+ is Estrogen Receptor Negative (ER-). That means there is no estrogen present on the surface of the cells, and estrogen is not required for growth of the cancer cells.

Different types of treatment can include: radiation therapy (also called X-ray therapy, radiotherapy, cobalt treatment or irradiation), chemotherapy, hormone therapy, biological therapy (sometimes called immunotherapy) and surgery. Treatment can be only one type or a combination of types. Regardless of which one or ones are used, healthy cells will be destroyed along with the cancerous ones. There really is no way to avoid that at this point in time (tomorrow may bring some new medical miracle). One reason for that is to try and prevent the spread, or metastasis, of the cancer. There are side effects, the most notable being nausea and fatigue. Both of us received great drugs and didn't have any nausea, except when we didn't follow directions. (Remember—there are two people you should always listen to and *never* lie to: your Physician and your Certified Public Accountant.)

Once you are diagnosed with cancer, your life changes, as do the lives of the people in your life. It is natural to feel depressed, angry, frightened, courageous, and to have concerns about your future. There is also the very real fear about medical costs—what will the insurance pay? If you don't have insurance, how will your treatment be paid? Write down questions to ask your health care providers. And most importantly, keep asking questions throughout treatment. If you don't understand something, ask what it means. Don't sit in silence. You are a member of this team, in fact, the key player in this drama, and have a right to know what's going on and why. Most doctors we have talked to are grateful when patients ask questions.

Cancer can have an impact on your life in a number of different areas. One of those is **sex**. We have devoted a whole section to that. Our body and our body images suffer in this cancer process, and it can take a long time to fully recover.

It is estimated today there are over five million people in the U.S. who have had cancer. It seems every day or every month, there is some new discovery of a drug to help, which means the chances of survival and recovery are also improving. Doctors use the term "remission" rather than "cure," because once you have cancer, it can come back again at some point in the future. The general rule of thumb is that if you can survive cancer with no recurrences, you have been "cured." There is still no guarantee, however, that you have been "cured." While statistics can give you the odds of survival, they are based on the mean, or average, of thousands, if not millions, of people. Your age, general physical condition, the type of cancer, the stage of the cancer and your response to treatment will determine more about your chance of recovery or remission than the statistics will show. This means that if you and your friend both have breast cancer, you both, regardless of the statistics, may have very different outcomes.

We live in an incredible age where countless researchers are working diligently to find the underlying causes, diagnoses, and treatments of cancer, as well as the best ways to prevent cancer from occurring in the first place. It used to be believed that people could "catch" cancer from someone else, but we now know that's not true. One estimate says that up to 73 million people will, at some point, contract cancer. Another estimate says that cancer will occur in about three out of every four families. Overall, rates for men are increasing, but decreasing for women. Rates for African-American males are increasing faster than for Caucasian males. The leading cause of death for both men and women is lung cancer. For women, lung cancer is worse than breast, cervical AND ovarian cancer COMBINED. Of special note is that 2/3 of women who contract lung cancer either never smoked, or quit smoking 10 years or more earlier. (No, this does NOT mean you should begin smoking.) Please read the Lung Cancer Alliance report, entitled *Out of the Shadows*, http://www.lungcanceralliance.org).

How is cancer caused? Researchers believe there are two causes: "initiators" and "promoters." Cigarette smoking has been proven to be an initiator: it starts the damage to cells that lead to cancer. For example, cigarettes contain a radioactive isotope—polonium 210. With every cigarette you smoke, polonium 210 settles in your lungs. It has been estimated that smoking 1 pack of cigarettes a day is the same as having 300 chest x-rays in one year (and the tobacco industry has known about this for close to 50 years, but chose not to address it or advertise it). Promoters in and of themselves do not cause cancer, but usually work in conjunction with an initiator. For example, alcohol can be a promoter for cancer in the mouth when combined with smoking. Researchers have determined that about 80% of all cancers may be related to our life styles (what we eat, drink and smoke) as well as our environment and workplace. This means **you can choose a lifestyle that would reduce the cancer risks you encounter every day.**

Of course, don't start smoking, and if you already have, STOP. Today! Immediately! Right now! If you think stopping is difficult, think about how difficult it will be to explain to your family and friends that you played a large role through a self-destructive lifestyle in causing your cancer. Smokeless tobacco is just as dangerous. Don't be fooled by the "smokeless" part.

There also appears to be a link between obesity and/or a high-fat diet that leads to some cancers. This includes pickled, cured or smoked foods. You should eat more grains, and fresh fruits and vegetables. Reduce your exposure to sunlight, alcohol, and watch out for carcinogens in cleaning products, lawn and garden products, even some skin lotions and sunscreens.

For a more in-depth discussion on this topic, please see: **http://www.memorialhospital.org/Library/general/cancer2.html,** or for more information on what cancer is, and the variety of ways it can be treated, go to the site at **http://www.cancerguide.org/pathology.html,** written by Edward O. Uthman, M.D.

Many resources are provided for you in the back of this book, but a few of them are worth highlighting here in this section as well. Each organization is dedicated to getting you the information you need, regardless of who you are or how you know cancer.

- American Cancer Society, 404-320-3333
- American Childhood Cancer Organization—AMCO (formerly, the Candlelighters Childhood Cancer Foundation), 1-800-366-CCCF
- Cancer Information Service, 1-800-4Cancer
- Childhood Cancer Canada (formerly Candlelight Childhood Cancer Foundation of Canada), 1-800-363-1062
- Leukemia and Lymphoma Foundation, 212-573-8484
- Make Today Count, 703-548-9674
- National Cancer Institute, 1-800-4-CANCER (1-800-422-6237)

Cancer and Stem Cell Research

In the U.S., steady increases in cancer survivors have been demonstrated over the past 30 years. Adults between the ages of 35–45 have shown the biggest increase in survivorship, but all ages have shown some improvement. According to Dr. Eric Kort, of the Helen DeVos Children's Hospital in Grand Rapids, MI, young peoples' cancer survivorship is also increasing. In terms of the general population, he attributes the increases in cancer survivorship to improvements in screenings, especially those for breast and colon cancer, and better treatments with the improvements in medicines.

Cancer has become the Number 1 most frequently diagnosed disease, replacing heart disease. On the web site, MLive.com, it was projected that in 2009, 1,479,350 people would be diagnosed with new cancer cases in the U.S.; of those, 562,340 will die from cancer. It was also reported that 41% of Americans could be expected to be diagnosed with cancer in their lifetime, and 21% will die from the disease. Further information may be found in the August 2009, issue of the journal, *Cancer Research*. *Breakaway from Cancer*, a website sponsored by Amgen and four non-profit organizations specifically established for the purpose of providing resource information for cancer patients and survivors, states that it is estimated of every one million Americans who are diagnosed with cancer, about 40% will be of working age. For more info, see: http.//www.breakawayfromcancer.com/index.html.

In the August 2009 Issue of the *British Journal of Cancer*, the author states that there is about a 3% increase in the numbers of cancer survivors in the U.K. In 1992, survivor numbers were about 1.2 million, and six years later in 2008, survivors numbered more than 2 million. Prostate and breast cancer patients have shown the greatest improvement in terms of their survival rates. Cancer survivorship in

England is a high priority. Northern Ireland, Scotland and Wales are implementing similar procedures by designing research studies to ascertain their survival rates. Currently, the data gathered document an unanticipated difference between two of the populations. Northern Ireland, which has the youngest population, has a much lower prevalence of cancer diagnoses than in Wales, which has a much older population, and has a higher prevalence of cancer.

The Future of Cancer Research

In looking into existing cancer research materials, Terry and Alexis were both astounded and overwhelmed by the volumes that have been done already, but were even more incredulous by all the research and trials that are currently underway. It truly is not an exaggeration to say that with every single passing day, new advances are being made with cancer, a fact that at this particular point in time, is more important than it ever has been to Tom, and to Terry. Tomorrow is not too soon for them. The discussion that follows will provide brief overviews of some of the more exciting and promising studies we found, and is in no way intended to be an exhaustive coverage of all that is occurring. So much good news is just beyond the horizon, survivorship may ultimately become the "expected outcome" for cancer victims everywhere. A Truism:

> *"Beyond every sunset, a new day comes within reach, bringing with it all the hope, new opportunities and successes your brain can possibly envisage, and render into action."*

Review of prior studies exposed a phenomenon that should be viewed as problematic. But perhaps, it should come as no surprise that it was found women are under-represented among cancer research subjects. We don't say this because we happen to be women. It is simply a fact. This holds true regardless of the type of cancer (except for breast cancer and those cancers relating specifically to men—prostate, testicular, etc.). This under-representation has continued despite the knowledge that there are not only biological differences (*vive le difference!*), but also social and cultural differences. Government-funded research tends to include more women, but the percentages are not significantly better when compared with privately-funded trials. Women are usually the primary child-care providers, which may be a barrier for their participation in clinical trials. Other factors may be fear and lack of knowledge. Further exploration of the gender disparity in cancer research participation rates between males and females needs to be conducted to identify why this occurs. Without clear understanding of the rationales for study subject selection, remedies cannot be put in place to assure the treatments and medical procedures for women are as timely, effective and "cutting-edge" as possible, or at least as advanced as they are for men.

Another area that needs greater focus in future cancer research is, without a doubt, in the area of genetic counseling and genetic testing. Despite the increase in using MRIs and ultrasounds along with mammograms, many women fail to be diagnosed with breast cancer. The reason for this is likely because the family history and genetic predisposition are unknown. Further complicating early diagnosis, the key to survival, is that it is now known that breast cancer is not just one disease, but demonstrates through a broad range of clinical presentations. Since it is already known that as women age, the risk of breast cancer increases, genetic testing could actually save lives by predicting a woman's propensity toward contracting cancer, so intervention and testing measures could be implemented early.

Probably the most notable need for genetic testing and genetic counseling is for two groups of Jewish women of Ashkenazi (originating in Eastern Europe) and Sephardic descent, who are at risk of hereditary breast cancer because of the BRCA1 and BRCA2 (**BR**east **CA**ncer) gene mutation. What is interesting, however, is the number of women of Mexican descent (or those identifying themselves as Hispanic or of Spanish descent) who are also showing up with the BRCA1 and BRCA2 gene mutations here in the United States. The likelihood is that in the 1500s, when the Spaniards were invading Mexico, Central and South America, Ashkenazi and Sephardic Jews were probably among the invaders. There were also Sephardic and Ashkenazi families who were escaping the Inquisition and went into Mexico for refuge. Either through rape or intermarriage, these genes, which can come down through both the male and female lines, have been passed on through the generations, while the Jewish heritage part has long been lost. People migrated from Mexico and arrived in New Mexico and Colorado. For those who carry the mutation for the BRCA1 gene, 50–85% of those women will develop breast cancer by age 70. Studies are currently underway to see whether the BRCA2 gene mutation carries the same risk. The gene may skip a generation before manifesting itself again. BRCA1 appears to increase the risk of breast and ovarian cancers; BRCA2 seems to be linked to a higher risk for male breast cancer. BRCA2 may also be linked to pancreatic, prostate and melanoma cancers.

Another gene, 185delAG, has also been discovered in Hispanic populations in the U.S. For those who are concerned about discrimination if irregularities are found as a result of the genetic testing, the Americans with Disabilities Act (ADA) may prove to be a safeguard. Other states and countries may also have regulatory procedures in place to prevent any subsequent discrimination for those affected with the gene. (For further information regarding genetic mutations, you may refer to: http://www.sharsheret.org, and download the transcript "Breast Cancer Genetics and the Sephardic Jewish Woman.")

Based upon your heritage or other background information, referral to a genetic counselor may be in order for you. The genetic counselor will compile a complete family history, and then determine the statistical probability your child or children may have a specific genetic mutation. You will then be prepared to implement appropriate early detection measures. If you cannot afford genetic testing, or your health insurance will not cover it, contact Myriad Genetics, to see if you qualify to participate in their hardship program. Another resource is Dr. Harry Ostrer, Director of the Molecular Genetics Laboratory of NYU School of Medicine.

As reported in the February 2010, issue of *Scientific American,* biotechnology may soon create a synthetic bio-organism that can surgically, but even more importantly, strategically, target specific cancer cells. Biomarkers, developed by LabCorp, analyze colon cells in the stool of patients for indicators of colorectal cancer. Biomarkers, which include PSA tests, are also being explored for other diseases such as schizophrenia, other cancers, inflammatory conditions, and heart disease. Studies are also being undertaken to help identify two or more diseases in people, because one biomarker may be effective for identifying one disease, but a different biomarker might have to be used to distinguish and/or diagnose any other illnesses that may be present with confidence.

Research currently being conducted by Dr. James J. Galligan at Michigan State University (MSU) focuses on the potential therapeutic uses of ATP—adenosine triphosphate, which is a nucleotide—a high-energy molecule essential in allowing cells to function and communicate with each other. Biologists are frequently cited for considering ATP to be the *"energy currency of life."* The premise of the study is that ATP will help people with chronic pain, one of the side effects of certain types of cancer, with irritable bowel syndrome (IBS) and with Crohn's disease. ATP might also be a natural cancer-fighting tool. Research into ATP initially conducted by Eliezer Rapaport in 1983, subsequently followed up by other researchers, appears to indicate that ATP inhibits the growth of tumors in the prostate, breast, ovaries, and esophagus. Further study must still be conducted to establish not only its efficacy, but to also discover the most effective means for capturing and utilizing ATP with all of its apparent limitless potential.

Preliminary findings from the research being conducted by Barbara Cromer, MD, with Case Western Reserve University, show that pesticides and plastics contain synthetic estrogens, which could be inducing girls to enter puberty earlier. The other concern isolated by the team is that the ingestion of cattle fattened with estrogens could cause girls to experience similar early onset puberty. If either of the two scenarios proves to be true, then girls in the next generation could be at increased risk for breast cancer in adulthood.

Cancer vaccines are also being researched. Provenge became the first therapeutic cancer vaccine approved by the FDA. This drug uses a body's own immune system against cancer tumors. Using a body's own immune system was first proposed back in the end of the late 1800s. In 1909, Paul Erlich posited that the body's own immune system actually destroyed the cancer cells that are almost always present in everyone. Early research seemed to support this idea. The idea was dropped in the 1950s when oncologists were experiencing better and more consistent results through surgery, the use of chemotherapy and eventually radiation. Researchers today have revived this concept because vaccines would be less invasive and actually hold greater promise for longer-range health. Vaccines could potentially use your own immune system to fight malignant tumors. There are three basic approaches to developing a therapeutic vaccine:

1. dendrite cells,
2. peptide cells, and
3. whole cells.

With Provenge, dendrite cells are taken from a patient's body, zapped with antigens that are cancer-specific (in this case, prostate cancer), and then reinfused into the patient every 2 weeks for 3 weeks. This buys a man, on average, up to 4 more months of life. To find the exact combination of proteins needed to develop effective vaccines will be a lengthy process. Once developed, it may take a vaccine as long as a year to show progress in attacking a malignant tumor. In comparison, chemotherapy can often show results in a matter of weeks. In the short term, the anti-cancer vaccines that are developed may be more effective with people in the earlier stages (stage 1 or 2) of their diagnosis. For the next several years, while vaccines are being perfected, people in the later stages (stages 3 and 4) may still need surgery, chemotherapy and/or radiation first before receiving the vaccine. Still and all, this is an exciting concept and one well worth continuing to explore.

The Swiss Medical Society for Psycholytic Therapy in Switzerland, headed by Dr. Peter Gassman, is exploring the therapeutic use of LSD—lysergic acid diethylamide-25—with patients who are terminally ill with cancer. While this study has an exceptionally small number of subjects participating, one man has reported the anxiety in being diagnosed with cancer he had initially experienced has already been eased. Completion of the study will determine whether LSD was found to be efficacious.

The April 2008, and again in April 2009, issues of *Scientific American* contained reports about researchers at Massachusetts General Hospital who are currently exploring ways to further refine a cancer diagnosis. As it stands now, people have to go through extensive blood work, biopsies, X-rays, etc., in order to determine the type of cancer they have and its extent of growth or stage of development. MGH is working on something they call "lab-on-a-chip," which will use only a teaspoon of blood to analyze the tumor cells. Since circulating tumor cells can be fewer than one in a million, especially in early stage cancers, this lab-on-a-chip should offer better diagnosis and real-time stage development of tumors. The chip is etched with silicon, and then fitted with microscopic columns; these columns act like miniature test tubes. The chip is also fitted with a pneumatic pump. There are 78,000 posts that extract the cancer cells from regular blood components. Tests are now being conducted on lung, prostate, pancreatic, breast and colorectal cancers. In addition to Massachusetts General Hospital, further information may be obtained from BioMicroElectro-Mechanical Systems Resource Center in Boston, MA, the December 20, 2007, issue of *Nature* and the July 24, 2008, *New England Journal of Medicine.*

As a sidebar in the April 2009 issue of *Scientific American*, it is noted that genetic differences in humans can often mean the difference between success and failure of the variety of cancer treatments. As medical researchers move toward more personalized cancer care, treatments could be adjusted, based upon each person's particular genetic structure. This would help each patient receive his/her proper dosage and type(s) of medication (chemotherapy, for example); this could potentially have the added benefits of reducing costs and potentially debilitating side effects. Also, in terms of genes, The Sanger Institute's Cancer Gene Census has issued a report stating ". . . there are 423 genes in the human genome that could be related to cancer," (*Discover*, May 2010).

Throughout the past decade, numerous studies have documented health treatments originating from the venom of snakes. The proteins in snakes, particularly poisonous ones like the Southern Copperhead Viper, may be a veritable slithering pharmacy. The brain of snakes may hold possible treatments for hypertension, convulsions, paralysis, and muscle weakness. The heart might hold promise to treat hypertension. The pancreas and salivary glands might work on blood clots. Muscles may be used for anaphylactic shock and disrupting nerve impulses, which lead to heart failure and suffocation. The proteins from the pancreas, heart, liver, brain, kidneys and venom of the snake may all be used as potential cancer treatments. Results from recent studies have shown the venom proteins have, in effect, frozen tumors into "suspended states of animation." The resulting suspended state has prevented malignant tumors from growing, and the cancer from spreading. Study results have documented the protein in the venom has actually slowed the rate of growth up to 70% in some subjects. Once again, it seems the potential for more effective cancer treatments may be imminent, this time from one of our most feared earthly companions. The snake, previously thought to present only danger to our lives, may now offer disease treatments and healing.

The November 2008, issue of *Scientific American* carried a report that indicated cancer vaccines are gaining new ground in fighting disease by redefining what they are supposed to do. Originally, they had been tested based on shrinking tumors, which proved fantastically unsuccessful. As mentioned earlier, how the problem gets defined, dictates the solution. The new area of research centers on how much longer a patient is likely to live. This was the case with the prostate cancer drug, Provenge. (It is intended for men diagnosed with Stage 4 metastic prostate disease, who have become hormone refractory). The problem seems to be that drug companies are unwilling (and for them, find it financially unfeasible) to develop adjuvants or compounds that might be helpful to another drug company. Researchers working for X drug company with a promising vaccine are unable to obtain compound Y from drug company Z.

In 2007, Susana Soares, then at the Royal College of Art, discovered that bees have an incredible sense of smell and memory. She devised a screening device and trained bees to remember a certain smell; when they recognized that smell, the bees then rushed into a plastic "bubble." This can potentially be used for diseases such as lung cancer, tuberculosis and diabetes. Bees are already used to detect land mines. Bees can be trained in as little as 15 minutes, compared to the weeks it takes for dogs to be trained to do the same thing.

John Kanzius, a retired businessman and radio technician in Erie, Pennsylvania, may have discovered a new way to treat some cancers. He discovered when nanoparticles from gold are injected into tumors, the nanoparticles become attached to cancer cells. He has developed the Kanzius RF Machine, which transmits radio waves that are focused on these nanoparticles. The nanoparticles release heat and destroy the cancer cells, while leaving the healthy cells alone. He developed this machine based upon his own experiences with leukemia and chemotherapy. Researchers at both the University of Pittsburgh and the M.D. Anderson Cancer Center are testing the Kanzius approach using the radio wave treatments on rabbits. Results to date have shown localized tumors and hepatic VX2 carcinomas have been successfully destroyed (*Discover* magazine, December 2008). The studies are still in process at this time.

Researchers at Children's Hospital in Boston, MA, discovered that people with Down syndrome rarely develop tumors. The researchers posited that people with this syndrome may have cancer-protective genes because of an extra copy of chromosome 21. Specifically, there was an additional copy of one of 231 genes on chromosome 21 called DSCR1. This gene inhibits the growth of the blood vessels needed by cancer cells to block a protein called calcineurin. Signs of potential Down syndrome usually don't appear until the second trimester of pregnancy, but researchers at Tufts Medical Center believe an antioxidant could be developed that might deter some facets of the syndrome. Additionally, it was found that targeted deletion of the calcineurin inhibitor DSCR1 resulted in suppressed tumor growth.

In another piece of research, it was reported that RNA, kin to DNA, might be more important than initially thought. RNA may determine things such as longevity and cancer. Further research has shown that chronic lymphocytic leukemia (CLL) was caused by the deletion of two microRNA genes. It was also found that microRNA genes in one tumor are totally different from those in another tumor. Researchers are now hypothesizing that future studies may show either increasing or decreasing the microRNA genes within a protein will lead to the development of new treatments for several diseases, including Alzheimer's, cancer, diabetes, heart disease, and schizophrenia.

John Pawelek and his colleagues at Yale University are exploring whether cancer metastasizes because the cells fuse with white blood cells, also known as macrophages. Their research has shown this is so in animals, and the research team members are now exploring whether this is true in humans. Metastasis is the leading cause of death from cancer. What is frustrating is that little is known about how cancer metastasizes. What is known is that macrophages freely roam around the body and enter most, if not all, body parts. Pawelek is working with cancer patients who have had a donor bone marrow transplant, because bone marrow provides white blood cells. Since the donor bone marrow is different from the patient's own bone marrow, it might be possible to determine whether tumor cells and macrophages do indeed link.

Malcolm Brenner, a geneticist at the Center for Cell and Gene Therapy at Baylor College of Medicine, in Houston, TX, is exploring the use of AdV—adenoviral virus—to treat and possibly cure EBV lymphoma, a rare form of blood cancer. Dr. Brenner uses common T-cells and turns them into AdV. The AdV in turn switches on the T-cells. Then he adds weakened Epstein-Barr virus, which the T-cells then go after, killing the cancer. Few, if any, side effects have been observed at this time. The dosage will vary from person to person—some may need only one or two treatments; others may need the injection once a month for the rest of their lives. This process is now being applied to other cancers, including neuroblastoma, which is especially virulent in children, and to melanoma and lung cancer.

Dr. Lawrence Lum, who was one of Terry's attending physicians at the Karmanos Cancer Center and professor at Wayne State University, is also exploring how to use a patient's immune system to become literally a cancer-killing machine. He is using two antibodies that will bind to T-cells and tumor cells, which will form a link between the immune system and the tumor, breaking up the tumor. Once the tumor has broken up, it will be eaten by other cells. This procedure will probably be used after microscopic surgery or after radiation or chemotherapy. The Leukemia and Lymphoma Society has endorsed Dr. Lum as the researcher most likely to make a dent in the worldwide battle against cancer.

Karmanos Cancer Institute and the Karolinska Institutet in Stockholm, Sweden, have collaborated on the development of a vaccine for Stage IV breast cancer, specifically for those who have the HER2-positive virus. Studies are still underway, but preliminary results have been encouraging. For further information about this study, contact Wei-Zen Wei, Ph.D., at Karmanos Cancer Institute, by calling 1-800-KARMANOS.

Biodegradable nanoparticles, which can deliver gene therapy for ovarian cancer, are being explored by Professor Robert Langer, at the Massachusetts Institute of Technology (MIT) and Janet Sawicki at the Lankenau Institute for Medical Research in Pennsylvania. At this stage, they are experimenting with mice but hope to begin human trials sometime in 2011. Nanoparticles are also being investigated at the Institute National de la Santé et de la Recherche Médicale in France by Georges Vassaux. These nanoparticles have been shown in mice to deliver gene therapy to cancerous cells. They will next focus on different tumors in other animals.

Sorry to lapse into technical jargon here (not that it hasn't happened before), but it is a necessity. Telomeres are located at the ends of chromosomes and repeat DNA sequences. With each division of a cell, these telomeres become shorter. Once they reach a certain degree of shortness, the cell dies. One thought is that if there could be a way to keep these telomeres longer, people could live longer and healthier lives (in fact, there has been a link shown between longer telomeres, diet, exercise and stress reduction). There are several researchers exploring how this might be accomplished. One more little piece of jargon: telomerase is an enzyme that maintains the telomeres in our body. Enzymes are proteins that living cells produce and help to produce biochemical reactions in our bodies. Now for the exciting part, the reason you needed those pieces of technical information. The possibility of a telomere therapy that could fight and kill cancer cells is conceivable. Telomerase usually doesn't exist in most of the cells in our bodies, but it is activated in cancer cells. Once activated, it helps cancer cells continue to divide and grow. If some kind of enzyme could be developed that prevents the telomerase from growing, it could cause the cancer cells to die. A company named Geron is in Phase I clinical trials right now to find just such a process that would kill the cancer cells, but not harm the healthy ones. There is one little problem, however. Using telomerase to stop the aging process could possibly increase the risk of developing some cancers, such as skin and breast cancer. Well, two steps forward, one step backward, puts us still ahead of the game!

In some cultures, dogs are man's best friends, and it may be proven to be a greater truth than anyone ever could have imagined. In very preliminary testing, French researcher Jean-Nicolas Cornu, MD, at Tenon Hospital in Paris, reported in June 2010, at the American Urological Association that it appears some dogs can be trained to sniff out chemicals in a man's urine that could detect early prostate cancer. These same researchers are also trying to determine whether dogs can detect cancers in the bladder, lungs and skin. The theory behind the research is that cancer tumors contain chemicals that have distinct odors; dogs can be trained to pick up the scents of these chemicals. Dogs used in this manner had fewer false-positives, recording a 95% accuracy rate, than even the medical standard, the PSA tests. Fewer than one third of men with high PSA scores are confirmed as actually having prostate cancer when the biopsies are performed. In addition, PSA tests do not determine whether the tumor is life-threatening or slow-growing. Does this mean that dogs, at some point in the future, will be running around doctors' offices or hospitals, sniffing people? No. It is planned that once the type of chemical the dogs are reacting to is identified, a sort of "electronic nose" might be able to be developed.

A study conducted under the direction of the lead researcher, György Horváth, MD, Ph.D., at the University Hospital in Göteborg, Sweden, also focused on the abilities of trained dogs and their seemingly unlimited powers to distinguish different types, and even grades, of ovarian cancer. Ovarian cancers appear to have a different odor to dogs than either cervical or endometrial cancers. Early-stage and low-grade ovarian cancers, however, have the same odor to dogs as those tumors that are far more advanced. This finding could lead to earlier detection. For further information, please see http://www.medicalnews today.com/articles/113085.php. Another study has shown that dogs, with minimal training, can detect the scents of both early- and late-stage cancers of the lung and breast.

Who would have thought that salivary glands might be useful in detecting some forms of cancer? Did you know your salivary glands produce about one quart of liquid each day? We didn't, either. What researchers have found is that there is a difference in saliva protein profiles between healthy people and those with certain types of cancer. Studies are underway to isolate what might cause this change, and how it might be helpful in making diagnoses. (As an aside, did you know saliva also contains compounds that help wounds heal faster? Perhaps we should emulate some of our favorite four-legged companions who lick their wounds to heal when they are injured.) (Ewww . . . .!)

Cancer cells are difficult to study in a laboratory because they mutate into different kinds of cells quickly, and are very difficult to kill in the body. There is new research being conducted at the Massachusetts Institute of Technology and at the Broad Institute which may help people with breast cancer. The researchers have found 32 chemical compounds (of some16,000) which might actually kill cancer cells. Of these 32 chemicals, they discovered salinomycin appears to be 100 times more powerful in killing the breast cancer stem cells in mice than Taxol or paclitaxel. It also appears that salinomycin reduces or prevents breast cancer cells from forming. Studies are currently underway to find whether this chemical is safe for humans or not. This discovery is potentially useful for pharmaceutical companies as they strive to develop effective strategies and medications for killing cancer cells, with little or no serious side effects.

LeRoy Hood is proposing a new approach—using genome sequencing, and recommends it be adopted in order to practice medicine. He has developed the P4 system—**P**redictive, **P**ersonalized, **P**reventive and **P**articipatory. What this could mean is that if you have a high percentage chance of developing a form of cancer (for example, by age 50 or 60), if you could take a preventive medicine at age 30 or 40, those odds might be reduced to less than 5%. This approach has the potential of de-escalating medical costs, which means that people living in poverty might also be able to avail themselves of the procedures.

Researchers at the University of California at San Diego have developed a nanoparticle that is fluorescent and glows inside the body. This glow makes it much easier to look for tumors and other organ damage that may be occurring within a patient. If the innovative glowing nanoparticles work as they should, they may facilitate earlier cancer diagnoses.

Another study being undertaken at the University of Michigan has shown that in mice, rapid freezing, called cryoablation, of breast cancer tumors prevented the spread of the cancer to the lungs. Cryoablation might also be effective in treating prostate cancer, kidney patients who are not candidates for surgery, and cancers that have spread to the liver and to bones. The U of M is currently taking part in a nationwide clinical trial to determine the effectiveness of cryoablation for women with early stage diagnosis of breast cancer.

The June 2010, issue of *Scientific American* contained a report on research being done by IBM in Haifa, Israel, concerning predictive modeling (originally used to prevent traffic jams). They are using a program called EuResist for HIV patients to predict the success rates of different cocktails over time. The analyses involve taking a person's HIV genotype and comparing the characteristics of that subject's health against a database of evolving treatment outcomes for over 33,000 patients with some 98,000 therapies. The research also has applications for breast or prostate cancer patients to help determine which treatment would have the greatest benefit. Within the same issue, but in a different article, mention is made of botulinum toxin, along with other "bioweapons" such as ricin and terrodotoxin, being developed by pharmaceutical companies, which might treat cancer and help to alleviate pain.

In the July/August 2010 issue of *Discover* magazine, an article reported on the research of Kun-Liang Guan at the University of California at San Diego and his colleagues, who are examining a process known as "acetylation." This process activates and deactivates proteins. While examining proteins in the human liver, they discovered more than 1,000 proteins had been acetylated, which means acetylation helps to determine how energy is metabolized. Problems with metabolization can lead to diseases such as diabetes, cancer, and obesity. Chunaram Choudhary, at the University of Copenhagen, has been looking at acetylated cancer cells. Perhaps acetylation may prove to be key in treating cancer and other diseases by turning proteins on or off.

The anti-cancer drug, Taxol, may also be useful in treating the microtubules in the brain. This drug may help repair brain micro-tubules which have suffered damage common from blunt force trauma injuries. Taxol may even be valuable in treating football players who are repeatedly hit in the head during games.

In another twist to cancer research, there appears to be a link between cancer and Alzheimer's disease. For Caucasians, those who have cancer may be 43% less likely to develop Alzheimer's. If you develop Alzheimer's, you may be 69% less likely to get cancer in the future. This may not be true, however, for other ethnic groups. There is some indication that minorities who develop cancer are likely to also develop Alzheimer's. Caution must be taken in drawing any conclusions though, because the numbers of minority participants in the study were too few to assure the findings are definitive. There is also research being conducted to see whether this cancer link holds true for other diseases that affect the brain, such as Parkinson's.

One of the most puzzling questions surrounding cancer is why it recurs, sometimes very quickly—which is what happened to Terry, even after having received massive doses of chemotherapy and radiation. According to an article published in *Cell* magazine, researchers at the Massachusetts Institute of Technology have been conducting a study on mice with lymphoma to ascertain why cancer cells recur, even after all of the treatments have been administered. To date, the study has made an invaluable discovery; it appears cancer tumor cells hide in the thymus, which is the organ that functions to produce immune cells, called T-cells. The thymus coats the cancer tumor cells that have migrated to it (the thymus), and protects them (the tumor cells) from the chemotherapy drugs. MIT is exploring whether the type of chemotherapy used for a patient should, and/or could, contain an agent that not only kills the tumor cells, but also blocks the thymus from protecting the cancer cells. Current chemotherapy treatments do not include this component. In tests conducted on mice, the tumors did shrink or disappear. However, more cancer cells were discovered in the thymus after chemotherapy was administered than were there before the treatment. This outcome is clearly problematic, but the research is ongoing, and will surely lead to more effective protocols in the future. (See *Cell*, Vol. 143, Issue 3, October 29, 2010, p. 355.)

Alnylam, a biotech company, announced in June 2010, that they had developed a drug that cut the blood flow in 62% of liver cancer tumors in 19 patients. They did this by using RNA. Again, sorry to lapse into technical jargon, but RNA makes single-stranded copies of the genes in DNA, which tells cells to make proteins. In cancer, excessive amounts of proteins are produced. The drug developed by Alnylam identifies which proteins should be shut off by the cell. The proteins to be shut off are those that help manufacture the new blood vessels, which feed the cancerous tumors. The drug is delivered into fatty tissue, which helps the liver get an even dose. If this research proves the drug is efficacious, it may not only stop most cancers from progressing, but it may also help with other diseases, such as high cholesterol, HIV, Huntington's, macular degeneration, and muscular dystrophy. If the research proceeds in a timely manner, the drug could be available in two to five years.

One of the more surprising findings from cancer research is that it appears having allergies may help in the fight against cancer, according to the November /December 2010, issue of *Science Illustrated*. Allergies arise in the immune system, which is fighting to expel unrecognized particles. Cornell University scientists conducted a review of the research since the 1950s, and discovered that **people with allergies** appear **NOT** to have developed cancer as readily as **those who do not have** allergies. The hypothesis is that the allergens force carcinogens out of the body that might later cause cells to become cancerous. If you sneeze and have watery eyes, they actually may be rejecting foreign particles which contain carcinogens. There is still quite a bit of controversy about this theory and more research is being conducted. The impetus behind the pursuit of the theory is to try to utilize various components of our own immune systems in the fight against cancer. Provenge, the new treatment approved by the FDA (April, 2010), works with the immune system of those with Stage 4 metastatic prostate cancer to kill cancer cells. It may be found that how allergies are treated should be re-considered, since they might prove to be an integral part of our natural defense mechanisms against cancer and other diseases.

Since cancer is on the rise in developing nations (partially because other diseases are declining not only there, but in the "developed" nations), people globally are increasingly working together, sharing resources and knowledge, which will have several positive effects. Such cooperation will increase the possibility of totally revamping the health care systems, along with improving the development of better diagnostics and improved chemotherapies, vaccines and palliative care. Unfortunately, most people in the developing parts of the world have little or no access to these treatments, but because medical staff members are working together, and not being so competitive and secretive, these protocols become available more quickly and more efficiently to those people, to all people. It is absolutely incredible that slides of biopsies can be shipped from Africa and sent to one of the top cancer research facilities in the U.S., Great Britain, Israel, Germany, or anywhere. We wouldn't be surprised if at some point in the very near future, the Internet could be used rather than have to wait for the biopsy to be sent to another country, delaying treatment. Did you know surgeries are now being performed via the Internet? A doctor in X country can see a patient in Y country, and through robotics, perform the surgery. Yes, it's true! And it has been successful! What other wonders await us?!? Even the greatest of our imaginations could hardly conceive what the future will hold for our children!

But finally, there appears to be an alarming trend that threatens the entire future of science, at least in the United States. We're not only talking about the dearth of kids taking science and mathematics classes, but also about the poor academic performance of those few who actually do take math and science classes. In part, we are also alluding to the conservative's stance on the evolution/creationism debate, and the repressive tactics used by some political administrations on scientists, especially in government.

The greatest threat, however, to science today is the lack of government funding, and the dependence of scientists on private agencies. In monitoring government spending over time, it was found that in 1965, the U.S. allocated funds for more than 60% of all scientific research and development (R&D) in the country. By 2006, the funding level figures had more than reversed, with our country's R&D being funded 65% by private companies and interest groups. This "reversal of fortune," or loss of funding (as it really is) relegates only one third of today's scientific research to being conducted by unbiased, objective scientists. What is occurring now is questionable and biased research that will most likely put favorable slants on the funding agent's—the companies'—product(s) or developments. This funding model is a little like asking the tobacco industry to conduct studies to "prove" that cigarette smoking is not dangerous to smokers, or to the rest of us. Livestock producers, for example, are now funding a study of the air quality for the antibiotic- and steroid-laden animals they house within their large-scale production facilities. What do you think the results will indicate? Pharmaceutical companies are now providing large amounts of monies to research departments in universities to "prove" their products are safe and effective. Just like with many sports programs at the university level, pharmaceutical companies ply medical students with "gifts" in order to get them to prescribe that company's products when the residents become doctors. After meeting with a "sales rep" for a pharmaceutical company, many residents change some of the medications they have been prescribing. It has also been found that one-third of Stanford University's medical administrators and department heads have financial conflicts of interest, as it relates to their own research.

In order to maintain the "status quo," many researchers are not permitted to pursue research that might stray from the "standard party line" or risk an unacceptable outcome for the financial security of the institution. Once a study is completed, a particular product may or may not prove to be beneficial for the intended consumer, but some way, the manufacturer must be able to make money on that new product to assure funding its research and development program. In other words, given current funding configurations, one primary goal of research must be concerned with making the money necessary for the continual financing of future research and development.

The third largest cause of death in the U.S. comes from medications that have been **properly** prescribed. Do you personally know how the development of the drugs you take was funded, or how the trials were conducted or how narrowly focused these trials were, or how comprehensive the data gathered were? Pharmaceutical companies also receive a lot of federal government funds. Early research is usually funded by the National Institutes of Health (NIH), and once the research begins to show some promise, pharmaceutical companies step in to continue the funding for completing the research. These companies also receive huge tax advantages; all research and development costs are tax deductible, as are marketing expenses. On top of that, pharmaceutical companies are entitled to seventeen years of exclusive rights to each medication's patent. Having that patent means that no other drug companies can manufacture or sell the particular medication, so the pharmaceutical company can offer it to the consumer at whatever price company representatives arbitrarily choose to set, within some boundaries, of course.

While an argument can be made that having private companies fund research leads to faster transfer of knowledge, quicker product development, more rapid clinical trials, and (potentially) increases in economic growth, the other side of that coin is that independence, integrity and objectivity, hallmarks of credible, pure research, might (will?) be lost. Commercial interests and profit margins may take precedence over verifiable research objectivity, academic autonomy, and "the public good," creating insurmountable conflicts of interest. In the case of GlaxoSmithKline's product, Avandia (Paxil), nearly 2/3 of the negative trials the product experienced were never published. When further investigated, it was discovered that children who had been prescribed Paxil, were two times more likely to present with pre-suicidal behavior. In the subsequent lawsuit, GlaxoSmithKline denied they had suppressed relevant data and, ultimately, allowed the results of the clinical trials to be posted online. Avandia was also shown to increase the risk of heart attacks by 43% percent of the adults who took Paxil. As a result of ensuing investigations, it was uncovered that the Food and Drug Administration (FDA) had known about the undisclosed negative findings for quite some time. Whistle-blowers both within the FDA and the academic setting have been pressured to withhold all information they possess regarding the drug and its potential risks and side effects.

Currently, the nation's pharmaceutical companies finance about 70% of all drug research. About 75% of the pharmaceutical funding goes to "for-profit" research firms, not even to educational or medical institutions. As mentioned earlier, the FDA had refused release of the prostate cancer drug, Provenge, until a further trial was given. Two of the voting board members who denied release of the drug allegedly had ties with a competing pharmaceutical company. All arguments, both those for increased federal funding, as well as those for continued privatization, cite "the public good" as their *raison d'être*. The concern we have is the apparent lack of any kind of balance in the institutional responsibility for our future scientific research between the private and public sector. How is it possible for institutions operating for profit to perform the medical and scientific research we need with veracity and integrity, strictly adhering to practices that ensure results in which we may be confident? Are we at the point where the Pandora's box of quick-return payoffs is replacing scientific integrity? There will be no either-or scenario soon, but we feel that serious reflection and consideration should be given, especially by the institutions of higher learning where medical research is conducted, that their motives for accepting funding do not impinge on the outcomes of their findings. Results—all results—must be reported accurately and must be absolutely independent of funding source interests. Their credibility and reliability must be maintained at all costs. It is extremely disconcerting even to think there could be integrity issues involved with any research, but reality has unmasked numerous alarming incidents, by both the public and the private sectors, that have given rise to public disillusionment and mistrust. Is it being too naïve to expect better from everyone involved?

The Future of Stem Cell Research

So—what do stem cells do anyhow? Why are they so valuable? What purpose do they serve?

In has only been relatively recently—since 1981—that stem cells were isolated, and the amazing potential is still just beginning to be realized. In terms of medical research, these past thirty years have brought about incredible—absolutely stunning—progress. Let's look first at a brief chronology of that evolution.

1981—Stem cells isolated in mice. For next 14 years, stem cell research continued in universities and medical facilities in countries all over the world.

1995—Stem cells isolated in rhesus macaque monkeys.

1998—First human embryonic stem cells isolated.

2000—Guidelines issued by the National Institutes of Health (NIH).

2001—Bush puts hold on federal funding for stem cell research; by July, two Republican senators want federal funding for stem cell research, but other Republican "leaders" oppose it; August—Bush lets 23 lines of stem cells be used, but of those, the vast majority prove to be contaminated or to have genetic mutations. The U.S. incurs a scientific "brain drain" as American researchers head overseas in order to be allowed to continue their stem cell research.

2004—South Korea clones a human embryo; New Jersey appropriates $9.5 million for stem cell research; November—California approves $3 billion over 10 years for stem cell research. Some American researchers, who had been overseas or who had worked in states that disallowed their research, begin to head to California to continue their work.

2005—South Korea streamlines the process to use fewer human eggs to produce useable embryos for stem cell research, which could lead to mass production. November—New Jersey approves an additional $150 million for stem cell research; the House passes a bill to ease Bush's restrictions for federal funding of stem cell research—bill passes to the Senate, but Bush promises to veto it. Connecticut approves $100 million over the next 10 years for adult and embryonic stem cell research; Connecticut governor signs a public act to permit stem cell research, but bans human cloning. Tennessee Republican Senator supports relaxation of the Bush restrictions. California researchers inject human neural stem cells to repair spinal cords in mice, which may help paralyzed mice walk again. Florida proposes an initiative to fund $200 million over 10 years for stem cell research; two days later, opponents petition to ban funding for stem cell research. South Korea research is challenged, saying it's "tainted." By December, South Korea will say all research is tainted, and by May 2006, the head researcher will be brought up on charges of fraud. New Jersey is the first state to finance human embryonic stem cell research and allocates $5 million to researchers.

2006—Maryland allocates $15 million for embryonic stem cell research. Bush vetoes a bill that expands federal funding of embryonic stem cell research. August—new technique is developed to remove a cell from an embryo, without harming the embryo. Missouri voters back a constitutional amendment to protect embryonic stem cell research.

2007—Studies conducted by two universities show that stem cells drawn from amniotic fluid donated by pregnant women might be equally as valid as embryonic stem cells. Iowa eases restrictions on stem cell research, and allows medical researchers to create embryonic stem cells through cloning. California allocates an additional $75 million to fund credentialed scientists at twelve non-profit and academic institutions. Senate passes a bill to expand funding for embryonic stem cell research, but the bill fails to achieve the 2/3 majority needed to override the Bush veto. An institute in Massachusetts shows that skin cells may be modified to act like embryonic stem cells. The House approves legislation to ease Bush's restrictions on federally funded stem cell research; the bill would allow the use of embryos from fertility clinics which otherwise would be discarded; the bill fails to get the majority needed to override the Bush veto. Bush again vetoes legislation that would permit stem cell research.

2008—Obama reverses restrictions on federal funds for embryonic stem cell research. More American researchers who had been overseas return to the U.S. to continue their work.

2010—November 9—U.S. Court of Appeals rules that federal funds for embryonic stem cell research may continue for now. The administration had argued that to stop research while the case proceeds through the court system would impede progress toward helping someone with a life-threatening illness. November 10—a woman with brain cancer is injected with neural stem cells to fight her cancer, the first in the world to do so; it will be months before any results are available. November 11—the first patient with a spinal cord injury is injected with stem cells that came from a donated human embryo; this was from a fertility clinic, which would normally have destroyed the embryo.

Stem cells may be obtained from a variety of sources: fetal cells, embryonic cells, embryonic germ cells and adult cells. Some researchers are also exploring whether or not fat cells can be used (if so, we want to be among the first to make a hefty donation). Stem cell research can help us understand more thoroughly how humans develop, and could also change how drugs are developed, thereby reducing the need for such expensive human clinical trials. Stem cells have been promoted as possibly being able to prevent, diagnose and treat people, not only with cancer, but with a variety of other illnesses as well: heart disease, diabetes, Parkinson's Disease, Alzheimer's Disease, multiple sclerosis, ALS, severely burned people, replace damaged organs, help replace atrophying muscles and tissues, cure or reduce the risk of sickle cell anemia, and even possibly to repair spinal cord injuries. Stem cells allow the body to heal itself. Stem cells can be "programmed" to develop into any of the 220 cell types within our bodies, such as glandular, blood, nervous system, pigment, and germ, just to name a few of the broad categories of cell types.

There is still considerable debate about whether (and when) to use embryonic stem cells or adult stem cells because both have their uses, but in very different ways. Embryonic stem cells allow researchers to know how the body is able to naturally grow, repair and regenerate tissue. It is only in the first few days of embryonic development that the stem cells can be transformed into any one of the 220 cell types. In a late-stage embryo, there is so much specialization that they become "multi-potent" cells that can only develop into specific tissues, but are unable to become "pluripotent" cells with the ability to become any kind of tissue. Adult stem cells right now are limited to growing into different types of their cells of origin, but new research is indicating this field may be broadening. Embryonic stem cells can be grown in cultures in the lab, while adult stem cells cannot be culture-grown as readily. The importance of this is that large numbers of stem cells are needed to do stem cell therapies. Whether stem cells live up to their advanced publicity remains to be seen, but the research being conducted will help researchers learn more about how humans develop, which may lead to the discovery of other therapies or cures.

The Bush (II) administration supported adult and umbilical stem cell research, but claimed there were 60 lines already in use by private researchers. Scientists, however, said there were only 11 usable stem cell lines. Of the 23 embryonic stem cells that were eligible for federal funding, the vast majority—some resources say as many as 20—were deemed damaged or had genetic abnormalities. The Obama administration rescinded the restrictions the Bush administration had imposed. In actuality, even if hundreds of embryonic stem cells were available, it wouldn't be enough. Remember, these embryonic stem cells would come from IVF embryos that would ultimately be discarded. Embryonic stem cells can be difficult to work with because some grow into liver cells (just as an example), others grow into blood, others into nerves or other tissues, such as heart cells. There is no way to determine which embryonic stem cells would grow into the actual area of the body in which a scientist wants to do research. It has been estimated that as many as 60% of people undergoing IVF would donate their unused embryos, if given the decision-making authority; another estimate projects there are as many as 400,000 embryos currently stored at fertility clinics across the country.

So what research into stem cells is currently being explored?

Shinya Yamanaka and his colleagues at the University of Kyoto were among the first, in 2006, to show how adult stem cells could be changed into "pluripotent" (iPS) stem cells, although research in this area has been on-going for nearly the entire thirty years since stem cells were isolated. Pluripotent stem cells are adult stem cells that have been returned to an embryonic state. They are easier to be programmed, but have problems making the transformation efficiently. Because iPS cells have the ability to change into any cell in the body, the inefficiency of the transformation is a critical problem to overcome. This unlimited capacity of iPS cells could mean that damaged organs can be repaired and other diseases can be treated. It takes about fourteen days for cells to become pluripotent. However, only 0.01 percent of iPS stem cells actually make the change into useful stem cells. A recent discovery by Duanquing Pei at the Guangzhou Institutes of Biomedicine and Health in China has found that vitamin C can boost the efficiency from 0.01 to 0.1 percent. While that may not sound like much, it is still a significant number that can be developed into iPS stem cells for different areas of the body.

If a person could donate his/her own cells to prevent, diagnose and treat a disease, there is less chance of rejection by the immune system, and a decreased need to take anti-rejection medications for the rest of his/her life. It has been found that iPS stem cells can be maintained indefinitely, which would be helpful in the development of cells for a specific disease or condition. There is also the potential to develop new drugs to treat various conditions. An unknown, at this point, is whether the iPS stem cells retain any kind of "memory" of the particular body cell from which they were taken. There is some concern being raised, however, about the use of pluripotent stem cells. The International Society for Stem Cell Research has raised a question about the hypothetical use of pluripotent stem cells to turn into either sperm or egg cells. This use could lead to cloning and other ethically questionable practices previously mentioned in this book.

Most everyone is familiar with Christian beliefs when it comes to the issue of stem cells. On one end of the spectrum, there is one side that says absolutely under no conditions should embryonic or fetal stem cells be used for research. This comes too close to "playing God." At the other end of the spectrum, another group says under certain conditions, such as just after a miscarriage, or with embryos that would be destroyed as a normal part of the in vitro fertilization process, fetal and embryonic stems cells may be used for research.

Islamic belief takes the middle ground when it comes to stem cell issues. As long as unborn babies are not being harmed, as long as there is no harvesting of fetuses, stem cell transplants and/or research is encouraged. There is a belief in the sanctity of life which applies to all medical research. Research that dedicates itself to the promotion of health and to increased longevity, but not at the expense of any other life, is to be encouraged. The use of organs after death to help another human being is O.K., because a living person is not being harmed. As with most religions, there is a wide range of opinions within Islam; the variations occur across the 72 different Islamic sects. It is believed, however, that you can find God in science. God gives you medicine, but you ". . . have to go to the mountain," so to speak. You have to seek out the medical experts, and not just wait for God to cure you. Prayer has to be supported and accompanied by taking action. Medical resources, including stem cell transplants, are one of the blessings of God. Spiritual and ethical answers require a combination of prayer and effort, and of finding the balance in all things.

Jewish belief also has a wide range of opinions. For Orthodox Jews, the Halachic (Jewish Law) tradition plays an integral part of determining medical issues, whether at the beginning of life or at the end. There is also a mandate to provide medical relief and healing wherever possible; this is called *pikuah nefesh*—the duty to save the life of a human being. As stated on the Torah website, ". . . good ethics—and good Jewish Law—require good facts." Halachic traditions make no distinction between stem cells and regular body cell tissues. The idea that using stem cells is "playing God" does not come into question. It is for Jews, in fact, a moral imperative. God is perceived as both a teacher, and a healer. Jewish law accepts medical intervention to correct defects. The issue is whether studying stem cells is to be used to treat a medical problem (such as exploring how to change genes to prevent Downs Syndrome or diabetes), or to improve upon God's creations by trying to produce people with only blonde hair and blue eyes or to clone another child. Within these examples, the former is acceptable, but the latter is not. Jewish tradition would allow the use of adult stem cells or umbilical cord stem cells to heal a disease.

In Jewish belief, for embryonic stem cells, once the embryo has been implanted in the uterus (around 40 days), it becomes a fetus. The harvesting of the fetus may NOT be used, even to save another life. The only exception to this directive is when it becomes necessary to save the mother's life, or when it has been determined the fetus will be born with a defect. Under no circumstances would it be condoned to conceive a child for the express purpose of obtaining stem cells, regardless of the circumstances. If an embryo has been developed to use for in vitro fertilization, and has not been transplanted into the mother and attached to the uterus, it may be used for stem cell research according to some Rabbis. The Halachic tradition considers it a sin not to use stem cell research, because of the law governing healing and the saving of human lives. Rabbi Mose David Tendler, a professor of Jewish Medical Ethics at Yeshiva University, has called stem cell research "the hope of mankind." Hadassah, The Women's Zionist Organization and the National Council of Jewish Women are also in favor of stem cell research. As technology and medical science advances, each will require a separate interpretation from the Torah. For a more in-depth discussion, see http://www.torah.org/features/secondlook/stemcell.html, and http://www.hods.org/English/m-issues/age-health.asp.

In the Sikh faith, a "Sikh" is a "disciple", a student of religion, someone who is to continue to learn and improve personal character throughout his/her life. One is to live by faith, hope and optimism, and to live without fear or hate. The greatest service for a Sikh is service to mankind. This is the true path of virtue. The wearing of a turban for a Sikh is to encourage a commitment to his/her beliefs and to show respect for others. There is the deep belief that all people belong to a single humanity, and women are treated as equals. The body is a vessel, a temporary abode for souls. You should not become attached to the body itself, but focus on the inner self. Our bodies are a gift to us from God for the soul's journey. Life and death are in God's hands. For

Sikhs, it is believed caution should be exercised when it comes to stem cell research. If embryos are used, where will this lead society? Will the practice be exploited? Will human trafficking occur because money might be involved? There is no real concern for using umbilical cords for research, because no harm is being done to any living being. A member of the Sikh faith would urge caution when it comes to abortion, primarily because it is unknown how society might judge this act, or whether the embryo might be sold. Use of a fetus from a miscarriage would probably not be a problem. Stem cell research conducted using animals raises concerns for someone of the Sikh faith. An animal is a living body.

For many faiths, ethical and spiritual questions inherent in stem cell research will remain topics for continued discussion, perhaps for decades to come. The blinding pace of scientific discoveries today will require ongoing review by Torah, Qu'ranic and Biblical scholars to interpret the extent to which the each new discovery is in accordance with the various doctrines teachings, beliefs and traditions of each faith.

Given the complexities and limitations of the knowledge that can be gleaned from stem cell research, it is an unavoidable fact that embryonic and fetal stem cells will continue to be needed. They can serve as a type of "reference point," or baseline data, for other areas of stem cell research. It may be that fetal stem cells are applicable for disease X; embryonic stem cells are applicable for disease Y; and pluripotent stem cells for disease Z. What is already apparent is that stem cells have the ability to revitalize and change, not only the medical field, but also the medicines being developed, the therapies to be used, the possibilities of a cure for some diseases, and even the world of research as we currently know it. There is such a vast potential to help people with an inestimable number of conditions.

Currently, numerous researchers are exploring the uses to which stem cells may be applicable. Just a few of those that appear to be very promising are described briefly over the pages that follow.

- Stem cells and cancer cells share one common attribute: they both are body-building cells. However, when cells, which normally help to build your body, run amuck, this rampant reproduction leads to cancer. The cancer cells mutate into a malignancy and become very specific forms of cancer. Normally there is a regular network in place to prevent cells from becoming cancerous, but once these networks are compromised, it's difficult to find the exact combination of mutations that caused the cancer. Stem cells do not have any restraints on them either, but the major difference is that with stem cells, the genomic potential is controlled, but in cancer, it's totally uncontrolled. (As an aside, cancer stem cells are a whole different breed of animal than the stem cells that are transplanted to help cancer patients).

- Replacement teeth: this is a difficult field to work with because of the relationship between the jaw, and which teeth have to go where. In a human embryo, teeth formation begins as early as ten days. These "buds" are formed between two embryonic tissues. As the jaw develops, signals are sent out that determine which tooth grows into which shape, and the kicker is—it can't be changed. This makes it difficult for stem cells to be placed in an adult's jaw and hope that the right tooth grows in the replacement spot. At this juncture, the adult jaw can't take the stem cells and program them into the correct tooth. But isn't it exciting to think it might be possible, particularly for those of us who are aging baby-boomers.

- In the February 2010, issue of *Scientific American*, it was reported that unspecialized epidermal stem cells in the embryo interact with cells in the dermis which can differentiate into hair follicles and different sweat glands. (Did you follow that? You should have seen the original sentence in the article.) Research is now being conducted in several places to determine how these epidermal stem cells are created and maintained, and how they become eccrine sweat glands in humans (humans have more eccrine sweat glands than animals do, which is why humans have watery sweat; it is far more efficient than an animal's oily sweat).

- Skin cells from the skin of ALS (amyotrophic lateral sclerosis, or "Lou Gehrig's disease," as it is known in the U.S., or "motor neuron disease" as it is known in the United Kingdom) patients have been turned into stem cells, which then were turned into motor neurons to help people with this crippling disease. This was achieved through research being conducted by a joint Harvard-Columbia University team of scientists. The study is intended to help understand how ALS develops, and might possibly help in screening medications to be used for treatment of the disease. The technology might also be useful for people with other degenerative diseases.

- Sickle-cell anemia—people with this disease have red blood cells, which normally carry oxygen, that are not the usual round shape, but rather crescent, or "sickle" shaped. These misshapen red blood cells have a difficult time going through the small blood vessels to deliver oxygen where it's needed. Frequent transfusions work for a period of time, but eventually the immune system learns to recognize the proteins and begins to attack the red blood cells. The body works to destroy the life-saving blood. Stem cell transplants have been used to alleviate this problem. A donor provides bone marrow, which contains non-infected stem cells. Chemotherapy drugs are used to destroy the bone marrow in the patient with sickle cell, and then the donated stem cells are inserted. The amazing thing is that the person who received the stem cells no longer has sickle-cell anemia—s/he has the blood of the donor. There is a however, however. This procedure does not work 100% of the time with 100% of the people. There are still inherent risks that must be addressed. Further complicating the issue is that currently there is no way to determine which patients will have success, or which ones won't. To date, results have shown bone marrow from a related donor has greater success than from an outside donor.

- Research is being conducted to see whether stem cells can be used to repair damaged hearts, help cancer go into remission, produce blood, generate nerve tissue, repair muscles, produce cells for the retina, stimulate tissue repair of the skin and cornea, and heal damaged spinal cords. Should these studies prove any of these hypothetical functions possible, we all triumph.

- Stem cell research is also exploring whether treatments can be developed for Parkinson's, Alzheimer's, arthritis, and paralysis.

In one preliminary trial, stem cells were used to help people with multiple sclerosis. Some neurological losses were reversed.

- Through funding by the U.S. Army, designs for replacement organs, such as the kidneys, heart and lungs, are being explored. The long-range goal is to determine whether arms and legs lost by soldiers in war can be regenerated. Can you just imagine what that would mean for our soldiers, the men and women who defend us at great expense to their bodies, or for anyone who might lose a limb?

- Japanese researchers have demonstrated the ability to regenerate organs that are inside the body itself. As yet, regeneration of appendages outside the body has not been successful.

- In 2007, a German doctor was treating a 40-year-old male patient, who not only had HIV, but also leukemia. Gene and cell therapies were used to create new stem cells, from which a stem cell transplant was performed. Following the transplant, the HIV could no longer be detected. The donor had been very carefully selected; he had a rare genetic mutation, which lacked an HIV receptor and made the new cells immune to HIV. The man was cured of HIV, and remains healthy to date. For people with HIV, however, the best course of treatment today continues to be the variety of drug "cocktails" doctors prescribe, unless there is some other complicating disease the patient has that needs to be addressed.

- At Advanced Cell Technology, stem cells have been used to treat or prevent blindness. This phase is in trial and has only been demonstrated on mice. The Pediatric Glaucoma and Cataract Family Association is using stem cells that exist in adult brains. In studies with rats, researchers have taken these stem cells and genetically modified them to produce (sorry, more technical jargon) neurotrophic factors called BDNF, and inserted them into the retina. There has been some success in lessening the extent of optic nerve damage with this procedure compared to a group that did not have the BDNF factor introduced. In Japan, a group of researchers (Negishi, Kubota, et. al.) found that embryonic stem cells could be used to support the regeneration of optic nerves. Speaking of blindness, Italian researchers have successfully reversed blindness caused by chemical burns by using the patients' own stem cells. This procedure was successful in 77% of the cases, including one man who had lost his sight over 60 years ago, and now has near-normal eyesight.

- Scientists are exploring the treatment of brain disorders with fetal cell transplants. The primary disease being targeted is Parkinson's. Muhammad Ali considered having his Parkinson's disease treated with fetal tissue in 1987. Recent initial findings seem to indicate that younger recipients fare better than older recipients. However, it may have been that there were some serotonin-secreting neurons that prohibited the effectiveness for older patients.

- Another trial involving stem cells is working with children who have Batten disease. Batten disease is a fatal condition where genetic mutations prevent patients from producing enzymes to clear cellular waste.

- Another children's trial using stem cell therapy focuses on a disease called Pelizaeus-Merzbacher (PMD). This disease is a genetic disorder that prevents the creation of myelin, which covers the axons of nerves. PMD causes a kind of crippling of the transmission of nerve impulses that slows physiological response time. This means, for example, that a child who touches a hot burner on a stove would most likely receive severe burns, because the "pull-back" or retraction reaction from the burner would be so slow as to cause deep burning of the dermal tissues.

- In the April 2009, issues of *Discover* and *Scientific American* magazines, mention is made of a preliminary trial using stem cell therapy to help people with multiple sclerosis. Northwestern University "stopped, and in some cases, reversed the effects of early-stage multiple sclerosis." This was originally published on January 30, 2009, online at *Lancet Neurology*. While this research was conducted using only a small number of patients and further research is needed, it is still an encouraging sign.

- Researchers are studying the use of embryonic stem cells to produce red blood cells. It is hoped sufficient quantities can be produced to use in blood transfusions. Currently bone marrow cells and the umbilical cords from newborn babies are being tested.

Both are in short supply and, at this time, are only useful to the donor. However, the hope is that this research will find a way to develop broader applications so that in a time of crisis, blood would never run out. Such a possibility would be especially useful in times of natural disasters, as well as during military engagements, which it seems, we humans will be forever bringing upon ourselves.

- Douglas Melton, co-director of the Harvard Stem Cell Institute, Cambridge, MA, has had a unique and interesting history with stem cells. Originally trained as a molecular biologist in amphibian development, Dr. Melton changed course at the peak of his career when his son, Sam, was diagnosed with Type 1 diabetes at six months of age, and began to focus on using stem cells to make insulin-producing cells. During the bleak years from 2000 through 2008, Dr. Melton practically kept the stem cell field alive by creating over 70 embryonic stem cell lines through the use of private funds, and then got them into labs for research, not only in the U.S., but around the world as well. Because of restrictions on stem cell research, many talented researchers from the United States moved abroad to continue their studies. Initially, the stem cell field focused on either embryonic stem cells that can grow into any one of the body's 200 tissue types, or cells from skin that were limited to a small number of tissues. Thanks to Dr. Melton, the stem cell field now has touched on regenerative medicine. He found a way to take cells and reprogram them to become another type of cell. Dr. Melton has now been able to watch Type 1 diabetes cells actually develop, and has gone farther afield in using non-stem cells to produce other cells. He has helped generate new ways of thinking about how to replace and repair damaged tissues. His huge body of research and discoveries could lead, in the future, not only to treating a disease such as diabetes, but also to curing it, so that people with the disease will no longer have to live out their lives being insulin-dependent.

- Along with the uses in regenerative medicine and cellular therapies for such diseases or conditions as diabetes, spinal cord injury or Parkinson's, stem cells may even have the potential to cure baldness, additional good news for those of us who are aging baby-boomers.

- Stem cells have been found in the thyroid gland at any age, with from six to eight renewals during each person's lifetime. What is not known is whether these stem cells originated in the thyroid or migrated from another location. It is also not known whether thyroid stem cells or universal stem cells can mutate, which could trigger tumor growth. It has been found that stem cells exist in higher quantities, but in an extremely small percentage, of goiters. Stem cells and cancer cells share a couple of common abilities—they can be both self-renewing and can grow indefinitely. Some researchers are exploring whether thyroid cancer is actually a stem cell disease. Cancer stem cells have been noted in some thyroid cancer cell lines. The possibility exists that stem cells from goiters could be used to treat some degenerative or myocardial diseases. At this time, however, it is unknown whether thyroid stem cells are a danger or a potential future resource.

- Stem cells are being explored as a treatment for severely burned skin or after some forms of radical surgery.

- Robert Lanza, rebel and risk-taker extraordinaire, has been working with hemangioblasts, multi-potent cells that are available in the embryo, and have now been found to be present in post-natal tissues of individuals, both the newborn and the adult female. (Please refer to the website at http://www.robertlanza. com/generation-of-functional-hemangioblasts-from-human-embryonic-stem-cells/ for information regarding his research.) During the second Bush administration, Dr. Lanza was prevented from using his stem cell research to help a 16-year-old boy regain his sight. He was also prevented from continuing research into using embryonic stem cells to reverse paralysis in a sheep that had spina bifida, intending, of course, to eventually apply the research to humans. At the same time, he was again prevented from helping a woman whose glial cells that support the functioning of the central nervous system, located in the cerebellum, which were rapidly degenerating. His research just might prevent limbs from being amputated, may help prevent blindness, and may even help prevent heart attacks. As an example, researchers injected hemangioblasts into a damaged limb, and there was nearly a 100% restoration of the blood flow to the limb within one month. By injecting the hemangioblasts into people who have had a heart attack, the death rate was cut in half. Dr. Lanza points out that there are more than eighty autoimmune diseases for which he is hoping to use hemangioblasts as progenitors in the immune system. He has used stem cells to make little kidneys, which have actually produced urine. Drugs are being explored that target cancer stem cells. This could revolutionize the treatment of leukemia and could possibly help stabilize and/or extend disease-free survival.

- Neither Alexis nor Terry were aware of what was being done with stem cell transplants for liver disease until a family member of a family member needed the information. A whole new world opened up. The X-Cell Center in Dusseldorf and Cologne, Germany, is a private clinic which is using autologous (self-donor) stem cells for degenerative liver disease. They are also exploring the use of stem cells in the treatment of cerebral palsy, spinal cord injuries, different forms of diabetes, Parkinson's disease, stroke, multiple sclerosis, macular degeneration, Alzheimer's disease, arthritis and heart disease. Hammersmith Hospital in London is using stem cells to try to reverse cirrhosis of the liver. A clinic in Japan is using autologous stem cells to treat liver fibrosis. The University of Minnesota in the U.S. is doing research in the areas of liver support and gene repair but the researchers estimate it will take five or more years to complete the studies; there are no human trials currently scheduled. The Oregon Health and Sciences University is studying macrophages, a type of white blood cell that destroys bacteria and tumor cells, and is also key in stimulating other cells in the immune system. The investigators hypothesize that it is actually the macrophages in bone marrow stem cells, and not the bone marrow stem cells themselves, that can cure a genetic liver disease. Currently they are using mice to test their hypothesis; there are no human trials expected in the near future. Researchers at the Beijing Institute of Transfusion Medicine in China are looking at hepatocytes, liver cells that make up 70–80% of the cells in the liver, from bone marrow or embryonic stem cells to improve therapies to treat liver disease. The University of Pennsylvania School of Medicine has found a protein marker in adult liver stem cells that can possibly be used for cell-replacement therapy. This is exciting because it means that in the not too distant future, these stem cells may be used to help people whose livers can no longer self-repair. At the University of California in San Francisco, one of the doctors hopes to transform some embryonic stem cells into new liver cells, especially for the treatment of young children. Johns Hopkins University in Maryland has shown that bone marrow stem cells can convert into liver cells and repair the organ. Newcastle University researchers in England have actually grown the first artificial liver through use of stem cells taken from the blood of a newborn baby's umbilical cord. This procedure has the added benefit of reducing the numbers of animals currently being used for research.

• Max Wicha, M.D., at The University of Michigan, is researching cancer stem cells. He has found that only about 1% of the millions of cells in a cancer tumor are cancer stem cells. The University of Michigan was the first institution to discover them in breast cancer tumors, and the U of M research team is now looking at adrenal, brain, breast, colon, head and neck, leukemia, lung, melanoma, myeloma, pancreatic, prostate and thyroid cancers. Dr. Wicha and his colleagues are trying to find a way to destroy, or, at least to control, the cancer stem cells. If these stem cells can be targeted and eliminated, it is possible the cancer will not spread to other areas of the body or recur at all anywhere. The cancer stem cells may also help predict how aggressive a person's cancer might be, and what treatment or protocols would be most likely to work best.

• In Italy, researchers helped to cure "bubble babies." Stem cells that contained the gene that is functional for this disease were inserted into the babies' systems, yielding profound results for the majority of infants.

• At some point in the future, stem cells may possibly be used to create your own personalized medical treatment. In combination with your genomes, your health care program would be tailored to your own particular genetic code, taking into consideration your personal lifestyle as well. Yearly examinations would be conducted to see whether you are becoming prone to cancer or any other diseases.

- Just in case you have not already heard, stem cells are also currently being explored to make meat. Yes—MEAT! It is estimated that up to 200 pounds of meat can be generated by just ONE stem cell. The In Vitro Meat Consortium, composed of scientists from Denmark, the Netherlands, Norway, Sweden and the United States, are exploring how to take a stem cell from an animal's muscle, force it to become a muscle cell, feed it nutrients, and then allow it to continue to grow and divide. A handful of animal umbilical cords could potentially make enough meat for all of the people on the planet for perhaps one full year. Just think of it . . . it could end world hunger and would revolutionize farming and eliminate the horrid, unhealthy and inhumane slaughterhouses. In the U.S., for example, up to 98% of our meat comes from "factory" farms. It has been estimated that it takes up to 5,000 gallons of water, 15,000 pounds of feed, and 284 gallons of oil for transportation costs to bring one cow to slaughter (the beef industry says it's 14 gallons of oil). With sufficient funding by world governments and the best and brightest of global scientific and mathematical minds, non-animal meat production that would eliminate the need for the wholesale slaughtering of our animals could become a reality in 10–30 years from now (10 years for ground meat; 30 years for more complex pieces of meat, such as steaks or roasts, etc.). See *Science Illustrated*, the November/December 2010, issue pp. 58–61, or go to http://www.invitromeat.org for more information. Now, after having read the February 2009, issue of *Scientific American*, "The Greenhouse Hamburger," by Nathan Fiala, we realized another consideration in support of the development of meat from stem cells. Just consider the impact on the environment. Our ingestion of meats and poultry eject more greenhouse gases than either industry or transportation put together. In fact, various estimates put it at between 14%-22% of the total emissions. To produce the annual beef diet of an average American creates greenhouse gasses equivalent to driving more than 1,800 miles in a car. Even the vegetables we buy at the grocery store contribute to greenhouse gases in the forms of the fuel required in the refrigeration and transportation of the farmers' produce. Admittedly, when we read about the research to produce meat out of stem cells, we were a bit squeamish, but even knowing that little bit about greenhouse gasses almost makes meat produced from stem cells palatable.

- Stem cell research and treatments for pets is also being conducted. In many respects, stem cell treatments for animals are light years ahead of that for humans. A company called Vet-Stem Regenerative Veterinary Medicine has developed a procedure that includes stem cell transplants for cats, dogs and horses. In horses, they can treat fractures, joint diseases and tendon and ligament injuries. They have treated dogs for osteoarthritis and orthopedic soft tissue injuries affecting the tendons and ligaments. Vet-Stem is also looking into the treatment of autoimmune diseases, cerebral and myocardial infarction, immune-related disorders, irritable bowel syndrome, muscular dystrophy, and treatment of liver failure. Only veterinarians who have completed Vet-Stem's Regenerative Cell Medicine Credentialing Courses are certified and approved for use of any of these protocols. Go to http://www.vet-stem.com and http://vetmedicine. about.com/od/diseasesandconditions/a/Vet_stem.htm. What is interesting is that research has also been conducted on other animals by using adipose-derived (fat) tissue. See http://www. vetlearn.com/ArticleDetails/tabid/106/ArticleID/1580/Default.as px, or the website at http://www.ncbi.nlm.nih.gov/pubmed/ 18183546

- For fun and, perhaps for decreasing the extent of your disbelief, go to the Microscope Imagining Station at the Exploratorium in San Francisco. There you and your kids can encounter the technology with your own eyes. You will be able to explore live mouse stem cells as they make their way toward becoming heart cells that can actually beat. Just think of the implications!

- And for those of you wondering if receiving a bone marrow transplant could fool a DNA test, the answer is—probably not. If there was a suspect in a case that had been cleared of a charge and who had had a bone marrow transplant, the inside of the cheek would be swabbed, or a skin sample taken. The results would reveal the true DNA.

- For a list of references about stem cell research, including cancers of the brain, breast, leukemia, lymphoma, multiple myeloma, ovaries, kidneys, retinoblastoma, sarcomas, and testicles (to name a few), as well as for end-stage bladder disease, corneal regeneration, coronary artery disease, Crohn's disease, diabetes, Epstein-Barr infection, heart disease, jawbone replacement and skull bone repair, limb gangrene, liver disease, lupus, multiple sclerosis, myasthenia, juvenile and rheumatoid arthritis, osteogenesis imperfecta, Parkinson's Disease, red cell aplasia, scleroderma, severe combined immunodeficiency syndrome, sickle cell and other anemias, spinal cord injury, stroke, thalassemia, etc., check out the website at, http://www.stemcellresearch.org/facts/asc-refs.pdf.

Many countries are participating in stem cell research. The parameters of the research can be very different though. What follows is a partial representation of the vast array of stances regarding stem cell research around the world, presented alphabetically by country.

- *Australia*—National laws have been enacted to ban cloning, but there is no consensus on stem cell research. The government will consult with researchers and community and medical groups before making a final determination. Stem cell research is allowed in certain parts of the country. However, no embryos developed for therapeutic use may be implanted in a womb, and must be destroyed within two weeks of development.

- *Belgium*—This country is an avid supporter of stem cell research and has been successfully extracting stem cells from embryos since 2005.

- *Brazil*—Stem cell research is permitted on embryos, which have been frozen for at least three years, and come from in vitro fertilization banks, which would normally have discarded them. In 2008, when Brazil's Supreme Court ruled that stem cell research was allowable, the practice was legalized.

- *Canada*—Research on discarded embryos from in vitro fertilization was legalized in 2006. However, at this point in time, embryos may not be created for the purposes of research.

- *China*—Research using embryonic tissue for stem cell research is banned in China. However, stem cells may be studied if drawn from the umbilical cord or placenta. The government also allows clinical trials for critically or terminally ill patients to participate in stem cell therapy.

- *European Union*—There is no direct funding for stem cell research that results in the destruction of the embryo. If research is approved, funding is directly given to the source. The vast majority of funds are allocated to adult stem cell research. The three top European nations that support stem cell research are Belgium, Sweden and the United Kingdom. There is a new law in Great Britain which allows researchers to create stem cells by cloning. If embryos are used, they must be destroyed after two weeks.

- *France*—In 2004 the French government opened a five-year window for researchers to conduct stem cell research by importing embryos that would have been discarded by in vitro facilities. In 2006, researchers were allowed to develop their own stem cell lines from extra embryos.

- *Germany*—Likely as a result of unethical Nazi experiments during World War II, Germany has one of the most restrictive stem cell policies in Europe. However, this was eased a bit in 2008, when the government allowed the use of stem cell lines developed before May 1, 2007. This exception was granted to help facilitate the study of stem cell therapies and treatments.

- *India*—There is a huge industry in stem cell banking in India that may be used by a patient for future medical treatment. Stem cells, however, may currently be used only for bone marrow transplants.

- *Italy*—There are strict limits in Italy when it comes to stem cell research. However, government policies do allow scientists to import already-existing stem cell lines.

- *Israel*—There are no laws in Israel that regulate stem cell research. Research into stem cells has been ongoing since the 1960s. Embryos may be used in stem cell research. Researchers have used embryos to grow heart cells that can actually beat on their own. Research is also being conducted that focuses on regenerative uses for stem cells in the areas of ALS, diabetes, Parkinson's disease and for spinal cord injury.

- *Japan*—Guidelines have been approved for stem cell research that includes the use of embryos. These embryos may only be taken from those used for fertility treatment that would otherwise be discarded. Kyoto University has also conducted research using bone marrow cells to withdraw adult stem cells. By combining these with bio-engineered substances, the university team has been able to regenerate nerves that had been damaged, fully restoring their functioning.

- *Mexico*—There are no regulations on stem cells in Mexico, even though there is a well-established stem cell industry in the country. Critically ill people from all across the world, including the United States, have been treated with stem cells for conditions such as autism and cerebral palsy. The lack of regulatory guidelines has been widely criticized by many doctors and researchers around the world.

- *Saudi Arabia*—Saudi Arabia has been very active in stem cell research. The research efforts officially began in 2002, when the Saudi government issued a proclamation that biotechnology was to become the "new oil" in the country. By 2003, it became legal to use embryos both for research and for therapeutic purposes.

- *Singapore*—Stem cell research has been ongoing in Singapore for many years. There are more than forty stem cell research groups in Singapore. A panel comprised of people in the fields of law, philosophy and science has been convened to examine ethical and moral issues surrounding biotechnology. By offering a plethora of incentives, the Singapore government has actively recruited researchers from around the world. It is legal to use embryos no more than two weeks old for therapeutic purposes.

- *South Africa*—In 2002, Mark Shuffleworth visited the International Space Station and studied stem cell development under zero-gravity conditions. In 2003, South Africa allowed the therapeutic cloning of embryos. In 2004, South Africa became the first country on the continent to create and operate a stem cell bank.

- *South Korea*—South Korea has led the way and been in the fore-front of stem cell research for many years. Policies regarding stem cell research are very flexible. Researchers have produced stem cells that are a perfect genetic match for all ethnic groups. This means that the stem cells may be individually matched, which reduces the risk of rejection by the immune system.

- *Spain*—Originally, Spain had determined that embryos frozen prior to 2003 could not be used. This law has been changed, and now, embryos frozen within two weeks of conception may be used both for research and for treatment. This law also permits the parents of a child with an incurable disease to conceive a new embryo, and then to use the stem cells of the new baby as a tissue donor for their sick child. This procedure is strictly moni-tored and may not be used until all other options have been tried. It is not meant to be a primary treatment. Spain became the third country in Europe to develop a stem cell bank. Spain has also developed three research centers specifically for con-ducting stem cell research and to further regenerative medicine.

- *Sweden*—This country not only has political support for stem cell research, but it also has wide public support as well. Sweden became the second European country to establish a stem cell bank.

- *Switzerland*—In a national referendum, approval was given for stem cell research through the use of embryos that were fertil-ized for in vitro purposes that would otherwise have been dis-carded. The government, however, does not allow embryos to be deliberately created specifically for conducting stem cell research.

- *Offshore* stem cell treatments are burgeoning. Countries such as the Dominican Republic and Thailand are experimenting with stem cell therapies that are not approved in the United States. American doctors are using the more flexible laws in these coun-tries to treat patients who can't get what they need in the United States. In the Dominican Republic, American patients receive autologous (self-donated) stem cells for a variety of conditions. It is very expensive—up to $64,000 in some cases, and insurance companies will not pay for what they consider to be experimental treatments. In the July 2010, issue of *Popular Science*, a report on a company, called Regenocyte Therapeutic, was included. The company reportedly harvests stem cells, flies them to Israel where they are given a platelet growth factor, and then are flown back to the Dominican Republic for transplant. Other companies, such as the XCell-Center in Germany, TheraVitae, with headquarters in Toronto, Canada, but operating in Thailand, and Beike Biotechnology in China are all using similar procedures. Some American doctors go overseas to conduct their research because of stringent, some say "strangling," review processes and trials required by the U.S. Food and Drug Administration. It is a delicate balancing act. How does a government agency, which is responsible for monitoring and overseeing that health care and pharmaceutical therapies assure safety for every person, and concurrently, NOT overburden or delay the development of life-saving treatments?

It is important to keep in mind that there are multiple stages in conducting the trials necessary for FDA approval, and expenses can top $100 million. In the United States, tissue use, such as that for skin grafts and bypass surgeries from a donor for personal use by that donor had not been regulated by the FDA, including stem cells. It was not until 2005 when stem cells, in use for decades, were put under government regulation if they had been treated with growth factors or other drugs. This is true whether they are autologous or donated for use by another person. Often, but not always, clinical trials conducted in some other countries do not go through the double-blind, random trials that are required in the United States, nor are there peer reviews or research published so that other scientists can try to replicate the processes and procedures. However, what is the line between good science and risk-taking to save a life? The question becomes: if the clock was ticking and you or someone you loved needed a potentially life-saving treatment not sanctioned by your government, would you not go anywhere possible to try and save that life, no matter how experimental or unverified?

Overall, stem cells have both a promising future and a rather dismal track record in terms of discoveries. Much of the research that has been and is currently being done revolves around using stem cells to cure diseases. While a lot of this has been unsuccessful, that doesn't mean that we should stop. One day, perhaps in the not-too-distant future, we will discover other uses for stem cells rather than curing diseases, and these uses will benefit all of human kind in one way or another. However, there is a relatively new process that shows great promise, and perhaps sooner than the other research being done. This is using skin cells, such as with people who have ALS, and then creating induced pluripotent (iPS) stem cells out of them. Mention has been made earlier in the book about iPS stem cells. What is unique about the research being done by Wendy Chung, at Columbia University in New York City, and in collaboration with Harvard University in Massachusetts, is that she and her team took these cells and created ALS in petrie dishes, or what has been termed "disease in a dish." This enables the researchers to really study how a disease goes wrong and as a result, develop truly effective drugs to combat various illnesses. Other researchers are now using this process to look at other blood diseases, juvenile diabetes, Parkinson's, sickle cell anemia and spinal muscular atrophy. In Germany, researchers have even made cardiac cells that actually beat just like a heart, which helps them study heart arrhythmias. Is this not unbelievable?

Much work remains to be done in stem cell research, but the promise over time is immense. The biggest boon might be for the relief from pain and suffering, as well as extended life. To think that today it is possibly just beyond the horizon makes this an amazing time to be living. But the question for some of us then becomes,

> *"Will it come soon enough? . . . in time for . . . whoever it is you love?"*

So—Someone You Love
Isn't Surviving Cancer . . .

. . . Now What?

Not everyone is as fortunate as we have been. Some people will die from cancer. Perhaps the two of us, at some point, will have our cancers recur. Perhaps you might also become one of "those" people, especially if your cancer metastasizes. Perhaps you love someone who won't survive. What can be done to help make that transition between final diagnosis and the end of life?

Whether or not you are the person who is dying, number 1 on the list is to be willing to talk about it, or to be willing to listen. That doesn't mean you force the issue. It means being willing to be open to a discussion about death. This should not even need to be said, but please do not barge into the person's living room or bedroom and say, "Now we are going to talk about death," or anything similar. And in the middle of a celebration is not the ideal time, either. There are those times when directness may need to be tempered with a little reflection and role reversal.

If you are the person who is dying, you may want to talk about it, but are afraid of upsetting your friends and family. If you are a family member or friend, you may be reluctant to bring it up for the same reason. *Please talk!* You need to do this; we all need to do this! If the person who has cancer wants to talk about it, *please listen.* That person needs to talk. Do NOT avoid the issue and run away. But also, respect the dying person's wishes if s/he is not ready to talk about it. You will have at least opened the door for future discussions to take place, when the time is right for both of you.

Next, talk about how you want your remaining days to be conducted. Remember you always have choices about how you want to live your life. Decide what's important to you, not only about the actual end of your life, but also what your priorities are for the time that remains. It is important to take care of the mundane details—where are the life insurance policies, title to the car, the safe deposit box key, the name of the mechanic for the car, who is good at home repairs? Does that mean spending more time with your family and friends in general, or only those of your friends and family to whom you are closest? Are you able to travel? What makes you laugh? Hospice provides people who can help you write your story (Janet, one of Tom's high school classmates, does this), how you want to be remembered, what was important to you or significant in your life (for example, how it was to grow up in the 1960s or during the depression, special memories of a treasured family member or friend, your greatest life achievement or most exciting experiences, etc.). It could be this is the time to start creative writing or participate in art therapy, not only for yourself, but also for your family. Live every moment you have left. Remember, you will be leaving your family and friends with *who you are*, giving them strength to cope when you are no longer either able to take care of things, or are not around to do them yourself.

Find a way to tell your story. Write things down, talk into a tape recorder, make a scrapbook of things you remember, and how you want people to remember you. This may also include stories that were told to you by your parents and grandparents. Think back over your life. If you have letters written to you by family or friends, these make great inclusions within a scrapbook. Write letters to the people who mean the most to you. Talk about the times you have spent together and how much they have contributed to your life. If this seems like too big a task to take on right now, ask a friend or family member to help you get started, to figure out how to set priorities. It makes a difference if you have been given two weeks or six months in what you say and do. Please don't be concerned whether things are spelled correctly, or the sentence is incomplete, or if you decide to illustrate your story, use stick figures if you have to. Most of us simply aren't Rembrandts, but look at how much a great many people admire the works of Pablo Picasso, Jackson Pollard and Salvador Dali. The important thing is that it will be from you, illustrated, as you want it to be for those you love.

Another way to tell your story is through photography. Terri Shaver, founder of the non-profit The Oldham Project, at http://www.

theoldhamproject.org or twitter.com/oldhamproject, provides free formal photographs for families who are facing a terminal illness. She began this project several years after she gave birth to a stillborn baby. While she and her husband had the opportunity to hold their daughter, there were no pictures taken of her. This left a big gap in her and her husband's lives. (She also works with "Now I Lay Me Down to Sleep," providing free photographs for parents who have had stillborn children.) Photographs can become an everlasting memorial, not only for the person with the illness, but also as a reminder of who the person was as a human being for those who remain. The Oldham Project works in conjunction with Hospice. The Oldham Project is located in East Lansing, Michigan, but you may want to contact the local hospice in your state or country to see if there is a similar program available where you are.

Find a way to live in the "now" of time. Enjoy the people who come to see you, the stories you share, the food you eat, a sunrise or sunset, the laughter of a child, and find things that make you laugh. Yes, you will be able to find them, even if right now it seems impossible and unfair. Yes, you may have to look and search deeply, but they are there. Find a way to focus on other areas rather than all the preparations. Others will take care of the details if you can give them some broad brush-strokes. Listen to your heart as it guides you through this next phase of your life.

When Tom's kids' maternal grandfather was dying of cancer (he had been given three to four months to live), the message had been passed on that no one was supposed to talk about his impending death. Linda's death was still painfully fresh in Terry's mind, the incompleteness of not being able to say goodbye was still achingly clear. We saw him about a month before he died. There was so much Terry wanted to say—what a wonderful influence he had been in her life, how much she had appreciated his sense of humor, the love he demonstrated to his family, his ability to treat everyone fairly, his depth of knowledge in some areas, his stories of his experiences during World War II, and all of his skills and abilities he so freely shared with his grandchildren and his great-grandchildren. Not talking about "it" became the elephant in the room. But it worked for him and his immediate family. He died the way he wanted. So sometimes, silence is perfect. Sometimes cancer can't be fixed, but if you are family or friend, simply being there can be enough. Or if you are the one who is dying, simply being there for your family and friends is enough. A Truism:

"Silence can be most eloquent."

Care at the End of Life

This chapter is written as much for us as it is for those of you facing this final battle, whether from cancer or another disease. A great deal of the content comes from a really helpful website called "Healthwise." We encourage you to access this website and respond to the questionnaires available there that can help you make informed decisions. Another truly helpful booklet is from the American Health Lawyers Association (AHLA) website at, http://www.healthlawyers.org, entitled "We All Need to Plan for the Future."

Regardless of how compassionate, knowledgeable, competent, qualified and experienced the doctors, nurses and support staff are, in spite of the excellence of the drugs and treatments that are administered, and despite the effectiveness of all the new drugs that researchers are constantly finding, the fact is that some people, many people, simply don't—or won't—survive cancer. They fight this magnificent fight for days or months or years, exhibit unbelievable fortitude and endurance, personify immense dignity and courage in the face of overwhelming odds, and somehow, find the inner strength to reach out and comfort those around them, and then . . . leave us.

As Doctor Beckrow said, "Tomorrow is promised to no-one." That's one reason to live life fully in the "now" and to cherish each moment. None of us knows how much time we have. Terry has promised her niece, Monica, to live until she's 112, but Monica's part has to be to live well into her 90s, which she could very well do if she would just stop smoking (update: she almost has! Hooray!!! That should give those of you who are smokers some hope and encouragement.). But— tomorrow is promised to no-one.

At the end of life, many decisions have to be made. First of all, you need to come to terms with how you feel about death. Are you afraid of dying? If so, then a trusted therapist or spiritual counselor or religious advisor should be contacted to work not only with you, but also with your friends and family. Another alternative, just in the beginning stages, concerns interesting research being conducted by Roland R. Griffiths (Johns Hopkins) and Charles S. Grob (as reported in the December 2010, issue of *Scientific American*). They are using a hallucinogenic drug, under exceptionally controlled clinical conditions, called psilocybin (hello, 1960s!) to treat people with advanced stage cancer. Some people participating in this research report a lack of the fear of death, of feeling a "oneness"—a sense of connectedness with all people and all things, a deep sense of sacredness or euphoria, even months after the last chemo treatment. Depending on the length of time you have remaining, you may have time to work with a therapist or spiritual advisor, but if time is short, you might want to explore a quicker option.

Some people may not want to work with a therapist or spiritual advisor, or use drugs. Regardless of the option or options chosen, the primary person who should have the most to say is the one who is facing impending death. This statement is not intended to discount those who will remain, or to ignore their very deep and real feelings of loss, impotence, hopelessness and heartbreak. But for the person that this disease or illness is impacting, here are a few additional thoughts to consider and talk over with a trusted person, one who will make sure your wishes will be honored. If your family and friends are objecting to your wishes, you may need to give your trusted friend or family member a Durable Power of Attorney, and make out a living will. Even if your life was lived impetuously, with a "come as it may" philosophy, you do need to plan your end—if it is in any way important to you.

In addition, some doctors feel uncomfortable talking about death with you, because they view themselves as having failed you, their patient, and your family. An interesting historical aspect is that in the past, medical schools did not prepare doctors with any training on how to talk to their patients about death and dying. Fortunately, this omission is being corrected, and medical schools now include this content within their curriculums. Good doctors do become emotionally involved with their patients, and the death of this living, breathing, vital person sitting in front of them can be as hard on the doctors, nurses and support staffs as it is on the families. In the cases of Terry and Alexis, some staff members at Red Cedar Oncology actually became a part of their families, and Terry and Alexis became parts of the families of some of Red Cedar's staff members. The deep connections made are likely to be enduring for all parties involved.

Another consideration to keep in mind is that some doctors may want to prolong your life as long as possible simply because of the threat of a malpractice lawsuit. Again, communication is absolutely essential. Before going in to talk to your doctor, write down all of your questions, including those not only about your physical condition and options, but also, any religious or spiritual concerns you may have. Your doctor may not be able to provide you with any counseling in this area, but it might help in making decisions regarding the final treatments you will receive.

Whichever of the options you choose, make sure you talk with your doctor and all of the potential persons who may be needed to carry out your final wishes. Your doctor will often have options that fit your personal philosophy of life through his or her knowledge of you as you have gone through treatment. When you have this discussion with your doctor, take the person along who has the Durable Power of Attorney. While it may complicate things, you might also want to take along the person who is objecting most to what you want. Sometimes, except in the case of the most stubborn of people, or those who are having the most difficult time letting go, having answers might help them cope. Whatever decisions you ultimately make, be sure your doctor and his/her associates know your wishes, including the doctor who takes over when your "real" doctor goes on vacation (yes, they need to do that for their own health and sanity). Put everything you want in writing. Leave nothing to chance. In this technological age, you could even make a video of your wishes.

Decide what kind of health care you want. If you stop breathing, do you want CPR or other heroic measures taken on your behalf? Make out an advanced directive, which includes a living will and a durable (medical) Power of Attorney (the terminology may vary from state to state or country to country). A living will details what you wish if you are unable to speak for yourself. A Durable Power of Attorney will name a person who will have the right to make treatment decisions for you at the end of your life, or if you are unable to speak for yourself.

Decide if you want any of your organs donated, either for study or for transplant (if you've had a stem cell transplant, you are ineligible). Talk with your doctor first to see if your illness precludes organ donation. If are able to donate organs and wish to do so, many states allow you to indicate this on the back of your driver's license. Or, you can fill out an organ donor card, which is a witnessed document that lists the organs you want to donate. Minors (youth under the age of 18) must have parent or guardian consent for their donation to occur.

Make out your will. You may not think you have much to leave, but if you don't, squabbles may arise that preclude your wishes from happening. If you have a will, update it. Determine who the executor is to be; this person will follow the wishes expressed in your will, from start to finish. Once the proceeds have finally been disbursed, the courts will close your estate.

What kind of care do you want? *Curative treatment* is: don't spare anything—do everything possible to maintain your life. You want every machine possible breathing for you, and every drug possible given to you to help you live. This would include the use of a feeding tube for administering artificial hydration and nutrition. There are several risks associated with artificial hydration and nutrition. For example, when Terry's Mom was dying, IVs were inserted to keep her free of pain. Swelling occurred, which meant the needle wasn't able to remain in the same place and it had to be reinserted. Her lungs filled with fluids and had to be emptied. On the other hand, if you are unable to eat or drink, artificial hydration can give you energy. If your condition isn't immediately life threatening and there is a good chance you may recover, use of feeding tubes could be a viable option for you.

Palliative care, on the other hand, doesn't try to prolong life. It looks at keeping you comfortable, and as pain-free as possible. Palliative care does not diminish the frequency with which you see your doctor, and you will still receive excellent medical care. Some of the questions you might want to ask yourself in making the decision about the type of care you should choose include: Is my life shortened by the illness I have? How important is it that my death be peaceful? What goals do I have yet for the remainder of my life? If my life is maintained or sustained, will the quality of the life I have left be enhanced? Is prolonging my life a realistic step to take? What is my long-term prognosis? Which choice of care affords me the greatest opportunity to leave this world with a sense of dignity? Which choice will be least difficult for my family to live with?

Other decisions need to be made that require you to answer more questions. Where do you want to receive care? . . . In the hospital? . . .

With Hospice? . . . In your home as long as possible and to the extent possible? . . . With your children? . . . In a nursing home? Who do you want to be primarily responsible for your care and medical decisions when are no longer able to do so?

Look for opportunities to talk with your family and friends about death. This is often awkward and uncomfortable. In American culture, we simply don't acknowledge death or talk about it. Other, more ancient, cultures fold death in as a part of life. When you talk about death with your family and friends, some people will be concerned about your religious or spiritual preparation for death. Some people will want to make sure you are as pain-free as possible. Some people will want to talk about your shared history, to remember the good times, to remember the laughter you shared. Some people will want to express their anger or their sorrow at this next stage of your life.

Before you get to the point of having to decide on either curative treatment or palliative care, is there a support group of people in the same position with whom you could freely talk? What services are available for your friends and family, both before and after your death? What financial issues should be considered? Should your will be amended to cover any unforeseen expenses that may arise?

What if you change your mind? That is entirely possible and in some cases, a very smart move. If so, make sure the person who has the responsibility of carrying out your wishes from your living will or Durable Power of Attorney knows about the changes you wish to make. Again, put everything in writing. If you've made a video tape, make a different one. And make sure your doctor knows.

And now comes, perhaps, the most difficult piece to talk about rationally: the dying process. Whether you are caring for someone who is dying or whether it is you, there are some common occurrences that tend to happen to most of us. People who are in the final stages of a disease, such as cancer, might experience one or all of the following symptoms as the time nears:

- Shows a decreased interest in eating.

- Has difficulty in either urinating, or in having a bowel movement.

- Experiences irregular body temperatures; some people either run a fever, or feel very cold.

- Exhibits behaviors indicative of a decrease in being socially involved with people, or caring what is going on in the outside world.

- Daily periods of being awake become much shorter, and energy levels decline; the body often becomes excessively weak.

- Breathing changes. Slow, deep breaths, turn into rapid breathing, which will alternate with short, shallow breaths, before breathing finally stops.

- Some people have visions of others they have known who have previously died, or see scenes from their past. For many people who are dying, these visions appear to bring them comfort, because they frequently seem to become much more peaceful toward the last moments of life.

It has been estimated that about 85% of dying people become comatose the last three days of their lives. Sight usually ceases at about the same time (it takes a lot of energy to see and keep your eyelids open). Hearing, however, remains keen up until almost the last breath. It is important that you keep talking during the final period of a person's life. Talk to him or her about memories from when they were young, stories they used to tell or something they said or did that helped you in your own life. Sing. Pray with him/her. Play his/her favorite music. Read passages out of one of their favorite books. If you are of a Christian faith and your friend is Jewish, it is fine to read from the Old Testament Psalms (according to Rabbi Jeffrey W. Goldwasser), if a Jewish Bible is not nearby. Write a letter and read it aloud. Reassure him or her that the family will be fine, and when it is time to leave, even though s/he will be missed, everyone will understand. In many cases, a person has a hard time dying until those reassurances have been given. If your faith or religion allows it, tell the person who is dying to look around—he or she might find other loved ones who have gone before them and are waiting to escort them Home; assure them death is nothing to fear, rather something to be celebrated with ultimate joy and awe. Tell him/her this last passage will soon take him/her to the place where s/he will be surrounded by peace and an eternal, unconditional love. Should you personally need to leave his/her bedside, either because of other responsibilities or even to answer the phone, and the person dies while you are gone, please don't feel guilty; realize that some people simply want to pass when everyone has left and everything possible has been said and done.

For many, the dying process can actually be a time of healing and for growth. It is a time to share memories, to heal and fix broken relationships, and what is equally, if not more important, to say good-bye. Terry's first concrete, palpable experience with death was when she was in junior high (called middle school today). She had gone through elementary school and junior high school with a boy of whom she was very fond; his name was Roger Evans. He was a kind and gentle soul, possessing a wonderful sense of humor and a smile that was at once shy and yet invited the world into his life. She and Roger quite often sat next to each other in school and helped each other with math. He played the cello, and Terry played the violin in music class. One day he was in school, the next day he wasn't. And then, she heard he had died. No time, no reason, no opportunity to say good-bye. Back then, and even now, kids were sheltered from death. Everything about Roger was all "hush-hush"—but by doing that, the children missed out on an opportunity to learn about an important part of life and, as a result, were never allowed to find or feel any kind of closure. Even today, what Terry still needs to do for herself is to find where Roger is buried, go there, and finally, have the chance at last, to say good-bye. This experience has remained an unfinished chapter, a mystic aching hole never filled throughout her life, one whose presence ebbed at times, but always resurfaced with a passion.

One of the most unquestionable truths at this stage is that Caregivers must take very good care of themselves. Caregivers have a critical role to play in this whole process and can become mentally, physically, emotionally and spiritually exhausted. They will have the need to seek help and comfort from your and their own circle of friends and family, to not feel like they are totally and completely alone in this devastating experience. While you as a caretaker are there to care for someone else, it's vitally important to take care of yourself, as well. An excellent book to read is Gail Sheehy's *Passages in Caregiving: Turning Chaos into Confidence.* Another resource developed by the San Diego chapter of Make Today Count provides a caregiver's "Bill of Rights." One of the doctrines they site unequivocally is that the caregiver has "the absolute right and the obligation" to take care of his or her own needs as a critical part of his/her role. (http://www.caregiverslibrary.org/Default.aspx?tabid=291.)

Caregivers also provide a large amount of informal time which is often not counted in cancer care costs. It may be that those who are caregivers have had to give up their jobs in order to care for the person who has cancer. In the September 4, 2009, issue of *Cancer*, it was reported that the National Cancer Institute had conducted a study in which they measured these donated or informal costs. The amount used to calculate these costs was $16.28 per hour. At those rates, informal caregiving costs for breast cancer were $38,334 (over a two-year period), for lung cancer were $72,702, for Non-Hodgkin's Lymphoma were $59,613, and for ovarian cancer were $66,210.

Often after a death, an autopsy ("to see for one's self") is conducted. If the death has been expected, there is usually no autopsy. If you do want your loved one to have an autopsy, be sure to determine the costs before proceeding.

Grieving is natural, normal and actually, healthy. There is no time limit for grieving. After a death, it is normal and healthy to be in denial, to feel shock, anger and guilt. Guilt can occur when the person who has died had a long illness, and those that remain are feeling glad the person is no longer suffering. Guilt can also occur when there is the feeling not enough had been done, that somehow or another, if "more had just been done," this loss would not have happened. Additionally, guilt may be felt if you were the person who had to choose to increase a medication to prevent excruciating pain, and as a result, the dying process was hastened. These guilt feelings are common during the grief process, but it is important for each of us to focus on the more positive aspects of all that was done for our loved ones, and on how we can celebrate the person that was a part of us, NOT on what "coulda, woulda, shoulda."

Some people are able to make a transition from grief to acceptance in as little as two years. Others can take much longer. Everyone grieves in a different way. Some people throw themselves into their work in order to cope. Some people resort to drugs, including alcohol. Others lose interest in life for a time, and fail to do even simple things, such as eat or bathe or provide for their young children. Survivors who grieve need to be patient with themselves, giving themselves the time necessary to go through this transition. Friends and family members of these survivors also need to be patient, and not say or carry an attitude of "Gee, it's been a year. You should be through this by now." What friends and family can help with is to watch the person who is grieving, and if that person seems to be having an inordinately tough time coping, help him/her get into grief counseling. Grief counseling is not for everyone, but can prove to be a tremendous help for anyone who seems to have become trapped within his/her loss.

Some websites with further information regarding end of life care and grief issues are listed below for your reference.

- http://www.dyingwell.org (for people who are facing death, their friends, families and caregivers)

- http://www.caringinfo.org (offers free resources and a help line for quality of life information)

- http://www.compassionatefriends.org (this one is intended for those of you who have lost a child)

- http://www.growthhouse.org (provides resources for life-threatening illnesses and end-of-life care)

- http://www.medicare.gov (Medicare information)

- http://www.nhpco.org (provides contact/service information about Hospice and palliative care)

- http://www.med.cornell.edu/public.health/ethics (from Cornell University; for patients, families, caregivers and medical professionals)

Steps to Take to Reduce Your Risk of Cancer or to Reduce Your Risk of Metastasis

The year 2010, became a banner year: it was the year cancer became the leading cause of death, replacing heart disease, which had reigned for about 100 years. Specifically, African-Americans will die at a higher rate of cancer than any other group in the U.S. A clinical trials database for a study by the Southwest Oncology Group, based on 20,000 patients, found that African-Americans with breast, ovarian and prostate cancers have a tendency to die earlier than cancer patients of other races, even if they get the same medical treatment and when their socioeconomic indicators are taken into consideration. African-American males face a 21% higher death rate for prostate cancer, and 61% of African-American females face higher death rates among those women diagnosed with ovarian cancer. These data indicate that in all likelihood, biological and/or genetic factors may account for differences in survival rates. There were no statistically significant differences found based on ethnicity for survival from other cancers, such as colon, leukemia, lung, lymphoma, and multiple myeloma. In a study conducted by the *Journal of Clinical Oncology*, it is predicted the incidence of cancer among minorities will be close to double by 2030, while Caucasian rates are expected to increase by about one third (31%).

Lifestyle changes are a must! We are not saying if you either already follow the suggestions detailed on the next few pages, or start to do them now, that you will definitely avoid cancer, or prevent it from recurring (metastasizing). We are simply saying that these suggestions will probably help you stay healthy, or at least stay healthier. As always, check with your physician, for any other advice s/he may offer.

1. *Know your genetic base for cancer.* Search for your family medical history. Because early detection is so key to cancer survival, check with family members to see if anyone has either died from cancer, or who may have died from cancer. Medical records from 100 years ago are sketchy at best, but you might find clues that could indicate cancer. Once you have this knowledge, share it with all your family. Keep good records of who had what and when, regardless of the disease. If you have had someone who died or contracted cancer on both sides of your family, be proactive and work with your doctor to be tested. If the doctor recommends tests, <u>take them all</u>. **<u>Don't leave anything to chance.</u>** Cancer is an opportunistic disease and can spread, even if you don't have symptoms. If you think something is wrong, camp out at your doctor's office until you get him or her to listen to you. Remember Alexis's experience—her doctor said she was "too young" to have a mammogram, regardless of her genetic background. In reality, according to Dr. Campbell, genetics accounts for between 1%-3% of diagnoses. The rest is probably life style and environmental conditions.

2. *Eat lots of fruits and veggies, preferably fresh,* but if not available, then frozen or canned (in that order). You should have a minimum of 5 servings (1/2 cup) of fruits and veggies every day. This may reduce your risk for colon cancer.

3. *Reduce, if not eliminate, your intake of red meat.* Yes, it's hard to give it up, especially in this fast food, hamburger-and-french fries world. Beef tastes good. And it does have some nutrients that help your blood manufacture iron. But if eating beef is simply a must in your diet, switch as much as you can to grass-fed beef and other meats. Grass-fed beef is lower in cholesterol, and tastes even better than corn-fed beef. Try not to have beef more than once or twice a month, and then no more than two ounces. Make sure the package of beef you buy in the grocery store says "<u>No Antibiotics</u>" and "<u>No Steroids</u>." "Organic" really doesn't say much, and "Natural" has absolutely no specific meaning whatsoever. Substitute fish and free-range chicken for animal protein, but beans would be an even better choice. <u>Stay totally and completely away from processed meats</u>—

bologna, pickled bologna, salami and hot dogs, to name a few. If you have to have hot dogs for your 4th of July picnic, try to buy kosher hot dogs, which are mostly all meat, or find some hot dogs that have been made from grass-fed beef. Research conducted at the University of Texas indicates that "well-done" meat increases your risk of bladder cancer by 94%. If you eat your meat medium-well, your risk is 46% lower. The findings indicated that cooking meat at higher temperatures and for longer periods of time actually created carcinogens.

4. *Drink alcoholic beverages in moderation.* Alcohol helps cancer progress more rapidly if you already have cancer. It has also been shown to increase the risk of getting cancer. Alcohol has been shown to increase the risk of head and neck cancers, breast cancer and cancer of the liver. Alexis will have a drink or two on the weekends. Terry might have a glass of wine every six months. There are some studies conducted by the French that show a glass of red wine can be beneficial, but you have to weigh that with their lifestyle—Europeans tend to be much more physically active, eat smaller portions of food, and have more free-range protein in their diets than Americans. And Europeans are less likely to get drunk than Americans; they tend to drink in moderation.

5. *Smoking—QUIT! Right Now . . . This Instant!* If you haven't started, *DON'T.* Stopping smoking is easier said than done, because not only are there addictive substances added to cigarettes, but the act of smoking becomes a very social habit. Research has now shown that cigarette smoke, whether first hand or second hand, causes—ready for this?—Immediate damage to your lungs and DNA. And damaged DNA can lead to cancer. Think you're safe by switching to smokeless tobacco? Think again. There is increased risk of fatal heart attack, fatal stroke, not to mention cancers of the mouth and throat. If you are a woman who has smoked 100 or more cigarettes *in your life*, you have significantly increased your risk of breast cancer, according to the Mayo Clinic. Research conducted by the Dartmouth Medical School and the National Cancer Institute has found that smokers in New Hampshire have increased bladder cancers since 1990. If you are a current or former smoker and

have head and neck cancer that is linked to the human papillo-mavirus (HPV), your prognosis is worse than for those who have never smoked. <u>You will also be five times more likely to have your cancer recur.</u> A European study has determined that smokers and children exposed to second-hand smoke have an elevated risk of developing bladder cancer. Even passive smoking can increase the risk of breast cancer by 27%. In pre-menopausal women, the risk with passive smoking for breast cancer goes up 68%, active smoking by 46%. A study in Britain has shown that if you are diagnosed with early stage lung cancer, stopping smoking may reduce your risk of the cancer recurring. Genentech researchers have found that in one particular patient who had a tumor removed from his lungs, there were over 50,000 genetic mutations. In this patient, <u>for every three cigarettes he smoked, one gene mutation occurred,</u> but gene mutations may occur with every cigarette you smoke. In public places where smoking has been banned, such as in workplaces, businesses, restaurants, etc., some studies were conducted to determine whether the cessation of public smoking in these enclosed environments made any difference in the health of those who were present on a daily basis. There was a 17% drop in heart attacks after only one year, and a 36% reduction in the number of new cancer contractions after three years, according to studies done in Europe and North America. In research published online in the *International Journal of Epidemiology* on February 15, 2011, Laura Blue and Andrew Fenelon reported that Hispanic immigrants who did not smoke (in fact smoked less than Hispanics born and raised in the United States) lived significantly longer despite economic disadvantages ("*Explaining low mortality among US immigrants relative to native-born Americans: the role of smoking*"). Regardless of what the tobacco industry says, there is a direct causal correlation, borne out by copious research, which shows cigarette smoking brings about lung cancer. ***If you won't quit for you, which is the real reason you should quit, quit for your children and other family members, who are DYING for you to have a cigarette!*** They are breathing in your second-hand smoke, which has been proven to be of even greater danger to them. In the April 2010, issue of *Scientific American*, <u>there is now the extreme danger of</u>

third-hand smoke. Cigarette smoke doesn't just linger in clothes, furniture, drapes, and in your mouth. The smoke from cigarettes can react with nitrous acid vapor, which comes from gas stoves, heaters, water heaters and cars. This reaction produces a chemical called tobacco-specific nitrosamines. These nitrosamines increase in volume several times after someone stops smoking even for a short while, such as a couple of hours. Once smoking has been completely stopped in an area, it can take up to a year or more for the carcinogens to leave your house, or restaurant, or place of business, dependent upon the density of the infusion. In the meantime, children are most at risk of absorbing this chemical into their systems. Studies are underway to determine the short- and long-range effects of this latest hazard, third-hand smoke. A Truism:

> *"What is the gift that NEVER stops GIVING . . . CANCER?"*
>
> *. . . A cigarette.*

Just ask yourself how frequently it is today that you know or hear about new cases of people who have been stricken with cancer who are not now, nor ever have been, smokers, but have inhaled second- and third-hand smoke. If you are honest with yourself, you know it is rapidly becoming the norm, rather than the exception.

6. *Always use sunscreens that contain blockers for both UVA and UVB rays.* Yes, even if you are of African descent. Blacks may be less likely to get skin cancer, but ironically, if they do contract the disease, they are more likely to die from it. Also, be sure to check the ingredients in your sunscreen. Many sunscreens contain potentially cancer-causing ingredients. Frequency analyses of cancer data are showing that non-melanoma skin cancers are appearing more on the left side of the face than on the right side. With a moment's thought, it becomes apparent why. People driving, whether to work or taking the kids to school, expose the left side of their faces to whatever rays are out on any given day. (We're wondering if the same holds true for people who drive from the right side of the vehicle?) What

makes skin cancers especially dangerous is that they can spread to bones and other bodily organs.

7. ***Check out your workplace exposure.*** We have all heard about asbestos and radon poisoning, and most workplace sites have complied with federal and local regulations prescribing the precautions that must be taken. Even building codes have been put into place to hopefully protect us. But you may want to verify compliance and check with your employer to have some measurements taken. And for those of you who spend lots of time in front of a computer screen at home and/or at work, you might want to check the emissions that emanate from it as well.

8. ***Exercise, yes we must!*** Groan! What a pain! Yuck! Ohhh, man! Gee whiz! &^%$^! While trying not to ignore all of the expletives going around, the fact is that this is one area of your life you can take complete control over and turn your body into a cancer-fighting machine. Terry keeps a rolodex of excuses of why NOT to exercise. (And just look where it got her.) <u>The key is to find something physical you like and really enjoy doing for an extended period of time, then stick with it!</u> Alexis likes biking and jogging, either on the treadmill or outside. Terry likes walking. Others of you may like Swimming, Racquetball, Cliff-climbing, Skiing, Skating—roller and ice, Golf, Basketball, or perhaps, Hang-gliding; the list of possibilities could be almost limitless. Just select one, and open yourself up to unlimited fun and feel-good days. <u>If you look, you will find something positive about doing the exercising</u>: Weight loss, Toning your body, Building endurance, Increasing your energy level, Improving your breathing, Having better **SEX (sorry, but it does happen)**, Sleeping better, Getting stronger, Helping to maybe prevent cancer and/or other diseases, or just finding yourself having a more positive attitude; this list can also go on and on. Recent research conducted in both Australia and at Johns Hopkins University has shown that exercise can reverse muscle loss in men who are receiving androgen deprivation therapy for prostate cancer. For these men, exercise improved their general health and their fatigue was reduced significantly. <u>Plan on exercising a minimum of four or five days a week, for a minimum of a half hour per day</u>, and make it as "hard" or challenging for

you as you are physically capable. Terry does mantras while walking and keeps an eye out for wild life (she has seen coyotes twice, a herd or gaggle or whatever-they-are of over 30 wild turkeys and a brand new hours-old baby fawn—absolutely awesome!). It makes the time go faster and the walking no longer seems like drudgery. Combining exercising with that new healthy diet you will already have started, and it will not be long before you will not recognize yourself, not in the mirror, not in how you feel, and not in how you think!

9. *Try to get at least 8 hours of sleep every night.* That is far easier said than done. We live in a fast-paced, highly intense world. We are prized for our abilities to work fast and multi-task; sometimes, we, unknowingly, compete with colleagues to see who can work the most hours in a day. The various stressors of the day can carry over into the night and haunt our dreams. If this is the case with you, <u>try some deep breathing exercises before going to bed. Find peaceful images to take the place of the worries you have.</u> This is a perfect time to concentrate on your self (note the space). If your significant other snores, move into another bedroom. Snoring, which usually includes sleep apnea, isn't good for him or her, either. There are surgeries that can reduce or eliminate the snoring, as well as a machine called a CPAP (yes, it's uncomfortable to wear). Moving out of the bedroom may turn out to be a good incentive to get your significant other to do something about it, thereby helping both of you. Just because s/he wants you to keep them company or warm during the winter is no reason to put your health at risk; leave the room if you must. A good night's rest combined with exercise has been shown to reduce the risk of breast cancer, especially.

10. *Get rid of plastic containers and switch to glass or metal.* The concern here is not so much to do with cancer, as it is with a byproduct called "bisphenol A" (or BPA). BPA is used to stiffen plastic bottles, the lining of cans and to make smooth paper receipts. The jury is still out, but evidence has been found that BPA is an endocrine disrupter, and has effects on both male and female development, prostate cancer, thyroid disease and cardiovascular disease. Fetuses are especially vulnerable to this and

other chemicals in every-day use. It is also estimated by the Centers for Disease Control and Prevention, that the urine in 93% of people ages six and older have BPA in their systems. This carries over into plastic wraps that are used when reheating foods. Alexis and Terry are gradually switching over to using waxed paper to reheat foods rather than plastic wraps to reduce our exposure to BPA. We are also eliminating the use of plastic bags to reheat foods. Senator Frank Lautenberg (NJ) and Senator Barbara Boxer (CA) introduced the Safe Chemicals Act of 2011 which would require companies to prove their products are safe before they are marketed.

11. *Make sure your sleeping environment is kept dark.* In a study conducted in Israel, an unexpected ancillary finding showed that women who live in brightly lit cities at night are 73% more likely to develop breast cancer. So, if any of you were looking for an excuse to keep your bedroom as dark as possible at night, this finding is a good one for you.

12. *If you have Type 2 Diabetes, check with your doctor to set up cancer screenings.* In a study conducted by Giovannucci, Harlan and Archer, reported in the June 16, 2010, online publication of *CA: Cancer Journal for Clinicians*, it stated that an association between diabetes (especially type 2) and an increased risk for cancers of the breast, bladder, colorectal, endometrium, liver and pancreas had been discovered. However, the study showed that there might be a decreased risk for prostate cancer. Risk factors for both diseases are age, poor diet, lack of exercise, and obesity. Further studies are already underway to explore these findings.

13. *Be very cautious of low-carbohydrate diets,* especially those that promote animal protein as opposed to vegetable sources. These diets have become quite popular in recent years. As mentioned earlier, eating a diet high in animal proteins does increase your risk of certain cancers, as well as causing higher risks for cardiovascular disease. High protein based on vegetables, however, seems to lower health risks, which can include heart disease and some cancers. The Nurses' Health Study and Health Professionals' Follow-Up Study recently concluded that

those who followed a low-carbohydrate diet based on animal protein were more likely to have a higher "all-cause" mortality, along with higher rates of cardiovascular and cancer mortalities. The same study also reached the conclusion that those who had a low-carbohydrate diet based on vegetables had lower all-cause and heart disease mortalities. Please check with your doctor or health care professional before embarking on any diet.

14. *Consciously make the effort to lower your intake of salt/sodium.* While no study, of which we are aware, has yet been conducted between high sodium or salt intake and cancer, there is a wealth of information documenting definite advantages to reducing sodium in your diet. In the United States, people consume copious amounts of sodium, mostly from processed and canned foods. Studies have shown that diets high in sodium lead to increased heart disease and high blood pressure. Recommended salt intake should be at or lower than 5.8 grams per day, but it would be better to limit it to about 3.7 grams per day. In the U.S., average sodium consumption for men is 10.4 grams/day, and for women, it is 7.3 grams. If people were to reduce their intake by 3 grams of salt per day, at the end of the year, new cases of coronary heart disease could be reduced by up to 120,000; stroke could be reduced by up to 66,000; heart attacks could be reduced by up to 99,000; deaths could be reduced by up to 92,000, and up to $24 billion in health care expenses could be saved each year. You've already survived cancer. Why put yourself at risk of another potentially crippling or life-threatening disease?

15. While this may seem a strange place to put this next section, it is crucial. *Educate your children, not only by following the suggestions above, but also by encouraging them, particularly your girls, to take classes in science and mathematics.* And the earlier you can get them excited about science, the better. Neither Pre-school nor Kindergarten is too early to begin; curiosity levels are extremely high during these early years. And it has been shown that infants as young as 8 months have a sense of probability, a necessary attribute in studying science. (As an aside, we also need to take a look at our educational system when it comes to teaching science:

schools teach science concepts abstractly while kids are looking at the real world; we need to somehow combine the two.) An article entitled "Start Science Sooner" appeared in the March 2010, issue of *Scientific American*. This article describes an approach to teaching science in Kindergarten called the "Scientific Literacy Project." The project is described at the following website: http://www.purduescientificliteracyproject.org. This approach combines both science and language so that another subject area does not have to be crammed into an already-full school curriculum. It is "low-tech"; one example of a science project is watching salt dissolve and if you wait long enough, once the water evaporates, you will see the salt crystals reform. Parents (and grandparents, aunts, uncles, cousins), this is something you could be doing at home right now. The University of Illinois has also developed an approach for grades 1–3; it is called "Integrated Science-Literacy Enactments and is available for review at http://www.uic.edu/educ/ISLE/. This project is particularly important in educating girls, who seem to get overlooked in science, and are the first to say they "aren't any good" at it. Studies done with Hispanic migrant girls show that if they get a high school education, they tend to leave the migrant stream, attain additional education, and do better financially, as do their children. The Perry Pre-School Project in Ypsilanti, Michigan, also demonstrated that children participating in an early childhood education program tended to graduate from high school at greater rates than those without the pre-school experience, fewer were on welfare, fewer had out-of-wedlock children, fewer ended up in prison, some went on for additional education, and most had better paying jobs than those who had not attended. Dr. Sohail Husain, a pediatric sub-specialist from the Yale University School of Medicine, provided this quote from the *Hadith* (sayings of the Prophet): "He (the Prophet) placed great stress on kindness to women, and would often say that if a father took it upon himself to educate his daughters and care for their upbringing, God would save him from the hell-fire." From the *Kanz al-Ummal,* "The Prophet once said, 'He who provides a good upbringing to three daughters shall go to Paradise.' A man asked, 'What if one has only two daughters?' 'He also shall go to Paradise.'

Another man asked, 'And what if one has only one daughter?' 'He, too,' replied the Prophet." Likewise from the *Ibn Majah—Kitabul Ilm:* "It is the duty of every Muslim man and every Muslim woman to acquire knowledge." And thanks to Ayesha for this Chinese proverb: "If you are planning for a year, plant rice. If you are planning for a decade, plant trees. If you're planning for a lifetime, educate people."

Whatever your ethnic background or faith, or even lack of faith, education is The Key to reducing and ultimately eliminating, the risk of cancer. Perhaps it will be **your** daughter or son, or your grandchild who finds the cure for cancer, AIDS/HIV, Alzheimer's, ALS (Lou Gehrig's disease), diabetes, Muscular Dystrophy, Multiple Sclerosis or Parkinson's. The list is limitless, but even greater are the possibilities unleashed by an educated human mind. It is truly just a matter of time . . . and hopefully, in time for you and the ones you love.

Alexis's Unexpected Angels

This section is dedicated to all of the unexpected angels in my life (as well as yours). Cancer rearranges not only your priorities, but your life, as well. You focus on everything. When that happens, it is even more amazing when a friend, stranger, co-worker, check-out lady or family member is put in your path for the explicit reason to comfort your soul, make you smile, help you hold it together, or just plain make you laugh, because you are not expecting it. Thus my title . . .

- Andrea, my friend, partner, confidant and soul mate. For every mile you drove me to chemo, for every minute you waited for a doctor to give you news on my condition, for having the strength and diligence to cut my hair and shave my head, for every time you looked at me—scared out of your mind and said, "Everything is okay," for all the long, endless hours we spent in the hot tub and all the decisions we made there, for every renegade turkey wrap and smile just because, I thank you. I wholeheartedly believe I would not have made it through this without you. You are my ever-present angel.

- Neequa—for your love, support, smile, hugs, advice, diligence and every time you stepped out of your comfort zone with me. Thank you . . . my sister angel.

- Mary H.—As you know, I was bound and determined to kick cancer's ass. I took eight weeks off school and jumped right back into a labor and delivery rotation at Battle Creek Health Systems. My first clinical was shortly before my second chemo treatment. Dressed in my "blueberry" uniform and a blue knit hat, I walked into the labor and delivery unit. My instructor, who is another angel, sent me to a prenatal class offered by the hospital. I met Ms. H. at that class. She was the instructor. We chatted briefly before the class about school and nursing. It was during one of the videos that I excused myself, and went to the bathroom. Let me remind you, I was looking rough. Cold, nauseated, no hair, pale, lightheaded (need I go on?!?). Mary followed me into the bathroom and immediately asked if I was all right. (I truly had to pee and take a deep breath.) Then she asked me what kind of cancer, and grabbed my hand. Her sincerity and honesty was exactly what I needed. I told her breast cancer and she told me, "Honey, I am a 10-year survivor. You are gonna be fine." She gave me a big hug and we both started crying. She let me exhale and told me she would be checking on me during my rotation, and she did. Every week, she would contact me or get a note to me, just letting me know she was thinking about me, was on my side, was hoping, praying and smiling for me. She gave me a shirt and a book on our last visit: *Top Ten Reasons to Be an RN* and Kris Carr's *Crazy, Sexy Cancer Tips*. I still have them in my special "Cancer Tote." Thank you for sharing yourself to help someone who didn't know how badly she needed to exhale . . . my unexpected cancer survivor angel.

- Ms. B.J. Roach . . . my friend. For every "just checking" phone call and all the comfort food, for all the care packages and being a listening ear for me or Andrea. Thank you for not only sharing yourself and your time, but for sharing the sacred place in your heart where your mom's memory resides. Thank you for sharing her story, her scarf and her strength, which I see every time I see you. Thank you for your gift of strength and giving . . . my unexpected sharing angel.

- Mrs. Macey Vanderwall—my clinical instructor, who knew when "rocking babies" was a good task for me; for reviewing my care plans and being patient with me and my chemo brain. Thank you for believing in me when I needed it the most. I meant what I said: "I will be a better nurse because of your influence." She's my unexpected instructor angel.

- Mrs. Vicki Hillborg, my labor and delivery classroom instructor who moved heaven and earth to make my dreams of continuing nursing school and beating cancer with chemo simultaneously happen. And for your understanding and prayers. Thank you, my unexpected instructor angel.

- Mrs. Theresa Dawson . . . Thank you for handling my cancer crisis without missing a beat. Your proactive response was an overwhelming boost to my "this will be all right" campaign. For helping me achieve both my Associate's and Bachelor's degrees, thank you. You are my unexpected advisor angel.

- My Mims, who dropped everything and put her life on pause to be near me. My mother's love is unfailing, unconditional and crosses barriers when necessary. Thank you for being my Mom. For that I am blessed . . . my "Mims" angel.

- The 2SE (2 Southeast) staff at Ingham Regional Medical Center. Though I never personally stayed on this floor, I have never felt a bigger healing presence than I do here. This is the Oncology floor at IRMC. The staff members all know me and my story, and I truly believe any one of them would drop everything at a moment's notice to help me. I have seen their passion every time I bring them a patient. "Bless their hearts," is one of my favorite sayings from that floor. To my healing place warriors . . . I thank you.

- My friend, Ray: Your spirit and friendship has truly and deeply blessed my soul and for that, you will forever be a part of my heart. Your courage, knowledge, strength and gift for treating and healing the mind, body and soul blesses every patient that you care for . . . My unexpected healing angel . . . Thank you.

- The bake sale warriors: To the women in the Emergency Department at Ingham Regional Medical Center who baked their asses off and raised one thousand dollars. That is amazing! My unexpected financial angels . . . Thank you.

- Food Fairies: To the girls who brought over loads, and I mean loads, of healthy, non-nauseating food that I would never buy myself that was sooooo good! Thank you for thinking outside of the box. My unexpected food angels . . . Thank you.

- Shelley Sawyer: For your love, concern, wonderful nursing assessment skills, positive attitude and healing hugs! My unexpected blessings angel . . . Thank you.

- To my family: Tim, Carol, Martin, Kaidyn, Kole, Dad and Carolyn: Thank you for being there, ever constant, ready for anything, willing to freely love. Thank you for all the talks, walks, hugs and tears. My family of angels . . . .Thank you.

- Mary at Wal-Mart: The checkout lady who still hugs me every time I see her. Thank you for caring about a stranger in need. My customer service angel . . . Thank you.

Terry's 9 Reasons Why Cancer Is a Gift

For some people, cancer is most definitely NOT a gift. It is a curse. It is the evil eye, the devil incarnate, the Destroyer. For Terry, however, it has been a gift, and for those of you who don't share that feeling, perhaps "opportunity" is a better word. In any case, do you remember the idea, "How the problem gets defined, dictates the solution"? Terry found that thought or belief to be even more of a truth than it sounds. You can choose your attitude

How do you make cancer a positive experience? You look for gifts (or opportunities, for those of you bristling at her insistence of this gift idea). What follows are a few of the reasons Terry knows her cancer has been a gift in her life.

1. *The outpouring of love and support from family and friends.* Sometimes we think we already know we have this and appreciate it, and we think we don't take it for granted, but we do—until something like cancer happens. Suddenly those you thought you knew drop the defenses and the facades of life, and just love.

2. *The recognition of the vastness of our untapped strengths.* We each are far stronger—physically, mentally, emotionally. psychologically, and spiritually—than we give ourselves credit for, as are our families, friends and colleagues. Having witnessed all of the occasions when people have risen outside of themselves and been able to do the most unexpected and extraordinary things on behalf of someone else gives cause for a celebration of life.

3. *The opportunity to meet and know some of the most incredible people, people I would never have known otherwise, those who truly have been the gifts that never stop giving.* Some were and are facing things much worse than I, and are doing it with such grace, dignity and humor that it takes your breath away and then, inspires you. Whenever I'm tempted to go on a pity party, which does happen, something or someone comes along and reminds me of how wonderful I really have it. Along with these people, have been the awesome, incredible and amazing medical staff teams. Tom once asked Dr. Rapson why she chose oncology. "Isn't it a depressing field? After all, very few of your patients will recover," he stated. Her response? "No, this is the most inspiring field I could have chosen; I learn so much from all of you, my patients," she said. Unbelievable!

4. *The knowledge that has been gained, and at some point, may be passed on to others for some kind of good.* Now, granted, all things considered, I wish Tom, Linda, Pat, Nicky, Rose, Rita, Erica, all the others and I had never had cancer. This kind of experience is one we can all do without. Except in the long run, you never know when this experience, and all the knowledge one gains through the battle, will become helpful to someone, somewhere, sometime, somehow.

5. *The spiritual growth that has occurred within me.* I have had the opportunity to read tons of books while undergoing chemo (when you're hooked up to an IV tree from 5 to 24 hours at a time, and there's absolutely nothing on TV, and you're tired of seeing the same movie for the sixth time, stretching your mind and learning can become wonderful events). I am finally beginning to understand some things going on inside of me, both intellectually and spiritually. My relationship with God has grown closer, and become more firmly an integral part of my life. I've explored the many questions I've had all my life about religion and Christianity. This has meant reading books upon which I'm sure the church hierarchy would frown. This has meant facing deeply held beliefs, examining them, putting aside those which now hold little relevance, being thankful for those beliefs from the past that still hold true, and embracing the new beliefs that now make much more sense. I learned that beliefs

can be, and should be, questioned, but faith is simply something that "IS." There has been this exhilarating sense of freedom in using my brains to do my own thinking. God gave me my brains. Why not use them to the best of my abilities?

6. *Free housecleaning services, both with the initial diagnosis and with the recurrence.* Deep down inside, when my cancer had returned, I hated the thought of having to go through more chemo (not that the chemo was really all that bad; just tiring and I'm not used to being without the energy to do things). I hated with a passion not being able to do things with the grandkids and great-nieces and -nephews. I hated not being able to meet people for lunch. I hated watching the cobwebs accumulating. I hated not being able to cook or bake, which is something I truly enjoy. But not to have to do housecleaning—maybe this whole thing has been worth it! All kidding aside, one of the great gifts of cancer was learning about Cleaning for a Reason, a national foundation established to help women who have cancer continue to live their lives in clean homes. If you refer to the following website, you can find out how to contact them and make arrangements for the services if you qualify (http://www.cleaningforareason.org). For right now, it is only for women. There aren't enough funds to go around to help men who have cancer. I received four free cleanings, which I had once a month, but they could have been spread over a year. That really took the pressure off. Once I had the stem cell transplant, the cleaning service became imperative for a short while, because I had to live in a clean, almost sterile, environment. What a blessing!

7. *This gift came as an evolution in my character courtesy of Becky, the blood pressure lady at Karmano's,* who was going through her own battle with breast cancer while studying to be a nurse and found she no longer had time to hate. Oh, of course, there are things that used to bother me, that I suppose still do. I'm still impatient with small-minded people and those who cannot understand the complete joy there is in everyday living, those who cannot see the gift in each day we are given. Cruelty, racism, injustice and unfairness also rank way up there on my irritation lists and must always be addressed. But to hate

a group of people, or to hate waiting in line, or to be angry with impatient people, or to ever presume to judge anyone for their actions, or to ridicule people for their ignorance, and then to react negatively to that—these things are (mostly) gone. I have two new criteria that determine whether or not to be upset:

1. *Fifty years from now will anyone remember this event or this situation?* And

2. *Will this change the course of world history?*

If the answer is "No" to either one of these two questions, it's not worth the effort to be angry, let alone ever to hate. That's not to say I still don't get frustrated at times (just ask the people at Sprint—poor Jay!). But once the initial phase passes, I can now put the frustration into perspective and deal with it in an appropriate way. . . . another gift that will keep on giving throughout my life.

8. In the last month, an additional gift has been revealed to me. All of us are composites or products of the people who have entered our lives, whether for just a few minutes or for most of our lifetimes. We are molded into who we are by our contacts, our interactions, and our interconnectedness with them. At the time, we are unaware of it. It may take 30 or more years before we realize the impact someone has had on us. When you enter teaching as a profession, you know you will be touching the lives of all those you teach as they enter into their futures. You have no way of knowing how things are going to turn out for your students. This is also true if you leave the classroom to take different positions in the school district. You are still impacting the lives of the next generation who will eventually take over your job. You become the "flame spotter" (to use Ayn Rand's term), those who will carry the torch into the future. Deep down inside, you are still a teacher. *Cancer gives you the opportunity to slow down, to think . . . to reflect . . . and to remember . . . then, to reach back.* In the last month, many people have reappeared to me from my past life of 30 to 40 years ago. And all these memories—of their kindnesses, their support, their patience, their professionalism, their knowledge, their car-

ing, their guidance, their generosity of spirit, their honesty,—it all came flooding back to me, and I realized how much I owed so many of them. It is a truly humbling experience, and yet, a most rewarding one, to be able to thank those people who contributed so much and helped me become the person I am today. I have sent out a little prayer to the Universe, asking that more of these incredible people come back into my life so I can express my gratitude to them, and acknowledge the debt I owe them for my life. Doctors, nurses and other health care people gave me back my life in one sense, but all of these other people gave me the life I have in another sense.

9. Another gift has manifested itself only recently. At least some of the pieces have started falling into place. As mentioned earlier, when you've been diagnosed with cancer, you become much more aware of how precious life is. It brings your life under personal scrutiny, and you begin to focus your thoughts on why you have lived. You also become more aware of what your legacy will be, asking yourself what your personal imprint on earth has been, of what ultimately your life has meant, of what you have done or need to do that lasts, that has or will make any significant difference in other peoples' lives. Certainly part of your legacy is held within your family and friends, who will carry a great part of you forward within their lives. But for most of us, I believe, we want there to be something else, something more, something that attests to our having been here at all. I am fully aware that all of us "little" people will never be considered to be great in the classical sense, but I do strongly believe each of us possesses greatness (however one chooses to define that) to varying degrees, and leave legacies behind that document the difference our lives have meant in this world. Finding that legacy is the hard part. Having and surviving cancer shall not be my legacy, ***but having cancer has contributed to the revelation of my legacy.***

While undergoing the stem cell transplant, this question came to me. What was my legacy going to be? Bits and pieces of disjointed ideas crossed my consciousness over the next year, but nothing felt "right." Then one day from out of nowhere, the phrase, "one teaspoon at a time," flashed across my memory. "Mountains can be moved, one teaspoon at a time."

Cancer is a huge mountain that has been tackled, one teaspoon at a time. Stem cell transplants are being tackled one teaspoon at a time. And then I met the four extraordinary women at the mosque, and their love for humanity made me feel as if I was in the presence of something much greater than myself, something that seemed to be both pulling and pushing me from within at the same time, perhaps from my very soul, saying that something simply had to be done. I started out trying to verbalize what was struggling to come out, saying that all of us on planet earth are faced with huge mountains to overcome, mountains of hate, of ignorance and of fear, and that we all have to band together to find a way to, once and for all, conquer these emotions. If there were two people working on this, rather than one, the mountain could be moved much more quickly and easily. ***Thus, "Two Teaspoons at a Time" was born.***

But the timing was still off. Fortunately Reema, one of the ladies at the mosque, and I hit it off and we discovered we shared many of the same beliefs, and ideas, and the same sense of urgency to create a legacy. She is young—in her 40s—and I am . . . well, into a couple of thirties, well into them! We are both from different cultures: we speak different languages, have different faiths, but somehow we reached across those vast divides to find what Reema calls the "thread of humanity." We are in the beginning stages of forming a non-profit organization called "Two Teaspoons at a Time." The idea, still in its neonatal stage, is to have two people sign up—***two very different people—who will pledge to be friends, to support, cherish, honor and nourish the other, and that between those two vastly different people, there will be unconditional love, respect and peace.***

It is likely that most of the people who sign up will be women. Women, after all, are the ones who pass on the culture, who raise their children to be good husbands or wives, good neighbors, good parents, who more often than not extend the hand of friendship to others. This is not to discount the influence or contributions fathers can and do have, but mothers are the most important influence in their children's' lives. This fact, however, in no way, precludes men from joining "Two Teaspoons at a Time." In fact, getting men to become a part of this may become one of our great challenges in making this a successfully functioning reality.

Reema has designed an incredible visual for the logo. Once we have enough people who have joined, we want to make donations to either individuals or organizations that espouse our beliefs, who are going the extra mile to bring peace to the world, and especially for the education of young women. Right now, we are still planning, still thinking, still creating, still dreaming, still needing to do all the paperwork necessary to make us viable. We are both right now still trying to find our "voice," our destinies. But stay tuned. Maybe in a year or so, you can use a search engine to find us. And maybe in a few more years after that, we can all be united as one thread of humanity. After all . . . All things are possible!

The Six Ls of Cancer

Be Able to . . .

Live—Cancer has taught us what it means to fully live—or at least how to approach it the vast majority of the time. To be able to appreciate the "now" of the moment, to "drink-in" the essences of all the people who come into your life, revel in the lessons they have to teach and incorporate them into your life, appreciate the joy of being able to get up in the morning, the joy of being able to do things again, being able to work, being able to open the doors to new experiences for children, to greet the day as one of unlimited possibilities. They are all just there—waiting for you to acknowledge their presence, pick them up and run with them.

Love—Cancer has taught us what it means to fully love and be loved. This is not only what our friends and family have demonstrated. The journey each of them has taken in support of us has demonstrated love in uncountable ways—taking us to doctors' appointments, sitting with us while getting chemo, providing positive thoughts to keep us going, bringing over food, visiting both at the hospital and at home, the laughter of little kids, bringing over inspirational books, doing fix-it jobs around the house, and more. We had always thought we fully loved our family and friends prior to cancer, and we did, but now this love takes on deeper and richer hues than ever before.

Laugh—Cancer has taught us the importance of laughter and having a sense of humor. A sense of humor is very different from wit. Lots of people will make funny remarks, but be unable to appreciate the humor of a situation. Nancy and Terry have laughs that go from the tips of their toes and erupt out of the tops of their heads. In a crowded restaurant, you will immediately be able to find us. We laugh loud and often. It was the same with Linda, Ricardo, Marc and Terry, when they used to go out to lunch. Our table is the one with the most laughter. Laughter has been shown to boost your immune system, lower cholesterol, lower blood pressure and reduce stress. Laughter can also help reduce the appetite hormone and is similar to an easy workout in the gym (no, you can't give up exercise, and no, it does not translate to actual weight loss; sorry). And laughing is so important when you are faced with a life-threatening illness. Laughter helps you make the situation a little more bearable. It takes you out of your self, out of wallowing in self-pity, out of wasting invaluable time, and into the realm of possibilities. It helps you reach out to people and embrace all they have to offer. Laughter can help battle depression and pain, both of which are common during and after cancer. You don't need to be totally serious all the time—at the initial diagnosis, yes. But after that, there will be plenty of opportunities to laugh, both at you, and at the situation.

Learn –Cancer has taught us the benefits of learning and subsequently passing on that knowledge to others to try and help them. We are all interconnected in one form or another. We are each a river flowing through life. Sometimes that river is turbulent; sometimes it is calm and serene. Sometimes we simply tumble over rocks for the sheer joy of living and learning. In the long run, we all flow into one main stream or ocean. Learning is like that. Sometimes we are alone in our learning, muddling along as best we can, but most of the time, it's because we connect with another river of learning that we really grow and finally, begin to see. What is gained from that knowledge goes into either a larger river or the giant body of knowledge. We have learned to take advantage of every learning opportunity, of every chance to question, to challenge, to reach out. What an incredible journey down our own river of learning and life this has been.

Leave—Cancer has taught us that sometimes we have to leave. Sometimes this means leaving a destructive relationship. Sometimes this means "tough love" when it comes to our kids. Sometimes it means letting our kids grow up and leave the nest. Sometimes it means leaving an old job with which we are so familiar and entering the uncertainties of a new job, new colleagues, and new work place, all requiring a new learning curve. We may have to leave long-time friends who insist on making us victims of our illnesses. We have to leave doctors when it's time for all of us to go our own ways, to follow our own paths. And sometimes we have to accept that our friends who have cancer or other terminal illness have to do their own leaving. This last one is so hard because we cling to life, no matter the ups and downs it takes, because the thought of not having that person in our lives is so painful, and we know that would leave such a great big gaping hole in our souls. But the greatest kindness, the greatest love we can give is to help them graciously cross that last bridge. It's not that we give our permission (that's a control mechanism) but rather, that we don't make it more difficult or hold them back, when it's their time to leave.

Let Go—Cancer has taught us that we have to learn to let go. As it says in Ecclesiastes:

> To every thing there is a season, and a time to every purpose under the heaven:
>
> A time to be born, and a time to die; a time to plant and a time to pluck up that which is planted.
>
> A time to kill, and a time to heal; a time to break down, and a time to build up;
>
> A time to weep, and a time to laugh; a time to mourn, and a time to dance;
>
> A time to cast away stones, and a time to gather stones together; a time to embrace, and a time to refrain from embracing;
>
> A time to get, and a time to lose; a time to keep, and a time to cast away;
>
> A time to rend, and a time to sew; a time to keep silent, and a time to speak;
>
> A time to love, and a time to hate; a time of war, and a time of peace.

Perhaps the ability to "Let Go" is the greatest challenge of The 6 Ls for our sense of self, our interconnectedness and a sense of completion. We will also face letting go ourselves when it is our time to die. Hopefully, we will have lived our lives in such a manner and to such an extent that we will leave with no, or at least very few, regrets, that there will be nothing left unsaid, and that any potential wounds will have long been healed, so we can breathe deeply and peacefully, let go, and quietly pass into death, what Albus Dumbledore in the Harry Potter series calls "the next great adventure."

In Closing

Three Years Later: Where We Are Now

For Alexis . . .

As of January 23, 2011, I am cancer free. I just passed my three-year anniversary since having been diagnosed, and having had the surgery. I am currently working as an RN, BSN in both an Emergency Department and an Intensive Care Unit. I am taking time off to enjoy my family and take weekend classes that don't require too much time away from home. I have not yet had a breast reconstruction, partly due to time constraints. My license plate now reads: SAVE2ND.

I distinctly remember some of the more interesting body change issues I have come across since my mastectomy. I had no idea how these little floppy "fruit roll up boobs" insulated my chest and kept me warm. I am forever and always chilly. I can feel every cold drink I have, and I have discovered that my new-found super power does not work with hot or warm liquids; it nearly initiates a rip-roaring hot flash.

There is also the curious. My shirts don't fit right. I very frequently go without my prosthetic boobs. I figure by the time I take a shower, get dressed, put on makeup and deodorant, bathroom break, contacts, brushed my teeth, . . . boobs are just not that high on my priority list. In all honesty, I am fine just being me (despite the fact that they are ten times better than any hand warmer I've touched!).

As always, I believe things happen in time, and with its passing, the meaning is revealed. It just hasn't been the right time for my reconstruction. It was the right time for me to get my closure tattoo, which is now a beautiful part of my back (a part that won't sag, sway or shift as I get older!) My partner, Andrea, is doing better after the scare in the I.C.U. in May 2010. Pea is a thriving 10 year old and, as always, has many questions. "When and how are your boobs gonna grow back?" has been the latest. I continue to state that I am not a "flag waver" for any cause. However, I have been blessed to have been put in the position I am in today. I have been blessed to have had cancer and to be a survivor. It is a topic about which I am very open and approachable, and will help anyone with his or her questions or concerns. I am a better nurse, better mother, better partner, and a better human being because of cancer. I allow it to be a part of my life, willingly. While it is one of my many identifiers, it is not what defines me. I am happy to further the fight against breast, or any cancer in order to prevent the loss of those people we hold dear.

For Terry . . .

Life has had its ups and downs, but mostly ups. One of the biggest concerns now is Tom's health. When we began the most current leg of our journey to see if Tom would qualify for Provenge, we were told that what usually happens is that Medicare will initially deny treatment (even though it has been FDA approved), and then will ask for more information. A month or three later, they may or may not approve Tom to receive the treatment. Further complications arose when it was determined Tom could not be on Taxotere if he were to be approved for Provenge; he also has to demonstrate three months of a rising PSA in order to qualify to receive it. Since he had received one treatment of Taxotere in November, his PSA had gone down, but Medicare will allow one dip, if medications, such as Taxotere, were administered to save a life.

In early January 2011, his PSA began to creep up and by the end of January, his PSA had jumped 20 points in a two-week period. Then his leg became swollen, along with some lymph nodes, and the recommended course of treatment was to put him back on Taxotere, which meant he might not qualify any time soon for Provenge. A CT scan was ordered to look at his chest, abdomen and pelvis to see if the prostate cancer was migrating to his kidneys and bladder, which could be causing the swelling in his leg. Then, despite our telling the Provenge doctor that Tom's cancer had already metastasized into both his bones and lymph nodes, after 3 months, the doctor told us Tom did not qualify for Provenge because of the metastasis into the lymph nodes. In May, 2011 a new drug was approved, Zytiga (formerly Abiraterone), and within 3 days, Tom was put on it (the drug is $5,000 a month; after another scare from Medicare they finally finally approved Tom to use the drug. Tom was used as a test case to demonstrate the real need for men to have this drug; it also helped for Dr. Pienta to go nuclear and mention "lawsuit" in his conversations. Clinical trials indicated that a person on Zytiga could be given another 4 months of life. We are also dealing with the lymphoma now spreading into his left leg, abdomen and groin. Tom's cancer has now spread into his ureters and bladder, and has had stents put in both ureters and a "percutaneous nephrostomy tube" inserted in his back to help his kidneys. The doctors do not know what is causing the lymphedema to spread.

Just as an aside, in completing the income tax forms for 2010, we found we had spent more than $9,300 in out-of-pocket medical expenses—a nice deduction. But that amount is a drop in the bucket compared to what the insurance paid for our treatments, for which we are and always will be, immensely grateful. We also found we had traveled 9,699 medical miles for trips to doctors' offices, hospitals, and for getting prescriptions. In September 2011, we are already ahead of last year's expenses for the same time 2010 time period. Every day we are grateful for having health insurance.

At one point we were dealing with three oncologists (Lansing, Ann Arbor and Grand Rapids), two urologists (Lansing and Ann Arbor), one internal medicine doctor (Lansing) and two radiation oncologists (Ann Arbor and Lansing). We were being asked to choose which doctor(s) we wanted. The dilemma was that we wanted to take advantage of all the specialists who are out of town, their knowledge and their resources, but in an emergency, we will, of necessity, fall back on the local doctors. We might not be able to wait to call the out-of-town doctor, wait for a phone call back, wait to see if the hospital will take us, and then drive 75 minutes to see what will, most likely, turn out to be an emergency room doctor anyway. And, at some point, the specialists will discharge Tom, and if we've burned our bridges with the local doctors, where will we be? We are still on this adventure and will be dealing with this for months to come. Tom still looks good, feels mostly good (except the Taxotere has messed with his taste buds), is in no pain whatsoever (talk about miracles and blessings!), and remains cheerful. He has developed neuropathy in his feet and partially up the right side of his leg. We take each day one at a time. Each day builds on the previous one in terms of knowledge and challenges.

As for me, I continue to do amazingly well. There are only minor daily irritations: fatigue (which is a side effect of the stem cell transplant), brownouts every time I stand up, occasional tingling in my fingertips and once in a great while, my toes, the occasional flare-up of Raynaud's when it's bitter cold outside, it takes longer to get rid of colds because my white blood cell count will always be lower for the rest of my life, my taste buds are still not back to "normal" (and might never be), my ability to concentrate when reading is still impaired to the point that even magazine articles can't be read from start to finish without taking a break. For the first time in my life, I have constant tinnitus, but strangely, am more susceptible to noises, especially high-pitched ones. Certain smells drive me around the bend. I now have a slight case of scoliosis and osteoporosis (neither of which are debilitating and do not interfere with my daily life; I am still a "full tilt" woman). It's hard to complete a task; I might start out folding the laundry, but then see a cobweb in the corner and on my way to clean the corner, I notice I had not finished putting away my crafts, but first I need to clean the stairway going upstairs. . . . Oh, the phone's ringing with a call from a district, another from a colleague, two more from friends, . . . Oh, and the prescriptions need to be called in and there's another call from the doctor's office with Tom's latest test results. And what junk can I throw away in the garage to make room for the pallets of books that will be arriving soon, but there are batts of insulation taking up the space on the garage floor that need to be put on the walls, and drywall which needs to be taped and mudded, but since it's close to zero outside, the mud might not set properly, so should I take care of the gardening things first, cleaning them and storing them for the winter? Maybe I better check to see if there's any work for MDE, but first I need to check my "To Do" list for today, and there's that item that has been there for a week now that still hasn't been done because I need to rerun the dryer to take out the wrinkles before I can fold the laundry. By the way, Alexis is experiencing the same kinds of things.

But all in all, this has been beyond an incredible journey, one I would NOT trade for anything. I have learned more patience, more compassion, to be both intro- and intra-spective, my faith in God has deepened, and every minute of every day is filled with wonder and joy. I no longer live my life in fear or dwell on the "What ifs" in life. My priorities in life have changed: family and friends (long-time friends, as well as those I haven't met yet) are now the most important parts of my life. The other important thing for both Alexis and me is to find the answers to a critical question for us now:"How can we help other people, whether or not they have cancer, but especially if they have cancer (we both chose helping professions and we are both "fixers")? This book is one of our answers. While I love my job and the people I am so very, very fortunate to work with, if I lose it all tomorrow, I know I will survive. There is a peace of mind, a sense of inner peace in all of this that I didn't have "BC" (before cancer). My life from now on will always have "new normals," which will all change, as my body and mind adjust for the next several years after chemo, radiation and the stem cell transplant (and as I age). I can choose whether to fight these changes, deny them, wish it wasn't so, or accept them with a measure of grace, and maybe some occasional grumbling and reluctance depending on what occurs, and see what new adventures will come my way as a result, what new positives I will encounter.

> *One of the many blessings that has come out of having cancer, one of my gifts, is drawing closer to Alexis. Alexis taught me that cancer means "finding your hope again." Every day is now filled with HOPE, and it is all because of cancer. What an amazing, wonder-full thing to have happen in one's life! How lucky can any one person get?*

And finally, Karen has come up with one last Truism:

> *"Of all the journeys you will take in your lifetime, none will ever . . . Give you so much, Take you so low, Raise you so high, Bring you so close, Show you so much, Make you so aware, Leave you so strong, Lift your vision so spiritually, Focus your life so purposefully, Move you so deeply, Change you so completely, and Target your efforts so selflessly . . . than this journey with cancer . . . survive or not, YOU WIN!!!"*

The Cancer Honor Roll

"Hero" can be defined in any number of ways, depending on the situation. It is most frequently used to refer to one who posseses or is endowed with great or extraordinary strength, ability, courage, nobility and achievements, or one who has certain qualities, such as nobility of purpose, boldness of vision, or who has given or has risked his/her life on behalf of another, of a cause and/or for a belief. What is often overlooked is the journey heroes often have to take. In Joseph Campbell's *The Hero with a Thousand Faces,* upon which the *Star Wars* films are based, the author identifies the stages a hero must go through as s/he undertakes her/his destiny. The first is the separation or departure from what is known and comfortable, what he refers to as the "call to the adventure." In this phase, there can be the refusal or denial of the call, or its acceptance. Once it is accepted, there is the appearance of "the assistance," in whatever form it may be provided by the powers overlooking the quest, to help the hero on his or her journey. This phase is followed by the "crossing of the threshold," and finally then, the "descent into the night" or darkness of the journey. The second stage involves "the trials or victories of undergoing the journey." In this stage, the hero must intensely search to develop an understanding of the underlying purpose of the trials that must be undertaken. The final stage is the "return, or the reintegration" back into what was formerly the familiar and comfortable, only this time, bringing with her/him, a form of "enlightenment." This enlightenment can also cause problems with what was previously known and comfortable, and ultimately, may become the one of the most difficult parts of the hero's journey. Misunderstandings may occur, especially for those the hero tries to help by sharing or using the new-found knowledge. The hero's journey is not one of "attainment, but of re-attainment, not discovery, but rediscovery." One of the things that is demonstrated to the person undertaking the journey is that all you have learned, all that has made you stronger, was within you all the time. This also fits the person, the hero, who has been diagnosed with cancer. We invite you to log on to our website, http://www.SoYouveSurvivedCancer.com and enter the name of a person who has either been diagnosed with cancer, or is a survivor. If you are unable to get to the website, please use the lines below to honor those you have loved and who have survived cancer.

In Memoriam

Like many heroes who undertake their adventure, some don't make it back. They answered the call to adventure, descended into the darkness or night of the journey, received enlightenment in one form or another, quite often rediscovering themselves in the process, and faced their situation with great courage and grace, and are now serving as the purveyors of new knowledge for those of us who remain.

Cancer is the true Equal Opportunity Employer. It does not discriminate and is no respecter of age, gender, ethnicity (not "race;" there's only one race and that's the human race), religion, sexual orientation or career. There have been and are many thousands of people diagnosed with cancer who have fought the good fight, but in the end, have lost their courageous battles against this disease. A Truism:

"Their valiant fights have enabled the rest of us to become survivors—-it is to them, each and every one of them, to whom we owe our lives."

Ours is a debt we can never repay, but there is something we can do; we can help others now, in their journeys with cancer.

We've come a long way in terms of better and earlier diagnoses, better and safer treatments, better and safer medications, better researchers and health care staff—but the fight is NOT over yet. It won't be over until there's a cure for all forms of cancer. That has become our daily prayer, and we ask you to join us. We also ask that you remember in your prayers the people who have gone "Home." We ask you to go to our website, http://www.SoYouveSurvivedCancer.com and enter the name of someone who fought the good fight, who served the cause by paving the way for those of us who did survive, but did not live to fight another day. Again, if you do not have access to the website, please enter the names below.

_____

_____

_____

_____

_____

_____

_____

_____

_____

_____

_____

Stem Cell Donation Information

Facts

- 30% of patients in need of a marrow transplant will find a donor in their family. There is a 1 in 4 chance that your brother or sister can be a donor. The remaining 70% turn to the National Marrow Donor Program.

- Searches occur through the National Marrow Donor Program for approximately *six thousand people* (men, women and children) *each day*. These people have leukemia, lymphoma, sickle cell anemia, other blood diseases or another life-threatening illness that can be treated by a bone marrow or cord blood transplant. For many, a transplant may be the best and only hope of a cure or survival.

- There are about seven million registered marrow donors and 70,000 cord blood units. Seventy-five percent of donors are Caucasian. This means that if you are Caucasian and need a transplant, you would probably find one.

- *If you are of African American, Asian, Hispanic, Middle Eastern, Native American, Pacific Islander or of multiple ethnic backgrounds descent, the chances are negligible that you will find a donor. The ethnic breakdown of donors is: 73% Caucasian, 10% Hispanic/Latino, 8% African-American, 7% Asian/Native Hawaiian/Pacific Islander and 1% Alaska/Native American Indian.*

- The National Marrow Donor Program has links worldwide to help others, as well as to access those donors to help people in the U.S.

What Does it Take to Become a Donor?

- 10 minutes to fill out paperwork and 4 Q-Tips to swab the inside of your mouth.

- If you are a member of an ethnic minority or of multi-ethnic descent, there is *no cost*.

- If you are Caucasian, the normal charge is around $100 in order to process the DNA testing, but funds can be secured to pay these fees. *All information is kept strictly confidential.*

Who Is Eligible to Become a Donor?

- Be between the ages of 18–60 and committed to helping a patient in need.

- You may not become a donor if you have been diagnosed with AIDS/HIV, lupus, multiple sclerosis, fibromyalgia, some forms of cancer or have had a heart attack, to name a few.

- Donors never pay for donating and are never paid to donate.

- If you are found to be a match for someone, you will be contacted.

- Please contact http://www.BeTheMatch.org for further information or to make a tax-deductible donation. Spanish language translations are available. Or contact Eric Trosko, 3100 West Rd., Suite 202, East Lansing, MI 48837, phone 1-800-471-3020, Ext. 101, or cell: 517-488-2670; http://www.marrow.org.

Appendix A

Alexis's Letter to Dr. X

Dear Dr. X,

My name is Alexis Hilliar and I was, until recently, a patient of yours. You have been my physician since 2006, and since I know you are leaving the area, I felt it necessary to write this letter to you. I believe I saw you in the office twice for my yearly gynecological/breast exams. Both times we discussed my "fibrous breasts", and how "lumpy" they were. I had had a baby (2001), and had lost approximately 100 pounds prior to becoming your patient. During both visits, I inquired as to when you would send me for a baseline mammogram. My concerns were obvious: fibrous breasts, and a history of breast cancer in the family, my mother. Waiting until I was 35 was the option you chose. December of 2007, I found a lump in my left breast. January 8, 2008, I was diagnosed with Stage II infiltrating ductal carcinoma. The lump had already created a secondary site in the same breast where the lump was found. Not shortly after, I had bilateral mastectomies and underwent 4 rounds of Chemo.

The reason for this letter is not anger, simply genuine concern. A mammogram would have found that lump before it had grown to the size it had when I found it. During this time when the Susan G. Komen foundation, a sea of pink ribbons, and "Save the Ta Ta's" t-shirts are common topics of conversation, we all know that being proactive is the key to saving lives. I have been blessed with a wonderful family, support system, and the wherewithal to do self breast exams every time I got in the shower. It and they saved my life.

I hope this letter, if nothing else, will make you pause, and take a moment to think the next time a young woman walks into your office and requests a baseline mammogram, especially if she has a Mother who has had breast cancer. Please, DO NOT discount the next 30-something woman who walks through your door. She may not have the strength, concern, or knowledge she will need to be diligent enough to do self breast exams when her own doctor tells her to wait until she is 35.

Respectfully,
Alexis Hilliar

Appendix B

Types of Cancer

Please note that there are some duplicates on this list; some people may know a cancer by one name, others may know it by a different name. In addition, some of these cancers may go by another name in a different country. For a direct link to these types of cancers, please go to one of the following websites. There you will find information about the risks for these types of cancer, what you can do to prevent them, types of screening, what the symptoms are, treatments currently in use, and what support is available.

http://www.cancer.gov/cancertopics/alphalist
http://www.oncolink.com/types/

Acquired Immune Deficiency (AIDS)-related Cancers
Acquired Immune Deficiency (AIDS) Lymphoma
Acute Lymphoblastic Leukemia—Adult
Acute Lymphoblastic Leukemia—Childhood
Acute Myeloid Leukemia—Adult
Adrenocortical Carcinoma
Adrenocortical Carcinoma—Childhood
Adenoid Cystic Carcinoma
Adrenal Gland Tumor
Amyloidosis
Anal Cancer
Appendix Cancer
Astrocytoma—Childhood
Astrocytoma—Childhood Cerebellar
Ataxia-Telangiectasia
Atypical Teratoid/Rhabdoid Tumor—Childhood
Central Nervous System
    Attenuated Familial Adenomatous Polyposis
Basal Cell Carcinoma (Skin Cancer, Nonmelanoma)
Beckwith-Wiedemann Syndrome
Bile Duct Cancer

Birt-Hogg-Dube Syndrome
Bladder Cancer
Bladder Cancer—Childhood
Bone Cancer, Osteosarcoma and Malignant Fibrous Histocytoma
Brain and Spinal Cord Tumors—Childhood
Brain Metastasis
Brain Stem Glioma—Childhood (Brain Tumor)
Brain Tumor—Adult
Brain Tumor—Central Nervous System Atypical Teratoid/
    Rhabdoid Tumor—Childhood
Brain Tumor—Central Nervous System Embryonal Tumors—
    Childhood
Brain Tumor—Cerebellar Astrocytoma—Childhood
Brain Tumor—Cerebral Astrocytoma/Malignant Glioma—
    Childhood
Brain Tumor—Craniopharyngioma—Childhood
Brain Tumor—Ependymoblastoma—Childhood
Brain Tumor—Ependymoma—Childhood
Brain Tumor—Medullablastoma—Childhood
Brain Tumor—Medulloepithelioma—Childhood
Brain Tumor—Pineal Parenchymal Tumors of Intermediate
    Differentiation—Childhood
Brain Tumor—Supratentorial Primitive Neuroectodermal Tumors
    and Pineoblastoma—Childhood
Brain Tumor—Visual Pathway and Hypothalamic Glioma—
    Childhood
Breast Cancer
Breast Cancer—Childhood
Breast Cancer—Inflammatory
Breast Cancer—Male
Breast Cancer—Metaplastic
Bronchial Tumors—Childhood
Burkitt Lymphoma
Carcinoid Tumor
Carcinoid Tumor—Childhood
Carcinoid Tumor—Gastrointestinal
Carcinoma of Unknown Primary
Carney Complex
Central Nervous System—Childhood

Central Nervous System Atypical Teratoid/Rhabdoid Tumor—
  Childhood
Central Nervous System Embryonal Tumors—Childhood
Central Nervous System Lymphoma—Primary
Cerebellar Astrocytoma—Childhood
Cerebral Astrocytoma/Malignant Glioma—Childhood Cervical
  Cancer
Cervical Cancer—Adult
Childhood Cancer
Cholangiocarcinoma
Chordoma—Childhood
Choriocarcinoma
Chronic Lymphocytic Leukemia (CLL)
Chronic Myelogenous Leukemia (CML)
Chronic Myeloproliferative Disorders
Colon Cancer
Colorectal Cancer—Adult
Colorectal Cancer—Childhood
Cowden Syndrome
Craniopharyngioma—Childhood
Cutaneous T-Cell Lymphoma (Mycosis Fungoides and Sezary
  Syndrome
Desmoplastic Infantile Ganglioglioma—Childhood
Dysgerminoma
Embroynal Tumors—Central Nervous System—Childhood
Endocrine Tumor
Endometrial Cancer
Ependymoblastoma—Childhood
Ependymoma—Childhood
Esophageal Cancer
Esophageal Cancer—Childhood
Ewing Family of Tumors—Childhood
Extracranial Germ Cell Tumor—Childhood
Extragonadal Germ Cell Tumor
Extrahepatic Bile Duct Cancer
Eye Cancer
Eye Cancer—Intrraocular Melanoma
Eye Cancer—Retinoblastoma
Eyelid Cancer

Fallopian Tube Cancer
Familial Adenomatous Polyposis
Familial Malignant Melanoma
Gallbladder Cancer
Gardner Syndrome
Gastric (Stomach) Cancer
Gastric (Stomach) Cancer—Childhood
Gastrointestinal Carcinoid Tumor
Gastrointestinal Stromal Tumor—GIST
Gastrointestinal Stromal Cell Tumor—Childhood
Germ Cell Tumor—Childhood
Germ Cell Tumor—Extracranial—Childhood
Germ Cell Tumor—Extragonadal
Germ Cell Tumor—Ovarian
Gestational Trophoblastic Tumor
Glioma—Adult
Glioma—Childhood Brain Stem
Glioma—Childhood Cerebral Astrocytoma
Glioma—Childhood Visual Pathway and Hypothalamic
Hairy Cell Leukemia
Head and Neck Cancer
Hepatocellular (Liver) Cancer—Adult (Primary)
Hepatocellular (Liver) Cancer—Childhood (Primary)
Hereditary Breast and Ovarian Cancer
Hereditary Diffuse Gastric Cancer
Hereditary Leiomvomatosis and Renal Cell Cancer
Hereditary Mixed Polyposis Syndrome
Hereditary Non-Polyposis Colorectal Cancer
Hereditary Non-VHL Clear Cell Renal Cell Carcinoma
Hereditary Pancreatitis
Hereditary Papillary Renal Cell Carcinoma
Histiocytosis—Langerhans Cell
HIV and AIDS-Related Cancer
Hypopharyngeal Cancer
Hypothalamic and Visual Pathway Glioma—Childhood
Islet Cell Tumor
Juvenile Polyposis Syndrome
Kaposi's Sarcoma
Kidney Cancer

Kidney (Renal Cell) Cancer
Kidney Cancer—Childhood
Lacrimal Gland Tumor
Laryngeal and Hypopharyngeal Cancer
Laryngeal Cancer
Laryngeal Cancer—Childhood
Leukemia—Acute Lymphoblastic—Adult
Leukemia—Acute Lymphoblastic—Childhood
Leukemia—Acute Lymphocytic—ALL
Leukemia—Acute Myeloid—AML—Adult
Leukemia—Acute Myeloid—AML—Childhood
Leukemia—B-Cell
Leukemia—Chronic Lymphocytic—CLL
Leukemia—Chronic Myeloid—CML
Leukemia—Chronic Myelogenous
Leukemia—Eosinophilic
Leukemia—T-Cell
Li-Fraumeni Syndrome
Lip and Oral Cavity Cancer
Liver Cancer—Adult (Primary; Hepatoma)
Liver Cancer—Childhood (Primary)
Lung Cancer—Non-Small Cell
Lung Cancer—Small Cell
Lymphoma—AIDS-Related
Lymphoma—Cutaneous T-Cell (Mycosos Fungoides and Sezary
    Syndrome)
Lymphoma—Hodgkin—Adult
Lymphoma—Hodgkin—Childhood
Lymphoma—Non-Hodgkin—Adult
Lymphoma—Non-Hodgkin—Childhood
Lymphoma—Primary Central Nervous System
Malignant Fibrous Histiocytoma of Bone and Osteosarcoma
Mastocytosis
Medulloblastoma—Childhood
Medulloephithelioma—Childhood
Melanoma
Melanoma—Intraocular (Eye)
Meningioma
Merkel Cell Carcinoma

Mesothelioma—Adult Malignant
Mesothelioma—Childhood
Metastatic Squamos Neck Cancer with Occult Primary Mouth
  Cancer
Muir-Torre Syndrome
Multiple Endocrine Neoplasia Type 1
Multiple Endocrine Neoplasia Type 2
Multiple Endocrine Neoplasia Syndrome—Childhood
Multiple Myeloma
Multiple Myeloma/Plasma Cell Neoplasm
Mycosis Fungoides
Myelodysplastic Syndromes—MDS
Myelodysplastic/Myeloproliferative Diseases
Myelogenous Leukemia—Chronic
Myeloid Leukemia—Adult Acute
Myeloid Leukemia—Childhood Acute
Myeloproliferative Disorders—Chronic
MYH—Associated Polyposis
Nasal Cavity and Paranasal Sinus Cancer
Nasopharyngeal Cancer
Nasopharyngeal Cancer—Childhood
Neuroblastoma—Childhood
Neurofibromatosis Type 1
Neurofibromatosis Type 2
Nevoid Basal Cell Carcinoma Syndrome
Oral Cancer—Childhood
Oral and Oropharyngeal Cancer
Oropharyngeal Cancer
Osteosarcoma and Malignant Fibrous Histiocytoma of Bone
Osteosarcoma—Childhood
Ovarian Cancer—Adult
Ovarian Cancer—Childhood
Ovarian Epithelial Cancer
Ovarian Germ Cell Tumor
Ovarian Low Malignant Potential Tumor
Pancreatic Cancer—Adult
Pancreatic Cancer—Childhood
Pancreatic Cancer—Islet Cell Tumors
Papillomatosis—Childhood

Paranasal sinus and Nasal Cavity Cancer
Parathyroid Cancer
Penile Cancer
Pharyngeal Cancer
Pheochromocytoma
Pineal Parenchymal Tumors of Intermediate
Differentiation—Childhood
Pineoblastoma and Supratentorial Primitive Neuroectodermal
    Tumors—Childhood
Pituitary Gland Tumor
Plasma Cell Neoplasm/Multiple Myeloma
Pleuropulmonary Blastoma—Adult
Pleuropulmonary Blastoma—Childhood
Pregnancy and Breast Cancer
Primary Central Nervous System Lymphoma
Prostate Cancer
Puetz-Jeghers Syndrome
Rectal Cancer
Renal Cell (Kidney) Cancer—Adult
Renal Cell (Kidney) Cancer—Childhood
Renal Pelvis and Ureter—Transitional Cell Cancer
Respiratory Tract Carcinoma Involving the *NUT* Gene on
    Chromosome 15
Retinoblastoma—Adult
Retinoblastoma—Childhood
Rhabdosarcoma—Childhood
Salivary Gland Cancer—Adult
Salivary Gland Cancer—Childhood
Sarcoma
Sarcoma—Alveolar Soft Part and Cardiac
Sarcoma—Bone (Osteosarcoma)
Sarcoma—Ewing Family of Tumors
Sarcoma—Kaposi
Sarcoma—Soft Tissue—Adult
Sarcoma—Soft Tissue—Childhood
Sarcoma—Uterine
Sezary Syndrome
Skin Cancer—Childhood
Skin Cancer—Melanoma

Skin Cancer—Non-melanoma
Skin Carcinoma—Merkel Cell
Small Cell Lung Cancer
Small Intestine Cancer
Small Tissue Sarcoma—Adult
Small Tissue Sarcoma—Childhood
Squamous Cell Carcinoma (Skin Cancer—Nonmelanoma)
Squamous Neck Cancer with Occult Primary—Metastatic
Stomach (Gastric) Cancer—Adult
Stomach (Gastric) Cancer—Childhood
Supratentorial Primitive Neuroectodermal Tumors—Childhood
T-Cell Lymphoma, Cutaneous (Mycosis Fungoides andSezary
   Syndrome)
Testicular Cancer
Throat Cancer
Thymoma and Thymic Carcinoma—Adult
Thymoma and Thymic Carcinoma—Childhood
Thyroid Cancer—Adult
Thyroid Cancer—Childhood
Transitional Cell Cancer of the Renal, Pelvis and Ureter
Trophoblastic Tumor—Gestational
Tuberous Sclerosis Syndrome
Turcot Syndrome
Unknown Primary Site—Carcinoma—Adult
Unknown Primary Site—Carcinoma—Childhood
Unusual Cancers of Childhood
Ureter and Renal Pelvis—Transitional Cell Cancer
Urethral Cancer
Uterine Cancer—Endometrial
Uterine Sarcoma
Vaginal Cancer
Vaginal Cancer—Childhood
Veterinary Oncology
Visual Pathway and Hypothalamic Glioma—Childhood
Von Hippel-Lindau Syndrome
Vulvar Cancer
Waldenstrom's Macroglobulinemia
Werner Syndrome
Wilms Tumor—Childhood

Appendix C

Cancer and Cancer Survivor Websites

When we started looking on the Internet for websites that might be helpful, there were literally millions upon millions upon millions of websites. The websites listed below are simply the ones we have checked out. The authors are not necessarily recommending these websites, but rather, they are intended for use as a springboard to other searches you might want to conduct. As with anything on the web, by the time this gets to print, some of these websites may no longer be in operation, despite the authors' best intentions to have the book be as current as possible. It is our intent that this listing simply demonstrate the wealth of information available on-line, but again, as with anything on the Internet, **PLEASE** check it out first (treat them all with skepticism), and *check with your doctor(s) before trying any of the recommendations generated from the sources listed*. This is especially true with medications. Please, also work with your physician(s), especially if you have any questions or concerns about what you find on these websites. These websites are *NOT* meant to take the place of the advice of your physician(s). Please, also be aware that listservs are anecdotal in nature, and not necessarily scientifically oriented

General Websites and Resources
100 Questions and Answers About Cancer Symptoms and Cancer Treatment
http://www.books.google.com/books?isbn=0763726125
101 Ways You Can Help Fight Cancer
http://www.myfamilywellness.org/MainMenuCategories/FamilyHealth-Center/Fighting-Cancer/101things.aspx
Advocacy Skills Training for Young Adult Cancer Survivors
http://www.springerlink.com/index/J414731370556U84.pdf
Aging with Dignity, *Five Wishes* and *Next Step Guide*
http://www.agingwithdignity.org/5-wishes.html
AIM DocFinder (State Medical Board Executive Directors):
http://www.docboard.org

Alabama

    Northwest Alabama Cancer Center http://www.nwalcc.org/

    Montgomery Cancer Center http://www.montgomerycancercenter.com/
University of, Comprehensive Cancer Center http://www3.ccc.uab.edu/

Alaska

    Alaska Regional Hospital http://www.alaskaregional.com/

    Fairbanks Memorial Hospital and Denali Center http://www.banner
health.com/Locations/Alaska/Fairbanks+Memorial+Hospital/_FMH_DC
_Home.htm

    Providence Cancer Center http://www.providence.org/alaska/pamc/
cancer/default.htm

    Rural Telehealth Network http://www.artn.org/index.php?option=com_
icalpro&Itemid=1&extmode=view&extid=70

Alternative (Complementary) Medicine

- American Cancer Society. *American Cancer Society Complete Guide to Complementary and Alternative Cancer Therapies.* Atlanta, GA. American Cancer Society 2009. See also http://www.cancer.org.

- Cavallo, Jo. *Prescription for Trouble: No Matter What the Prognosis, Experts Say Alternative Medicine Is Never a Replacement for Conventional Cancer Treatment.* Cure, Vol. 6, No. 2, Spring 2007, p. 27. http://www.curetoday.com

- Complementary Therapies Program at the University of Michigan Comprehensive Cancer Center. http://www.mcancer.org

- M.D. Anderson Cancer Center. *Patients Talk About . . . Complementary Therapies and Cancer.* http://www.mdanderson.org/department/cimer.

- National Cancer Institute. *Thinking About Complementary and Alternative Medicine—A Guide for People with Cancer.* http://www.cissecure.nci.nih.gov/ncipubs/. See also http://www.cancer.gov/cancertopics/treatment/cam

- National Center for Complementary and Alternative Medicine http://nccam.nih.gov/

- Office of Cancer Complementary and Alternative Medicine at the National Cancer Institute http://www.cancer.gov/CAM

- Quackwatch http://www.cancertreatmentwatch.org

- Unconventional Cancer Therapies http://www.bccancer.bc.ca/HPI/UnconventionalTherapies/default.htm.

American Academy of Medical Acupuncture 323-937-5514
    http://www.medicalacupuncture.org

American Association for Retired Persons http://www.aarp.org

American Bar Association http://www.abanet.org/women/probono.html

American Cancer Society 1-800-ACS-2345http://www.cancer.org
  http://www.cancer.org/docroot/SHR/content/SHR_1_CSN.asp
  http://www.cancernetwork.com/survivorship/display/article/10165/11645
  70?pageNumber=4 http://www. oncochat.org
  http://www.cancer.org (keyword—"insurance")

American Cancer Society Cancer Action Network
  http://www.action.acscan.org/cancer_survivors_network

Anderson Network http://www.mdanderson.org/departments/andersonnet

American Board of Medical Specialties 1-866-ASK-ABMS
  http://www.abms.org

American Cancer Society http://www.cancer.orgTTY: 1-866-228-4327
  • *Sexuality and Cancer: For the Man Who Has Cancer and His Partner*
  • *Sexuality and Cancer: For the Woman Who Has Cancer and Her
    Partner*

American Cancer Society Man to Man Support Groups
  http://www.cancer.org/docroot/CRI/content/

American Foundation for Urologic Disease/Prostate Health Council
  1-800-242-2383, http://www.afud.org

American Institute for Cancer Research http://www.aicr.org

American Medical Association Physician Select
  http://www.ama-assn.org/aps/amahg.htm

American Society of Clinical Oncology 1-703-299-0150 http://www.asco.org

Angel Flight http://www.angel-flight.org

APIAHF National Cancer Survivor Network
  http://www.apiahf.org/programs/ncsn/index.htm

Approved Hospital Cancer Program (Commission on Cancer of the American
  College of Surgeons) http://www.facs.org/public_info/yourhealth/aahcp.html

Arizona
  Cancer Survivor Network Meetings
  http://www.sierravistacancercenter.com/events/04262007CancerSurvivor
  NetworkMeetings.htm
  University of Arizona Cancer Center http://www.azcc.arizona.edu
  University Medical Center, Tucson http://www.azumc.com

Arkansas
  Arkansas Cancer Research Center, Little Rock http://www.uams.edu
  Central Arkansas Radiation Therapy Institute http://www.carti.com

Bealer's Buddies http://www.musc.edu/catalyst/archive/1998/co5-1buddy.htm

Berkley, Benjamin. *My Wishes: Your Plan for Communicating and
  Organizing the Essential Information Your Family Needs*, Naperville, IL:
  Sphinx Publishing, 2006

Best Hospitals Finder (US News & World Report)
  http://www.usnews.com/usnews/nycu/health/hosptl/tophosp.htm
  http://www.usnews.com/usnews/nycu/health/hosptl/speccanc.htm

Block, R.A. Cancer Foundation http://www.blochcancer.org

Blood and Marrow Transplant Newsletter http://www.brntinfonet.org/
  letter.html

Body Image and Psychosocial Adjustment in Adolescent Cancer Survivors
  http://www.jpepsy.oxfordjournals.org/cgi/reprint/22/1/29.pdf

Bone Marrow Foundation, brochure, 1-800-365-1336; English and Spanish
  http://www.bonemarrow.org

Boughton,, Barbara. *Facing the Future: Planning for a Good Death*. Cure;
  Vol. 2, No. 1, Spring 2003, p. 51 http://www.curetoday.com

Boughton, Barbara. *Saying Goodbye with Love*. InTouch, vol. 4, No. 2,
  March 2002, p. 35.

Breast Cancer Care http://www.breastcancercare.org.uk

Breast Cancer Screening for Pediatric Cancer Survivors
  http://www.crmagazine.org/archive/Crpodcasts/Pages/BreastCancer
  ScreeningforPediatricSurvivors.aspxm

California

  Cancer Prevention Institute of California
  http://cancer.stanford.edu/outreach/cpic.html

  Cedars-Sinai Comprehensive Cancer Center, Los Angeles
  http://www.csmc.edu

  City of Hope, an NCI-designated Comprehensive Cancer Center
  http://www.cityofhope.org/Pages/default.aspx

  Sanford-Burnham Medical Research Institute
  http://www.sanfordburnham.org

  San Jose, Bay Area Breast Cancer Network http://www.babcn.org/here.htm

  Stanford University Hospital http://www.cancer.stanford.edu

  UCLA Jonsson Comprehensive Cancer Center http://www.cancer.ucla.edu/

  University of California Davis Cancer Center
  http://www.ucdmc.ucdavis.edu/cancer/

  University of California Irvine http://www.healthcare.uci.edu

  University of California San Francisco http://www.ucsfhealth.org

  University of Southern California, Norris Comp. Cancer Center
  http://www.uscnorriscancer.edu

CancerCare for Kids, http://www.cancercare.org/get_help

Cancer Care, Inc. 212-712-8400 (administration), 212-712-8080 (services)
  1-800-813-HOPE (4673) http://www.cancercare.org, http://www.cancer
  care.org/hhrd/hhrd_financial.htm (financial assistance) info@cancercare.org
  Also part of this organization: Cancer*Care* for Kids

Cancer-central.com http://www.cancer-central.com/

Cancer Council Australia http://www.cancer.org.au/home.htm

Cancer Help http://www.cancerhelp.org.uk

Cancer Information Network http://www.cancerlinksusa.com/support

Cancer Index http://www.cancerindex.org

Cancer Rehabilitation http://www.cottingco.com/CancerConference07/index.html

Cancer Research Foundation of America's Healthy Eating Suggestions http://www.preventcancer.org/whdiet.cfm

Cancer Research Institute 1-800-99-CANCER http://www.cancerresearch.org

Cancer Source Book for Nurses http://www.books.google.com/books?isbn=0763732761

Cancer Staging http://www.medical-dictionary.thefreedictionary.com/cancer+staging

Cancer Supportive Care (financial assistance) http://www.cancersupportivecare.com/pharmacy.html

Cancer Survivor Dating and Social Network http://www.cancermatch.com

Cancer Survivor Retreats http://www.cancer-infos.com/cancer_survivors_retreats

Cancer Survivors Bill of Rights http://www.healthandage.com/public/health-center/40/article home/1737/The-Cancer-Survivors-Bill-of-Rights.html

Cancer Survivors' Fund http://www.cancersurvivorsfund.org/SuccessStories/SoniaPotter.htm

Cancer Survivors Network http://www.csn.cancer.org/
http://www.networi.nature.com/groups/cancer_resource/forum/topics/2542
http://www.wellsphere.com/wellpage/cancer-survivor-stories
http://www.cancersurvivorsproject.org/reading_list.aspx@first=11&last=15&fmt=3.html

Caring4Cancer http://www.caring4cancer.com

Caring Connections http://www.caringinfo.org/

Caring for Someone who Is Dying. Hospice Foundation of America

Caregiver websites

    Care Connection http://www.careconnection.com

    Caregiver http://www.caregiver.com

    National Family Caregivers Association http://www.thefamilycaregiver.org

    New Health Partnerships http://www.newhealthpartnerships.org

Carney, KL, "What is Cancer Anyway? Explaining Cancer to Children of All Ages," 1998

Carrier, Ewa, *100 Questions & Answers about Bone Marrow and Stem Cell Transplantation*, Sudbury, MA: Jones and Bartlett, 2004

Centers for Disease Control and Prevention (CDC) 1-404-639-3534, 1-800-311-3435 http://www.cdc.gov

Chemotherapy and You, National Institutes of Health, National Cancer
Institute, NIH Publication No. 07-7156, 1-800-4-CANCER
http://www.cancer.gov

Childhood Cancer
http://www.biomedexperts.com/.../Secondary_sarcomas_in_childhood_
cancer_survivors_a_report_from_the_Childhood_Cancer
http://www.ucsfhealth.org/childrens/special/s/100903.html
http://www.beyondthecure.org/

Childhood Cancers Home Page—National Cancer Institute
http://www.cancer.gov/cancertopics/types/childhoodcancers

Childhood Cancer Survivor Study http://www.jco.ascopubs.org/cgi/content/
full/27/14/230

Childhood Ovarian Cancer http://www.forums.curesearch.org/Show
Post.aspx?PostID=374

Children's Oncology Group http://www.survivorshipguidelines.org/

CIGNA http://www.cigna.com/healthinfo/shc12.html

Cleaning For a Reason Foundation http://www.cleaningforareason.org/

College Scholarships for Young Cancer Survivors www.cancer.org/docroot/
SPC/content/SPC_1_College_ScholarshipsList.asp

Colorado
Breast Cancer Support Resources Directory http://www.breastcancer
colorado.org/04supportorganizations/supportorgcolorado.shtml
University of Colorado Cancer Center http://www.uccc.info/
for-healthcare-professional/cancer-center/index.aspx

Common Ground, Dave Corby 303-690-3900
http://www.commonground.org.

Connecticut
The Yale Cancer Center http://www.yalecancercenter.org

Conquering Cancer Network http://www.conqueringcancer.net/resources_
community.html

Corporate Angel Network (possible free flights for cancer patients)
http://www.corpangelnetwork.org/news/press/12-27-05%20raffle.htM

Crowe, Karen, *Me and My Marrow: A Kid's Guide to Bone Marrow
Transplants*, Deerfield, IL: Fugisawa Healthcare Inc., 1999 (ages 10–18);
http://www.astellas.us/docs/meandmymarrow.pdf

Cure Magazine, Special Issue, Vol. 7, No. 4, 2008, *Where Are We Now?*

Cure Media Group. *HEAL. Living Well After Cancer.* http://healtoday.com

Dana-Farber Cancer Institute (Lance Armstrong) http://www.dana-farber.org/
pat/surviving/survivorship-education/default.html

Data Bases

http://www.brntinfonet.org—Blood and Marrow Transplant Information Network

http://www.cancer.gov—"NEWS Center"

http://www.cancer.org—"ACS News Today"

http://www.cancereducation.com—"Patient & Family Center"

http://www.cancerpage.com/news/

http://www.healthology.com—webcasts and transcripts

http://www.medlineplus.gov—Top of every health topic page

http://www.oncolink.com—"Cancer News"; also questions and Answers Databases

http://www.patient.cancerconsultants.com—"Cancer News"

http://www.peoplelivingwithcancer.org—"News Center"

http://www.plwc.org—People Living with Cancer Medical Illustrations; click on "Library"

http://www.pubmed.gov—Medical textbook, *Cancer Medicine*

http://www.virtualtrials.com—Clinical trials and treatments for brain tumors

http://visualsonline.cancer.gov—NCI Visuals Online

DCCPS:OCS Post Treatment Resources
http://www.dccps.nci.nih.gov/OCS/health.html

Delaware Medical Center of Delaware http://www.ChristianaCare.org

Dictionary of terms relating to cancer http://www.mcancer.org/thrive

District of Columbia—See Washington, D.C.

Eating Hints for Cancer Patients Before, During and After Treatment, National Institutes of Health, National Cancer Institute Publication No. 08-20791-800-4-CANCER, http://www.cancer.gov

Emmert, S.D. *The Consumer's Practical Guide to Funerals, Burials & Cremation*. Baltimore, MD: American Literary Press, 2005

End of Life Care: An Information Resource Guide. Michigan Department of Community Health http://www.michigan.gov/mdch

End-of-Life Care http://www.cancer.net

Eurekalert http://www.eurekalert.org

Exercise for Cancer Survivors http://www.living.health.com/2008/08/26/exercise-for-cancer-survivors/

Facing Forward: Life After Cancer Treatment" http://www.cancer.gov

Family and Medical Leave Act http://www.dol.gov/dol/esa/public/regs/statutes/whd/fmla.htm

Families of Children with Cancer, Inc., http://focwc.org/ourkids/links/default.asp

Fatigue Coalition http://www.ncbi.nlm.nih.gov.

FinAid! http://www.finaid.org/scholarships/cancer.phtml

Firefighter Cancer Support Network http://www.firehouse.com

Florida

> H.Lee Moffitt Cancer Center http://www.moffitt.org

> Shands Hospital at the University of Florida http://www.shands.org

> Sylvester Comprehensive Cancer Center http://www.sylvester.org

Foley, Sallie. *Sex Matters for Women: A Complete Guide to Taking Care of Your Sexual Self.* New York, NY: The Guilford Press, 2002.

Fred Hutchinson Cancer Research Center http://www.fhcrc.org

Free ACS Cancer Survivors Network Downloads http://www.rocketdownload.com/popular/downloads/american-cancer-society-cancer-survivors-network.html

Gallo-Silver, Les L. *Reawakening Physical Intimacy During Cancer Treatment.* Coping; Vol. 20, No. 2, March/April 2006, p. 38

Genetics http://www.cancer.med.upenn.edu/causeprevent/genetics

Georgia,

> Emory University Hospital http://www.emoryhealthcare.org

> Northside Hospital http://www.northside.com/medical_services/cancer_support.aspx

> St. Joseph's Hospital, Atlanta http://www.stjosephsatlanta.org/cancer_center/cancer_survivors_network/index.html

Gilda's Club http://www.gildasclub.org

Goshen Health System http://www.goshenhealth.com/main.asp?id=768

Gould, Stephen Jay, *The Median Isn't the Message*

Great News Network http://www.greatnewsnetwork.org/index.php/news/article/docs_grow_new_jawbone_for_cancer_survivor

Guam

> University of Guam Cancer Research Center http://www.crch.org/PDF/innovations/INNOVATN_52.pdf

Guidelines for Long-Term Follow-up of Pediatric Cancer Survivors http://www.stjude.org/stjude/v/index.jsp?vgnextoid=2dc10307f6e70110VgnVCM1000001e0215acRC

Guide to Protecting Your Health after (Bone Marrow) Transplant: Recommended Tests and Procedures http://www.cibmtr.org

Harpham, WH, "When a Parent Has Cancer: A Guide to Caring for Your Children," 1997

Harpham, Wendy Schlesi. *Happiness inn the Storm: Facing Illness and Embracing Life as a Healthy Survivor.* New York, NY. W.W. Norton and Co., 2005

Hawaii

> Cancer Research Center of Hawaii http://www.crch.org

Maui Memorial Medical Center Foundation http://www.mauihospitalfoundation.org

Health Care Costs and Cancer Survivors http://www.reuters.com/article/healthNews/idUSTRE51442Y20090205

Health Care Financing Administration (Breast Cancer and Medicaid programs) http://www.hcfa.gov/medicaid/bccpt/default.htm

Health Insurance Association of America (HIAA), 1-202-824-1600 http://www.hiaa.org

Health Insurance Guidance and Tips for Survivors http://www.beyondthecure.org/future/insurance/survivor/guide-lines.html

Health Resources and Services Administration, Hill-Burton Program, 1-800-638-0742; 1-800-492-0359 (Maryland area, only), 1-301-443-5656 http://www.hrsa.gov/osp/dfcr/about/aboutdiv.htm

Healy, Bernadine. *Living Time: Faith and Facts to Guide Your Cancer Journey*. New York: Bantam Dell Publishing Group, 2008

Helping Childhood Cancer Patients Grow Up http://www.sciencedaily.com/videos/2005/1208-helping_cancer_survivors_grow_up.htm

Holland, Jimmie C., and Lewis, Sheldon. *The Human Side of Cancer: Living with Hope, Coping with Uncertainty*. New York: HarperCollins, 2001.

Hospice Foundation of America http://www.hospicefoundation.org/

Hospice Net http://www.hospicenet.org/

Hospital Select (AMA and Medical-Net, Inc.) http://www.hospitalselect.com/curb_db/owa/sp_hospselect.main

Hospital Web (Dept. of Neurology, MA General Hospital): neuro— http://www.mgh.harvard.edu/hospital/web.shtml

Idaho
    North Idaho Cancer Center http://www.hospitalsoup.com

Iliana's Love Page http://www.ileanalovespage.ning.com

Illinois:
    Robert H. Lurry Comp. Cancer Center of Northwestern University http://www.cancer.northwestern.edu
    Rush-Presbyterian-St. Luke's Medical Center http://www.rush.edu
    University of Chicago Cancer Research Center http://www-uccrc.uchicago.edu
    University of Chicago Childhood Cancer Survivors Center http://www.uchicagokidshospital.org/specialties/cancer/survivors/
    University of Chicago Hospitals http://www.uchospitals.edu

Imsurvivor (childhood cancer) http://www.imsurvivor.com/xn/detail/1414236:Topic:8484

I'm Too Young for This http://www.imtooyoungforthis.org/community/i2y-orgs2.shtml

Indiana University Medical Center http://www.indiana.edu

Interfaith Family, Rabbi Earl A. Grollman http://www.interfaithfamily.com/ life_cycle/death_and_mourning/How_to_Talk_to_Your_Kids_about_Deat h.shtml

International Breast Preservation Foundation http://www.breastpreservation foundation.org/resources

International Cancer Alliance (ICARE) 1-800-ICARE-61, 1-301-654-7933, Fax—201-654-8684 http://www.icare.org/icare

Iowa
   University of Iowa Hospitals and Clinics http://www.uihealthcare.com/ uihospitalsandclinics

I've Lost Someone Special to Cancer http://www.ivelostsomeonespecialto cancer.synthasite.com

Jan Jarvis Access My Library http://www.accessmylibrary.com/coms2/ summary_0286-9575342_ITM

Kansas
   Kansas City Cancer Center http://www.kccancercenter.com/content. aspx?id=40600&section=search
   University of Kansas Cancer Center http://www.cancer.kumc.edu

Kentucky
   Markey Cancer Center http://www.ukhealthcare.uky.edu/markey

Kids Cancer Network http://www.conqueringcancer.net/resources_online support.html

Kids Cancer Care http://www.kidscancercare.ab.ca/

Kids Kicking Cancer313-557-0021 http://www.PowerPeacePurpose.org

Kids Scope http://www.kidscope.org (help kids who have parents with cancer)

Kornmehl, Carol. *Best News About Radiation Therapy: How to Cope and Survive*. Howell, NJ: Academic Radiation Oncology Press, 2003

Lance Armstrong Foundation http://www.livestrong.org

Laken, Keith. *Making Love Again: Hope for Couples Facing Loss of Sexual Intimacy*. Sandwich, MA: Ant Hill Press, 2002

Landay, D., "Be Prepared: The Complete Financial, Legal, and Practical Guide for Living with a Life-Challenging Condition." 1998

Lee, Elizabeth. *In Your Own Time: A Guide for Patients and Their Caretakers Facing a Lasting Illness at Home*. New York: Oxford University Press, 2002.

Leukemia and Lymphoma Society http://www.leukemia-lymphoma.org

Librarians' Internet Index http://www.lii.org/cs/lii/view/subject/3332

Lilleby, Kathryn U., *Steve's New Blood*, Pittsburgh PA: Oncology Nursing Press, 2000 (one for kids ages 6–10, another for kids ages 10–17)

LiveStrong http://www.livestrong.org

Long-Term Follow-Up Care for Pediatric Cancer Survivors
http://www.pediatrics.aappublications.org/cgi/content/abstract/123/3/906

Louisiana

Louisiana State University, Stanley S. Scott Cancer Center
http://www.ssscc.lsuhsc.edu

Ochsner Cancer Center http://www.ochsner.org/services/cancer

Tulane Cancer Center http://www.som.tulane.edu/cancer

University of Louisiana, Feist-Weiller Cancer Center
http://www.feistweiller.org

Macmillan Cancer Support http://www.macmillan.org.uk

Maine

Central Maine Comprehensive Cancer Center http://www.cmmc.org/
pc-cancercare.html

Maine Center for Cancer Medicine & Blood Disorders
http://www.mccm.org

Maine Medical Center Cancer Institute http://www.mmc.org/mmc_body.
cfm?id=3195

Make the Difference Network http://www.mtdn.com/tamikaandfriends

Making Every Bite Count (DVD), University of Michigan Comprehensive
Cancer Center Nutrition Program http://www.mcancer.org

Marie Curie Cancer Care http://www.mariecurie.org.uk

Maryland

Frederick Cancer Research and Development Center
http://www.web.ncifcrf.gov

Johns Hopkins Hospital http://www.hopkinsmedicine.org

Johns Hopkins Ovarian Cancer Center http://www.ovariancancer
center.org/patients/profiles.cfm

University of Maryland, Greenebaum Cancer Center http://www.umgcc.org

Massachusetts

Brigham and Women's Hospital http://www.brighamandwomens.org

Dana-Farber Cancer Institute http://www.dana-farber.org

Massachusetts General Hospital Cancer Center
http://www.msg.harvard.edu/cancer

Mayo Clinic www.mayoclinic.com/health/cancer/DS01076/TAB=resources

M.D. Anderson Cancer Center, University of Texas
http://www.mdanderson.org/

Medicaid Information http://www.hcfa.gov/medical/medicaid.htm

Medical Media Associates. *Intimacy* (audiovisual; Woman to Woman Series),
2001

Medline Plus http://www.medlineplus.gov

Memorial Sloan-Kettering Cancer Center
http://www.mskcc.org/mskcc/html/338.cfm

Michigan

Barbara Ann Karmanos Cancer Institute http://www.karmanos.org

Henry Ford Hospital http://www.henryfordhealth.org

Michigan Hospice & Palliative Care Organization
http://www.mihospice.org/

Michigan State University http://www.olin.msu.edu/msustudentcancer
supportnetwork.php

University of Michigan Comprehensive Cancer Center
http://www.cancer.med.umich.edu

William Beaumont Hospital http://www.beaumonthospitals.com

Minnesota

Mayo Clinic http://www.mayoclinic.com

Ovarian Cancer Alliance http://www.mnovarian.org/survivor_
exchange.htm

University of Minnesota, Masonic Cancer Center
http://www.cancer.umn.edu/cancerinfo/NCI/CDR438960.html

Minority Survivors of Childhood Cancers
http://www.biomedexperts.com/.../Minority_adult_survivors_of_
childhood_cancer_a_comparison_of_long-term_outcomes_health

Missouri

Barnes-Jewish Hospital http://www.barnesjewish.org

Montana Cancer Family Network http://www.cancerfamilynetwork.org

Mothers With Cancer http://www.technorati.com/blogs/motherswithcancer.
wordpress.com?reactions&page=2

Multicultural Cancer Information Service http://www.macdivgp.com.au/MC
SD/MCSD210.html

Multinational Association of Supportive Care in Cancer http://www.mascc.org

Music and Imagery (CD), Casselman and Gunnell http://www.mcancer.org

MyHopeSpace http://www.myhopespace.com/index.php?page=blogs

National Bone Marrow Transplant Link http://www.youtube.com

"New Normal: Life After Bone Marrow/Stem Cell Transplant"; also
http://www.nbmtlink.org

National Cancer Institute 301-435-3848 (Public Information Office)
http://www.nci.hih.gov
http://www.cancernet.nci.nig.gov/genesrch.shtml (genetics)
http://www.als.nci.hih.gov/finding/centers/html/map.html (Cancer Ctrs.)

"Eating Hints for Cancer Patients Before, During and After Treatment

"Taking Time: Support for People with Cancer and the People Who
Care About Them"

National Center for Complementary and Alternative Medicine
1-888-644-6226 http://www.nccam.nih.gov

National Coalition for Cancer Survivorship 1-800-877-NCCS-YES
http://www.canceradvocacy.org/news/press/2006/cancer-advocacy-now.html

National Comprehensive Cancer Network 1-888-909-NCCN
http://www.nccn.org

National Financial Resource Book for Patients: A State-by-State Directory
http://www.data.patientadvocate.org/

National Library of Medicine 1-888-346-3656 http://www.nlm.nih.gov

National Marrow Donor Program 1-888-999-6743 http://www.marrow.org
English, Spanish, Mandarin

National Society of Genetic Counselors http://www.nsgc.org

National Survivor Volunteer Network http://www.health.msn.com/health-
topics/skin-and-hair/articlepage.aspx?cp-documentid=100107417

National Teen Network http://www.candlelighters.ca/cgi-bin/htsearch?
words=survivor

Nebraska

Southeast Nebraska Cancer Center http://www.sncc-of-lincoln.com

University of Nebraska, Eppley Cancer Center
http://www.unmc.edu/cancercenter

Needy Meds (financial assistance to purchase drugs)
http://www.needymeds.com

Network of Strength: So When Do You Officially Become a Cancer Survivor?
http://www.orums.networkofstrength.org/index.php?showtopic=357&st=20

Nevada State Health Division Cancer Registry
http://www.health.nv.gov/VS_NVCancerRegistry.htm

New England Journal of Medicine http://www.content.nejm.org/

New Hampshire

Norris Cotton Cancer Center http://www.cancer.dartmouth.edu

New Jersey

Robert Wood Johnson Medical School Cancer Institute,
ComprehensiveComprehensive Cancer Center http://www.cinj.org

Special Report Commission on Cancer Research http://www.state.nj.us/
health/ccr/documents/adultsurv.pdf

New Mexico

University of New Mexico Cancer Research & Treatment Center
http://www.cancer.unm.edu

New York

Albert Einstein Cancer Center http://www.einstein.yu.edu/cancer

Columbia-Presbyterian Cancer Center http://www.cumc.columbia.edu

Memorial Sloan-Kettering Cancer Center http://mskcc.org

Memorial Sloan-Kettering Survivor Network
http://www.mskcc.org/mskcc/html/64245.cfm

Mount Sinai Medical Center http://www.mountsinai.org

New York Hospital-Cornell Medical Center http://www.med.cornell.edu

New York University, Kaplan Cancer Center http://www.ci.med.nyu.edu

Roswell Cancer Institute http://www.roswellpark.org

University of Rochester Cancer Center http://www.urmc.rochester.edu

Western New York Breast Cancer Network
http://www.bcnwny.org/SurvivorStoryMarcia.html

North Carolina

Duke University Comprehensive Cancer Center http://www.cancer.duke.edu

North Carolina Breast Cancer Resource Directory
http://www.bcresourcedirectory.org/directory/11-survivorship_index.htm

University of North Carolina Lineberger Comp. Cancer Center
http://www.unclineberger.org

Wake Forest University Baptist Medical Center http://www.wfubmc.edu

North Dakoka—there are no NCI-designated cancer centers in North Dakota; the nearest are Iowa, Minnesota and Wisconsin. In doing a web search, there were no facilities that we were comfortable listing. That does not mean there aren't any qualified, excellent services in North Dakota.

Nutrition

- American Cancer Society. *The American Cancer Society's Healthy Eating Cookbook: A Celebration of Foods, Friends and Healthy Living.* 1999. http://www.cancer.org

- American Institute for Cancer Research (several publications) http://www.aicr.org; also *Food for the Fight* (audiovisual)

- Bloch, Abby. *Eating Well, Staying Well: During and After Cancer.* Atlanta, GA: American Cancer Society

- *Cancer Center Recipes Just for You.* http://www.mcancer.org/

- CancerRD http://www.cancerrd.com (written by 3-time cancer survivor, Diane Dyer)

- Caring4Cancer http://www.caring4cancer.com/go/cancer/nutrition/

- Gilletz, Norene. *The Low Iodine Diet Cookbook: Easy and Delicious Recipes & Tips for Thyroid Cancer Patients.* Your Health Press, 2005

- Greer, Julia B. *the Anti-Cancer Cookbook: How to Cut Your Risk with the Most Powerful, Cancer-Fighting Foods.* North Branch, MN: Sunrise River Press, 2008

- Osbourne, Michael, et. al., *The Strang Cancer Prevention Center Cookbook: A Complete Nutrition and Lifestyle Plan to Dramatically Lower Your Cancer Risk.* New York, NY: London,, England: McGraw-Hill, 2004.

- Physicians Committee for Responsible Medicine. *Healthy Eating for Life: To Prevent and Treat Cancer*. New York, NY: John Wiley & Sons, Inc., 2002

Office of Minority Heath, US Government http://www.omhrc.gov/templates/content.aspx?ID=5090

Ohio

    Cleveland Clinic http://www.my.clevelandclinic.org/cancer

    Ohio State University Comprehensive Cancer Center—Arthur G. James http://www.jamesline.com

    Toledo Hospital http://www.promedica.org

    University Hospitals of Cleveland http://www.uthospitals.org

Oklahoma

    Oklahoma University Cancer Institute http://www.oumedicine.com/academictemplate_landing.cfm?id=90

Oklahoma Women's Network http://www.oklahomawomen.blogspot.com/2009/02/breast-cancer-survivors-sought-for.html

OncoLink Network
    http://www.linkinghub.elsevier.com/retrieve/pii/S0897189703000089

Oncotalk:improving oncologists' communication skills
    http://www.oncotalk.info

Oregon Health Science University Hospital http://ohsu.edu

Path of Pink http://www.pathofpink.org

Pediatric Cancer Foundation http://www.pcfweb.org/

Pediatric Cancer Survivorship: The Costs Associated with the Cure
    http://www.hemonctoday.com/article.aspx?rid=29103

Pediatric Oncology Resource Center http://www.acor.org/ped-onc/

Pennsylvania

    Abramson Cancer Center http://www.oncolink.upenn.edu/

    Allegheny General Hospital http://www.wpahs.org

    Fox Chase Cancer Center http://www.fccc.edu

    Genetics http://www.cancer.med.upenn.edu/causeprevent/genetics

    Pittsburgh Cancer Institute http://www.upci.upmc.edu

    Thomas Jefferson University, Kimmel Cancer Center http://www.kimmelcancercenter.org

    University of Pennsylvania Cancer Center http://www.penncancer.com/cancerprograms_detail2.cfm?id=32

    Wistar Institute Cancer Center http://www.wistar.org

Planet Cancer (for young adults)
    http://www.planetcancer.org/html/connect.php?sec_Id=4&cat_Id=26
    http://www.pennhealth.net/feature/jun08/cancer.html

Planning for Your Peace of Mind: A Do-It-Yourself Guide to Medical and Legal Decisions. State of Michigan http://www.michigan.gov

PTSD Among Mothers of Pediatric Cancer Survivors http://www.jpepsy.oxfordjournals.org/cgi/content/abstract/23/6/357

Pregnant with Cancer Network http://www.pregnantwithcancer.org

Puerto Rico

> H. Lee Moffitt Cancer Center http://www.moffitt.org
>
> NCI National Cancer Institute http://www.ncccp.cancer.gov
>
> Puerto Rico Cancer Center at the University of Puerto Rico http://www.md.rcm.upr/edu/ccpr/eng

Radiation: Kornmehl, Carol. *Best News About Radiation Therapy: How to Cope and Survive.* Howell, NJ: Academic Radiation Oncology Press, 2003

Recognizing and Celebrating Milestones http://www.cancer.net/portal/site/patient/menuitem.169f5d85214941ccfd748f68ee37a01d/?vgnextoid

Re-Mission: Game for children with cancer http://www.re-mission.net/site/community/links.php

Rhode Island

> Rhode Island Cancer Council, Inc. http://www.ricancercouncil.org/resources/facilities.php
>
> Rhode Island Comprehensive Cancer Center, The Miriam and NewportHospitals http://www.lifespan.org

St. Jude's Children's Research Hospital http://www.stjude.org

Samoa, American

> American Samoa Community Cancer Network http://www.crchd.cancer.gov/cnp/pi-tofaeono-description.html
>
> Lyndon B. Johnson Tropical Medical Center http://www.asmca.org M.D. Anderson Cancer Center http://www.mdanderson.org
>
> NCI Cancer Center http://www.nci.nih.gov/cancertopics/factsheet/NCI/cancer-centers

Sankar, Andrea. *Dying at Home: A Family Guide for Caregiving.* Baltimore: Johns Hopkins University press, 1999.

Schepens Eye Research Institute http://www.schepens.harvard.edu

Science Daily http://www.sciencedaily.com

ScholarshipLink http://www.scholarshiplink.com/student-aid/scholarships/scholarship-cancer/

Senior Super Stores http://www.seniorsuperstores.com

Setting the Standards for Life After Childhood Cancer http://www.emaxhealth.com/1/51/30511/setting-standards-life-after-childhood-cancer.html

Social Security Administration, Office of Public Inquiries, 1-800-772-1213, 1-800-325-0778 (TTY) http://www.ssa.gov

Social Support and Long-Term Adjustment for Adult Pediatric Cancer Survivors http://www.allacademic.com/meta/p190964_index.html

South Carolina

Hollings Cancer Center http://www.hcc.musc.edu

Medical University of South Carolina Department of Radiation Oncology http://www.radonc.musc.edu

South Dakota—there are no NCI-designated cancer centers in SD

Sanford University of South Dakota Medical Center http://www.sanfordhealth.org

Stewart, Susan K., *Autologous Stem Cell Transplants: A Handbook for Patients*, Highland Park, IL: BMT Newsletter, 2007

Stupid Cancer http://www.stupidcancer.com (I'm Too Young for This! Cancer Foundation)

Survivorship: *Facing Forward: Life After Cancer Treatment* http://www.cancer.org

Surviving Childhood Cancer: Growing Up Too Fast http://www.socialworktoday.com/archive/mayjun2008p20.shtml

Survivors Network (adult survivors of childhood cancer) http://www.doi.wiley.com/10.1002/10970142(19930515)71:10+%3C33 54::AID-CNCR2820711737%3E3.0.CO;2-2

Talking About Cancer http://www.talkingaboutcancer.com/about

TC-Cancer.com http://www.tc-cancer.com/forum/showthread.php?t=9000

Tennessee

St. Jude's Children's Research Hospital http://www.stjude.org

Vanderbilt University Medical Center http://www.mc.vanderbilt.edu

Vanderbilt Trauma Survivors Network http://www.mystsn.org

Texas

Arlington Cancer Center http://www.acc-tx.com

AtlantiCare, University of Texas http://www.atlanticare.org/cancer/livingwell/links.php

Lewisville Organizes Housecleaning for Women with Cancer http://www.greatnewsnetwork.org/index.php/news/.../lewisville_foundation_organizes_housecleaning_for_women_in_cancer

University of Texas M.D. Anderson Cancer Center http://www.mdanderson.org/

Thiboldeaux,, Kim, and Golant, Mitch. *The Total Cancer Wellness Guide: Reclaiming Your Life after Diagnosis*. Dallas, TX: BenBella Books, 2007

Top 50 Cancer Survival Inspiration Blogs http://www.radiologytechnician schools.net/top-50-cancer-survival-inspiration-blogs

Ulman Cancer Fund for Young Adults http://www.ulmanfund.blogspot.com/
2009/01/imerman-angels-and-collaboration.html

United Seniors Health Cooperative (USHC), 1-800-637-2604, 1-202-479-6973
http://www.unitedseniorshealth.org

United States Administration on Aging http://www.aoa.gov

USDA Dietary Guidelines http://www.usda.gov/cnpp

US TOO International,1-800-808-7866, 1-630-323-1002, Fax 1-630-323-1003
http://www.ustoo.com

Utah
    University of Utah Huntsman Cancer Institute http://www.hci.utah.edu

Vermont
    Cancer Center http://www.vermontcancer.org/index.php?id=495

    Cancer Survivor Network http://www.vcsn.net

    State Cancer Plan http://www.vtaac.org/2008-activities-report.pdf

    Vermont Comprehensive Cancer Center http://www.vermontcancer.org

Veterans Affairs, Department of 1-800-827-1000 (reaches local VA office);
202-273-5400 http://www.va.gov

Views of Childhood Cancer Survivors http://www.doi.wiley.com/10.1002/
10970142(19930515)71:10+%3C3354::AIDCNCR2820711737%3E3.
0.CO;2-2 www.ncbi.nlm.nih.gov/pubmed/8490882

Virginia
    Massey Cancer Center http://www.massey.vcu.edu

    University of Virginia Health Sciences Center
    http://www.healthsystem.virginia.edu

    University of Virginia Cancer Center Support Coping Kids
    http://www.healthsystem.virginia.edu

Volunteer Match http://www.volunteermatch.org/search/?k=survivor&v=true

Washington
    http://www.cheshirerelay.org/survivors.htm

    http://www.tacomahealthcoalition.ning.com/ (Health coalition for
    communities of color)

    http://www.canceradvocacy.org/news/press/2006/cancer-advocacy-now.html

    http://www.seattlecca.org/fred-hutchinson-survivorship-access

    Fred Hutchinson Cancer Research Center http://www.fhcrc.org

    University of Washington Medical Center http://www.uwmedicine.
    washington.edu

Washington D.C.
    Lombardi Cancer Center http://www.lombardi.georgetown.edu

    Washington Cancer Institute http://www.whcenter.org

    Young Adult Cancer Survivors http://www.yacsdc.org/partners_
    resources.html

Weinstein-Stern, Deborah, *Mira's Month*, Highland Park, IL, BMT
    Newsletter, 1994 (for kids whose parents are undergoing BMT)
Wellness Community, The. http://www.thewellnesscommunity.org
West Virginia
    Cancer Care Center of Southern West Virginia http://www.camc.org
    Edwards Comprehensive Cancer Center http://www.edwardsccc.org
    Mary Babb Randolph Cancer Center http://www.hsc.wvu.edu
    St. Mary's Regional Cancer Center http://www.st-marys.org
UPMC Cancer Center Support Group http://www.upmccancercenters.com/
    supportgroups/supportgrpresults_newsearch.cfm
Winston's Wish http://www.winstonswish.org.uk
Wisconsin
    Radio Network http://www.wrn.com/gestalt/go.cfm?objectid=56664
    E9D-9ABE-A5D5-E5A06914C5800DD2
    University of Wisconsin Hospital and Clinics http://www.uhealth.org
    University of Wisconsin Comprehensive Cancer Center
    http://www.cancer.wisc.edu
Women's Cancer Center
    http://www.womenscancercenter.com/info/articles/daily.html
Wyoming
    Big Horn Basin Radiation Oncology Center http://www.bhbasin
    cancer.org
    Bill and Joanne Price Medical Arts and Cancer Treatment Center
    http://www.westparkhospital.org/area_clinics.html
    Northern Rockies Radiation Oncology Center http://www.nrroc.org
    Welch Cancer Center http://www.sheridanhospital.org/welch
    cancercenter
    Wyoming Department of Health http://www.wdh.state.wy.us/wcsp/new.asp

Cancer-Specific Websites

Anal Cancer

American Cancer Society http://www.cancer.org/docroot/cri/content/cri_2_4_
    1x_what_is_analcancer_47.asp
American Society of Colon and Rectal Surgeons
    http://www.fascrs.org/patients/conditions/anal_cancer/
Cancer Answers http://www.canceranswers.com/Anal.Cancer.html
Mayo Clinic http://www.mayoclinic.com/health/anal cancer/ds00852/
    dsection=symptoms
MedlinePlus http://www.nlm.nih.gov/medlineplus/analcancer.html
National Cancer Institute http://www.cancer.gov/cancertopics/types/anal

New York University Medical Center
http://www.med.nyu.edu/crs/info/anorectal10.html

Bladder Cancer

Bladder Cancer Advocacy Network http://www.bcan.org/stay-informed/
newsletter/ask-the-doctor-winter-2009

Inspire http://www.inspire.com/groups/bladder-cancer-advocacy-network/
discussion/who-are-we-patient-victim-survivor-what

Bone Cancer

Adult Bone Cancer Survivors http://www.abc-survivors.net/

American Cancer Society http://www.cancer.org/docroot/cri/content/cri_2_4_
1x_what_is_bone_cancer_2.asp

Bone Cancer FAQ http://www.cancerindex.org/ccw/faq/

M.D. Anderson Cancer Center http://www.mdanderson.org/patient-and-
cancer-information/cancer-information/cancer-types/bone-
cancer/index.html

Mayo Clinicwww.mayoclinic.com/health/bone-cancer/ds00520

National Cancer Institute http://www.cancer.gov/cancertopics/factsheet/
Sites-Types/bone

Bone Marrow Transplants

Bone and Marrow Transplant Information Network www.bmtinfonet.org

Bone Marrow Foundation, 1-800-365-1336 www.bonemarrow.org, English
and Spanish

Carrier, Ewa, *100 Questions & Answers about Bone Marrow and Stem Cell
Transplantation*, Sudbury, MA: Jones and Bartlett, 2004

Crowe, Karen, *Me and My Marrow: A Kid's Guide to Bone Marrow
Transplants*, Deerfield, IL: Fugisawa Healthcare Inc., 1999 (ages 10–18)

Leukemia & Lymphoma Society http://www.leukemia-lymphoma.org

Lilleby, Kathryn U., *Steve's New Blood*, Pittsburgh, PA: Oncology Nursing
Press, 2000 (one for kids ages 6-10, a second for kids 10–18)

National Bone Marrow Transplant Link http://www.nbmtlink.org

National Marrow Donor Program, 1-888-999-6743 http://www.marrow.org,
English and Spanish

Stewart, Susan K., *Autologous Stem Cell Transplants: A Handbook for
Patients*, Highland Park, IL, BMT Newsletter, 2007

Stronach, Keren, *Survivors' Guide to a Bone Marrow/Stem Cell Transplant:
What to Expect and How to Get Through It*, Southfield, MI: National
Bone Marrow Transplant Link, 2002, http://www.nbmtlink.org

Weinstein-Stern, Deborah, *Mira's Month*, Highland Park, IL: BMT Newsletter, 1994 (for kids whose parents are undergoing BMT)

Williams, Susan, *Inside Stem Cells: A Look at Blood and Marrow Transplantation*, Cure (magazine), Vol. 3, No. 2, Summer 2004, p. 41

Brain Cancer

American Brain Tumor Association http://www.abta.org

Brain Cancer Survivors http://www.cnn.com/2008/HEALTH/05/21/ tumors.irpt/index.html

Brain Tumor Society http://www.tbts.org

CancerCare, *Brain Tumors: Current Treatments and Hope for the Future*, http://cancercare.org

National Brain Tumor Foundation http://www.braintumor.org

National Cancer Institute, *What You Need to Know about Brain Tumors*, https://cissecure.nci.nih.gov/ncipubs/

Patient Education Institution, *Brain Cancer Interactive Tutorial* http://www.medlineplus.gov; click on "Interactive Tutorials"

Stark-Vance, Virginia, *100 Questions & Answers about Brain Tumors*, Sudbury, MA: Jones and Bartlett, 2004

StemSave http://www.community.pennwelldentalgroup.com/video/stemsave-important-to-a-brain

Breast Cancer

Bonner, Dede, *The 10 Best Questions for Surviving Breast Cancer: The Script You Need to Take Control of Your Health*. New York: Simon and Schuster, 2008

Breast Cancer Care http://www.breastcancercare.org.uk

Breast Cancer Interactive Tutorial http://www.medlineplus.gov

Breast Cancer Network of Western New York http://www.bcnwny.org/BreastCancerLinks1.html

BreastCancer.org http://www.breastcancer.org

Breast Cancer Survivors' Network, Inc. http://www.thebreastcancersurvivorsnetwork.org

Breast Cancer and MS Survivor http://www.woai.com/content/raceforthecure/story/Breast-cancer-survivor-inspires-as-she.../mqQKZpNWGEGOD_LHN5SmbQ.cspx

Breast Friends (for young survivors) http://www.breastfriends.com/survivor_support/

Brown, Zora. *100 Questions and Answers About Breast Cancer*. Sudbury, MA: Jones and Bartlett Publishers, 2007

Cans For Cures http://www.cansforcures.org/links.asp

Childhood Cancer Survivors Miss Needed Mammograms
http://www.reuters.com/article/healthNews/idUSTRE50Q7R020090128

Cleavage Creek's Charity Wine http://www.trendhunter.com/trends/cancer-survivors-for-charity-cleavage-creek-cellars-wine

See also Colorado above

Dia de la Mujer Latina1-866-54MUJER http://www/diadelamujerlatina.org

First 48 Hours: Breaking the News to Your Children, Beth Brophy
http://www.healthcentral.com/breast-cancer/just-diagnosed-674-143.html

Health Care Financing Administration (Breast Cancer and Medicaid programs) http://www.hcfa.gov/medicaid/bccpt/default.htm

Ivengar Yoga http://www.healthline.com/blogs/cancer_treatment_survivorship/2006/10/iyengar-yoga-for-breast-cancer.html

Kaelin, Carolyn M. *Living Through Breast Cancer: What a Harvard Doctor and Survivor Wants You to Know about Getting the Best Care While Preserving Your Self-Image.* New York, NY: McGraw-Hill, 2005

Lange, Vladimir. *Be a Survivor: Your Guide to Breast Cancer Treatment.* Los Angeles,, CA: Lange Productions, 2007

Living Beyond Breast Cancer http://www.lbbc.org/

Male Breast Cancer http://www.cancer.org, http://www.cancer.gov

Male Breast Cancer Listserv http://listserv.acor.org/acrhives/malebc.html

MAMM Magazine http://www.mamm.com

MBROS Consumer's Guide to Breast Reconstruction
http://surgery.med.umich.edu/plastic/

National Cancer Institute—*Surgery Choices for Women with Early-Stage Breast Cancer* http://cissecure.nci.nih.gov/ncipubs/

National Lymphedema (travel tips)
http://www.medicinenet.com/script/main/art.asp?articlekey=50499

See also New York, Western above

North Carolina Breast Cancer Resource Directory http://www.bcresourcedirectory.org/directory/09support_patient_survivor.htm

Numeroff, Laura. *Kids Speak Out About Breast Cancer.* Samsung Telecommunications America and Sprint PCS, 1999

Path of Pink http://www.pathofpink.org

Pennsylvania Breast Cancer Coalition http://www.pabreastcancer.org/support/displayco.php?coid=101

Pink Link http://www.pink-link.org

Previvors and Survivors http://www.previvorsandsurvivors.com /

Scripps Nurse-Supported Programs Pairs Breast Cancer Patients with
Sharsharet: Linking Young Jewish Women in Their Fight Against Breast

Cancer (and soon to include ovarian cancer) 1-866- 474-2774 http://www.sharsharet.org

Sisters Network, Inc (African-American) 1-866-781-1808 http://www.sistersnetworkinc.org

Susan G. Komen Foundation http://www.komen.org/

Survivors http://www.nursezone.com/nursing.../Scripps-Nurse-Supported-Program-Pairs-Breast-Cancer-Patients-with-Survivors_21770.asp

Sexual Health Network http://www.sexualhealth.com/article/read/disability-illness/cancer/373/

Sponsor a Breast Cancer Survivor (International) http://www.wcbcf.ca/dev/wp-content/uploads/2008/01/d4-wcbcf-delegate-sponsorship.pdf

Waiting Room Magazine (International) http://www.waitingroommagazine.com/resources.php

WomenStories. *Psychosocial Video Series.* WomenStories: Buffalo, NY 2001 http://www.womenstories.org

Young Survival Coalition http://www.youngsurvival.org

Cervical Cancer

American Cancer Society http://www.cancer.org/docroot/FPS/content/FPS_1_Cervical_Cancer_Survivors_Determination_Inspires_Others.asp

Eyes on the Prize http://www.eyesontheprize.org/stories/dx.html

Mayo Clinic http://www.mayoclinic.com/health/cervical-cancer/ds00167

National Cancer Institute http://www.cancer.gov/cancertopics/types/cervical

National Cervical Cancer Coalition http://www.nccc-online.org/community/stories.html

Wall of Hope http://www.wcn.org/wall_of_hope/cervical_cancer/

Childhood/Young Adult Cancer

Alliance for Childhood Cancer http://www.allianceforchildhoodcancer.org

American Brain Tumor Association, *Alex's Journey.* Des Plaines, IL:

American Brain Tumor Association, 1994 (ages 9–14; also a video) http://www.abta.org/kids/home.htm

American Cancer Society http://wwww.cancer.org

Apel, Melanie Ann. *Coping with Leukemia.* New York, NY: Rosen Publishing Group, 2001 (includes section for teenaged siblings)

Ask Kids http://www.askkids.com/resource/Talking-about-Cancer-with-Children.html

Association of Cancer Online Resources http://www.acor.org

Cancer.net http://www.cancer.net/portal/site/patient

Cancer.gov http://www.cancer.gov

Cancer BACUP (British) http://www.cancerbacup.org.uk

Candlelighters.org1-800- 366-2223 http://www.candlelighters.org/

Coloring books http://www.candlelighters.org,
http://www.leukemialymphoma.org

Crowe, Karen. *Me and My Marrow: A Kid's Guide to Bone Marrow Transplants*. Deerfield, IL: Fugisawa Healthcare, Inc. 1999

CureSearch.org http://www.curesearch.org

Families of Children with Cancer, Inc., http://focwc.org/ourkids/links/default.asp

First 48 Hours: Breaking the News to Your Children, Beth Brophy
http://www.healthcentral.com/breast-cancer/just-diagnosed-674-143.html

Field,, Molly. *Through and Beyond: 13 Teenagers Share Their Battles with Cancer*. Wicasset, ME: Molly Field, 1998

FinAid http://www.finaid.org/scholarships/cancer.phtml

Gill, Kathleen A. *Teenage Cancer Journey*. Pittsburgh PA: Oncology Nursing Press, 1999

Gordon, Apel Melanie *Let's Talk About: When Kids Have Cancer*. New York: Power Kids Press, 1999

Keaton Raphael Memorial http://www.childcancer.org

Kids Cancer Care http://www.kidscancercare.ab.ca/

Kids Kicking Cancer 313-557-0021 http://www.PowerPeacePurpose.org

Kimmie Care Dolls http://www.kimmiecares.com

Klett, Amy *Amazing Hannah: Look at Everything I Can Do!* Candlelighters 2002; http://www.candlelighters.org (also have other books)

Interfaith Family, Rabbi Earl A. Grollman http://www.interfaithfamily.com/life_cycle/death_and_mourning/How_to_Talk_to_Your_Kids_about_Death.shtml

Journal of Clinical Oncology http://jco.ascopubs.org/cgi/content/abstract/23/16/3733

Lilleby, Kathryn U. *Stevie's New Blood*. Pittsburgh, PA: Oncology Nursing Press, 1999. (one for ages 6–10, the other for ages 10–17)

Listserv: 4Youth (discussion group for children/teens who are cancer survivors) http://www.acor.org, http://listserv.acor.org/archives/4youth.html

Macmillan Cancer Support http://www.macmillan.org.uk

Making the Grade: Back to School After Cancer for Teens. New York, NY: Leukemia and Lymphoma Society, 1999

Marie Curie Cancer Care http://www.mariecurie.org.uk

Musicians Against Childhood Cancer http://www.bluegrassclassic.com

My Hair's Falling Out . . . Am I Still Pretty?. Necessary Pictures Film & Media, 1992 (physician who had cancer as a child)

National Children's Cancer Society http://nationalchildrenscancersociety.com

OncoLink (Scholarships) http://www.oncolink.org/resources/article.cfm?c=6&s=29&ss=74&id=927

PED-ONC Resource Center http://www.acor.org/ped-onc

People Against Childhood Cancer http://www.curechildhoodcancer.ning.com

Rose, Ellen. *Ellen Rose's Story.* Boston, MA: Brain Tumor Society

St. Baldrick's Foundation http://www.stbaldricks.org/

St. Jude Children's Research Hospital http://www.stjude.org

ScholarshipLink http://www.scholarshiplink.com/student-aid/scholarships/scholarship-cancer/

She Knows http://www.sheknows.com/articles/804653/hot-to-talk-to-your-kids-about-death http://www.sheknows.com/articles811082/when-a-child-fears-dying

Siblings of Children with Cancer

- American Cancer Society—*When your Brother or Sister has Cancer*
- Cavallo, Jo. *Shadow Survivors: A Childhood Cancer Diagnosis Often Makes Well Siblings Feel Like They're Battling the Disease, Too.* Cure, Vol. 5, No. 4, Fall 2006, p. 66.
- Cancervive. *Kids Tell Kids: What It's Like When Their Brother or Sister Has Cancer.* Los Angeles, CA: Cancervive, 1998. Contact SuperSibs (below)
- Dodd, Michael. *Oliver's Story: For "Sibs" of Kids with Cancer.* Kensington, MD. Candlelighters Childhood Cancer Foundation, 2004. http://www.candlelighters.org
- National Cancer Institute—*When Your Brother or Sister has Cancer: A Guide for Teens* https://cissecure.nci.nih.gov/ncipubs/
- Sibling Support Project http://www.siblingsupport.org/
- Sonnenblick, Jordan. *Drums, Girls and Dangerous Pie.* Ketchum, ID: DayBlue Publishers, 2004. Contact SuperSibs (below)
- SupSibs—*Parent Guide.* 1-866-444-7427 http://www.supersibs.org, http://www.supersibs.org/pdf/for-you/guide-for-parents.pdf

Stupid Cancer http://stupidcancer.com (I'm Too Young for This! Cancer Foundation)

Sunrise Day Camp http://www.sunrisedaycamp.org

Talking with Children about Cancer

- Ackermann, Abigail & Adrienne. *Our Mom Has Cancer.* Atlanta, GA: American Cancer Society, 2001.

- American Cancer Society. *It Helps to Have Friends: When Mom or Dad Has Cancer*; *Because . . . Someone I Love Has Cancer: Kids' Activity Book*
- Ammary, Neyal J. *In Mommy's Garden: A Book to Help Explain Cancer to Young Children*. Lehighton, PA: Canyon Beach Visual Communications, 2004. Also available in Spanish.
- CancerCare. *Helping Children When a Family Member Has Cancer*. http://www.cancercare.org/about_us/connect_booklets.php
- Cancervive. *Kids Tell Kids What It's Like When Their Mother or Father Has Cancer*. Los Angeles, CA. Cancervive,, 1998 (video)
- Cancer Family Care. *What About Me? A Booklet for Teenage Children of Cancer Patients.*
- Carney, Karen L. *What Is Cancer Anyway? Explaining Cancer to Children of All Ages*. Wethersfield, CT. Dragonfly Publishing Co.,, 1999
- Clifford, Christine and Lindstrom, Jack. *Our Family Has Cancer, Too!* Duluth, MN: Pfeifer-Hamilton Publishers, 1998
- Collins, Leigh and Courtney, Nathan. *When a Parent Is Seriously Ill: Practical Tips for Helping Parents and Children*. Metairie, LA. Jewish Family Service of Greater New Orleans, 2003.
- Gupta, Nelly Edmondson. *Taking Care of the Kids: When a Parent Has Cancer, Raising Children Poses Special Challenges . . . and Rewards*. InTouch, Vol. 4, No. 2, March 2002, p. 23.
- Hamilton,, Joan. *When a Parent Is Sick: Helping Parents Explain Serious Illness to Children*. Nova Scotia, Canada. Pottersfield Press, 2001.
- Hannigan, Katherine. *Ida B: and Her Plans to Maximize Fun, Avoid Disaster and (Possibly) Save the World. New York, NY: Greenwillow Books, 2004.*
- Kids Konnected. 1-800-899-2866, 2701 Cabot Rd., Ste. `01, Laguna Hills, CA 92653. http://www.kidskonnected.org
- Kidscope, 3399 Peachtree Rd. Suite 2020, Atlanta, GA 30326; http://www.kidscope.org
- National Cancer Institute. *When Your Parent Has Cancer: A Guide for Teens*. https://cissecure.nci.nih.gov/ncipubs/
- Ness, Eric. *Straight Talk: Kids React Differently to a Parent's Diagnosis*. Cure, Vol. 7, No. 1, Spring 2008, p. 16.
- Numeroff, Laura. *Kids Speak Out About Breast Cancer*. Samsung Telecommunications America and Sprint PCS, 1999

- Russell, Neil. *Can I Still Kiss You? Answering Children's Questions About Cancer*. Deerfield Beach, FL. Health Communications, 2002
- Schnipper, Hester Hill. *Growing Pains: How to Cope When Your Teenage Daughter Cannot*. MAMM, Vol. 3, No. 9, July/August 2001, p. 22
- University of Virginia Cancer Center Support Coping Kids http://www.healthsystem.virginia.edu
- *What Do I Tell the Children? A Guide for a Parent with Cancer*. http://www.cancerbacup.org.uk
- Yaffee, Risa Sacks. *Parenting Through Cancer: There Should Be an Open Exchange Between Children and a Parent with Cancer*. Coping Magazine; Vol. 14, No. 2, March/April 2000, p. 74.

Teens Living with Cancer. http://www.teenslivingwithcancer.com/

Trillin, Alice. *Dear Bruno*. New York, NY: The New Press, 1996

Wescott, Patsy. *Living with Leukemia*. Austin, TX: Raintree Steck-Vaughn Publishers, 2000 (ages 4-12)

Winston's Wish http://www.winstonswish.org.uk

Clear Cell Cancer

American Cancer Society http://www.cancer.org/docroot/cri/content/cri_2_4_1x_what_is_kidney_cancer_22.asp

Cancer Survivors Network, American Cancer Society http://csn.cancer.org/node/143886

Inspire http://www.inspire.com/groups/ovarian-cancer-national-alliance/discussion/clear-cell-adenocarcinoma-anyone/

Johns Hopkins Pathology http://ovariancancer.jhmi.edu/clearcellca.cfm

National Institutes of Health http://dccps.nci.nih.gov/acsrb/pubs/des_pubs/clear_cell/understanding.html

Resource Guild for DES-Exposed Daughters and Their Families http://dccps.nci.nih.gov/acsrb/pubs/des_pubs/clear_cell/clearcellcancer.html

The Oncologist® http://theoncologist.alphamedpress.org/cgi/content/full/11/10/1089

Wise Geek http://www.wisegeek.com/what-is-clear-cell-carcinoma.htm

Colon Cancer

Stage 4 Colon Cancer Survivors Needed http://www.cancercompass.com/message-board/message/all,31993,0.htm

Colorectal Cancer

American Cancer Society http://www.cancer.org/docroot/cri/cri_2x.asp?
    sitearea=lrn&dt=10

Colon Cancer Forum http://ehealthforum.com/health/topic99429.html

Colon Cancer Alliance http://www.ccalliance.org/

Colorectal Cancer Network http://www.cancerlinksusa.com/colorectal/
    index.asp

Fred Hutchinson Cancer Research Center http://www.endcoloncancernow.
    org/about/stories.html

Mayo Clinic http://www.mayoclinic.com/health/colon-cancer/ds00035

National Cancer Institute http://www.cancer.gov/cancertopics/types/colon-and-
    rectal

On Top of Cancer http://www.ontopofcancer.org/colon_cancer_support_
    group.php

Endometrial Cancer—See also Uterine Cancer

American Cancer Society http://www.cancer.org/docroot/cri/content
    /cri_2_4_1x_what_are_the_key_statistics_for_endometrial_cancer.asp

Cancer Information Network http://www.cancerlinksusa.com/uterus/index.asp

Cancer Survivors Network http://www.stanford.wellsphere.com/wellpage/
    endometrial-cancer-survivors

Eyes on the Prize http://www.eyesontheprize.org/stories/dx.html

M.D. Anderson Cancer Center http://www.mdanderson.org/patient-and-
    cancer-information/cancer-information/cancer-types/uterine-
    cancer/index.html

On Top of Cancer http://www.ontopofcancer.org/uterine_cancer_support
    _group.php

Women's Cancer Network http://www.wcn.org/

Hodgkin's Disease

American Cancer Society http://www/cancer.org

Cancer.gov http://www.cancer.gov

Leukemia & Lymphoma Foundation. *Hodgkin's Lymphoma.*
    http://www.leukemia-lymphoma.org

Listserv: http://www.acor.org

Lymphoma Research Foundation. *Understanding Hodgkin's Lymphoma: An
    Introductory Guide for Patients.* 1-800-500-9976 (free copy)

Lymphoma Research Foundation of America.1-800-500-9976
    http://www.lymphoma.org

National Cancer Institute. *What You Need to Know About Hodgkin's
    Disease.* http://www.cancer.gov

Leukemia

American Cancer Society: http://www.cancer.org; click on topic:
- Leukemia- Acute Lymphocytic (ALL)
- Leikemia—Acute Myeloid (AML)
- Leukemia—Chronic Lymphocytic (CLL)
- Leukemia—Chronic Myeloid (CML)
- Leukemia—Chronic Myelomonocytic (CMML)

Ball, Edward D. *One Hundred Questions & Answers About Leukemia.* Sudbury, MA: Jones and Bartlett, 2008

Children's Cancer Network http://www.childrenscancernetwork.org/News/Children's_Cancer.pdf

Leukemia & Lymphoma Foundation. *(Several publications, audiovisuals and some free materials)* http://www.leukemia-lymphoma.org

Leukemia & Lymphoma Society http://www.leukemia-lymphoma,org

Leukemia Research Foundation1-847-424-0600 http://www.leikemia-research.org, http://www.lrf.org.uk

National Cancer Institute. *What Everyone Should Know About Leukemia.* http://www.cancer.gov.

Liver Cancer

American Cancer Society http://csn.cancer.org/node/155458, http://www.cancer.org/docroot/CRI/content/CRI_2_4_1X_What_are_the_key_statistics_for_liver_cancer_25.asp

Blog for a Cure http://livercancer.blogforacure.com/weblog/2006/12/03/0001

Cancer Help UK http://www.cancerhelp.org.uk/type/liver-cancer/treatment/statistics-and-outlook-for-liver-cancer

Cancer Information Network http://www.cancerlinksusa.com/liver/inanswer.asp

Inspire http://www.inspire.com/groups/lung-cancer-survivors/discussion/metastatic-liver-cancer/?reply_sort=desc

M.D. Anderson Cancer Center http://www.mdanderson.org/patient-and-cancer-information/cancer-information/cancer-topics/survivorship/index.html?cmpid=google_survivorship_ppc&gclid=CJ6Sh6XxwKECFUI65QodQGt0_Q

SpringerLink http://www.springerlink.com/content/p18541665g760825/

University of Michigan Canton Health Center, 1-800-865-1125

Lung Cancer

American Cancer Society (several publications) http://www.cancer.org

CancerCare—several publications http://www.cancercare.org

Henschke, Claudia I. *Lung Cancer: Myths, Facts, Choices—and Hope*. New York, NY: W.W. Norton & Co., 2002

Lung Cancer Alliance, 888 16th St., NW, Suite 800, Washington, DC 20006 e-mail: info@lungcanceralliance.org, http://www.lungcanceralliance.org

Lung Cancer Online http://www.lungcanceronline.org/support/psychosocial.html

National Cancer Institute. *What You Need to Know About Lung Cancer*. http://www.cancer.gov/cancerinfo/wyntk/lung

Parles, Karen. *100 Questions & Answers About Lung Cancer*. Boston, MA: Jones and Bartlett, 2006

Patient Education Institute. *Lung Cancer Interactive Tutorial*. http://www.medlineplus.gov

Lymphedema

American Journal of Nursing http://journals.lww.com/ajnonline/Fulltext/ 2009/07000/Post_Breast_Cancer_Lymphedema__Part_1.30.aspx

Dr. Susan Love Research Foundation http://www.dslrf.org/breastcancer/content.asp?CATID=0&L2=1&L3=5& L4=0&PID=&sid=131&cid=507

Female Care http://femalecare.net/womens-health/obesity-increases-lymphedema-risk-for-breast-cancer-survivors/

Lymphovenous-Canada http://www.lymphovenous-canada.ca/ bclymphedemastudy.htm

National Institutes of Health http://www.ncbi.nlm.nih.gov/pubmed/ 19064976

National Lymphedema Network http://www.emaxhealth.com/1/51/30511/ setting-standards-life-after-childhood-cancer.html

Lymphoma

American Cancer Society http://csn.cancer.org/node/136135

The Cancer Blog http://www.thecancerblog.com/

Coping with Cancer Magazine http://www.copingmag.com/cwc/index.php/ cancerType/lymphoma/

FinAid http://www.finaid.org/scholarships/cancer.phtml

Everyday Health http://www.everydayhealth.com/blog/zimney-health-and-medical-news-you-can-use/do-lymphoma-survivors-face-a-higher-risk-of-a-second-cancer/

Hope Begins in the Dark http://www.hopebeginsinthedark.com/

Leukemin & Lymphoma Society http://www.leukemia-lymphoma.org/ all_page?item_id=8623

LymphomaInfo.net http://www.lymphomasurvival.com/

Lymphoma Survival http://www.lymphomasurvival.com/

Lymphoma Survivors Network http://www.inspirezone.org/cancer/ survivors.html

On Top of Cancer http://www.ontopofcancer.org/lymphoma_support_ group.php

Two-Time Cancer Survivor Scales Mt. Everest http://www.thedenverchannel. com/news/4495340/detail.html

Melanoma

Actors' Network Hack n' Smack http://www.hacknsmack.org/survivor.php

American Cancer Society http://www.cancer.org/docroot/FPS/content/FPS _1_Melanoma_Survivor_Relishes_Every_Day.asp

CancerGuide http://cancerguide.org/kshapiro_story.html

Cancer Survivors' Fund http://www.cancersurvivorsfund.org/SuccessStories/ SoniaPotter.htm

Melanoma Hope Network http://www.melanomahopenetwork.org/ TwoCol.asp?SID=6006

National Coalition for Cancer Survivorship http://www.canceradvocacy.org/ community/survivor-profiles/brooke-hamilton.html

On Top of Cancer http://www.ontopofcancer.org/melanoma_support_ group.php

Myeloma

American Cancer Society http://csn.cancer.org/forum/168

Cancer Blog http://www.thecancerblog.com/category/multiple-myeloma/

Cancer Information Network http://www.cancerlinksusa.com/myeloma/ index.asp

Coping with Cancer Magazine http://www.copingmag.com/cwc/index.php/ cancerType/myeloma/

Livestrong http://www.livestrong.com/groups/group/myeloma-survivors/

Multiple Myeloma Survivors' Stories http://www.acor.org/mm/

M.D. Anderson Cancer Center http://www.mdanderson.org/patient-and- cancer-information/cancer-information/cancer-types/melanoma/index.html

National Coalition for Cancer Survivorship http://www.canceradvocacy.org/ toolbox/multiple-myeloma/

National Institutes of Health http://www.ncbi.nlm.nih.gov/pubmed/ 15322968

On Top of Cancer http://www.ontopofcancer.org/multiple_myeloma_ survivor.php

Neurological Cancers
University of Michigan Canton Health Center, 1-800-865-1125

Oral, Neck and Head Cancer
100 Questions and Answers About Head and Neck Cancer
   http://www.books.google.com/books?isbn=0763743070
American Dental Association—Oral Cancer Information for Patients and the
   Public http://www.ada.org/public/topics/cancer_oral.asp
Bioportfolio Limited—Search Screen for Oral Cancer News
   http://www.bioportfolio.co.uk/Health_News/Oral_Cancer.shtml
Greater Amsterdam Cancer Registry http://www.ikcnet.nl/uploaded/
   FILES/IKA/kankerregistratie/overleving/3.xls
International Association of Oral Oncology http://www.internationacademy
   oforaloncology.org/)
Journal of Oral and Maxillofacial Surgery http://www.joms.org/
Mouth Cancer Foundation: Initiative of the Restorative Dentistry Oncology
   Clinic http://www.rdoc.org.uk
Oral Cancer Foundation http://www.oralcancerfoundation.org
Oral Oncology http://www.elsevier.com/locate/oraloncology
Restorative Dentistry Oncology Clinic http://www.rdoc.org.uk/
Società Italiana di Patologia e Medicina Orale—Oral Cancer http://www.
   sipmo.it/app/prvt/VediFile.d/File92/FAQ%20ca%20iper.pdf (Italian)
Support for People with Oral and Head and Neck Cancer
   http://www.spohnc.org/nsvn.html,
   http://www.breakawayfromcancer.com/psace.php
   http://www.oralcancerfoundation.org/multimedia/index.htm
University of Manitoba—Oral Cancer Self Evaluation
   http://www.umanitoba.ca/outreach/wisdomtooth/exam.htm
West of Scotland Cancer Awareness Project
   http://www.woscap.co.uk/nhsstaff/default.asp?p=da51
Yul Brynner Head and Neck Cancer Foundation http://www.headandneck.org/

Ostomy
European Ostomy Association, http://www.ostomyeurope.org
International Ostomy Association, http://www.ostomyinternational.org
   Lebanese Ostomy Association, http://www.arabostomy.com
Ostomy Association of Greater Lansing (MI), 1988 Willoughby Rd., Mason,
   MI 48854; 517-676-1835 or 517-282-4539
National Ostomy, http://www.meetanostomate.com
United Ostomy Associations of America http://www.uoaa.org

Winnipeg Ostomy Association, http://www.ostomy-winnipeg.ca

Ovarian Cancer (see also Maryland, Johns Hopkins above)

Eyes on the Prize http://www.eyesontheprize.org/stories/dx.html

The Sidney Kimmel Comprehensive Cancer Center At Johns Hopkins http://www.ovariancancercenter.org/survivors/

Minnesota Ovarian Cancer Alliance http://www.mnovarian.org/young_ survivors.htm

Ovarian Cancer Support Group http://www.ontopofcancer.org/ovarian_ cancer_support_group.php

Whisper Network http://www.ovationsforthecure.org/whispernetwork/?cat=5

Young Survivor Network http://www.tcdailyplanet.net/article/2008/05/15/ ovarian-cancer-young-survivors-older-women-s-disease.html

Pancreatic Cancer

PanCAN http://www.pancan.org/Patient/support.html

Pancreatic Cancer Action Network Store http://www.kintera.org/ AutoGen/ECommerce/Product

Pancreatic Cancer Support Network http://www.thesurvivorsclub.org/support-center/health/cancer/pancreatic-cancer.html

Penile Cancer

AlterNet http://www.alternet.org/health/80007

American Cancer Society http://csn.cancer.org/node/154736

Dana-Farber Cancer Institute http://www.dana-farber.org/pat/surviving/ default.html

GazetteLive http://www.gazettelive.co.uk/news/teesside-news/2008/06/10/ cancer-survivor-joe-speaks-out-as-warning-to-other-men-84229-21048561/

National Cancer Institute http://www.cancer.gov/cancertopics/types/penile

On Top of Cancer http://www.ontopofcancer.org/penis_cancer_support _group.php

Penectomy http://www.menshealth.about.com/od/cancer/a/Penectomy.htm

The Independent http://www.independent.co.uk/life-style/health-and-families/features/penile-cancer-a-taboo-im-just-glad-to-be-alive-1942837.html

University of Minnesota, Masonic Cancer Center http://www.cancer.umn. edu/cancerinfo/NCI/CDR438960.html

Prostate Cancer

Advanced Prostate Cancer Alliance. *Living with Advanced Prostate Cancer: When PSA Rises During Hormone Therapy.*

American Cancer SocietyMan to Man Program http://www.cancer.org

American Foundation for Urologic Disease/Prostate Health Council http://www.cancer.org/docroot/CRI/content

American Prostate Society 1-410-859-3735 http://www.ameripros.org

American Urological Association Foundation 1-866-RING AUA (US only) 1-410-689-3700, Fax—1-410-689-3800 http://www.auafoundation.org, http://www.urologyhealth.org

Cancer.net http://www.cancer.net

Cancer Survivors Network http://www.prostatepros.com/page/read/ Survivorship-Resources/37

CaPcure (The Association for the Cure of Cancer of the Prostate) 1-800-757-CURE http://www.capcure.org

Condom Catheters http://http://www.drugs.com/cg/how-to-care-for-your-condom-catheter.html, http://www.seekwellness.com/incontinence/ manage-incontinence-with- catheters.htm

Conquer Prostate Cancer Now http://www.conquerprostatecancernow.type pad.com/

See Also Delaware Online above

Department of Defense Center for Prostate Disease Research http://www.cpdr.org

Ellsworth, Pamela, Heaney, John A. and Gill, Oliver. *100 Questions & Answers about Prostate Cancer.* Boston, MA: Jones and Bartlett Publishers, 2003

Harvard Medical School—Prostate Knowledge http://harvardprostateknowledge.org

Krahn, Leona. *Not Alone: Couples Sharing Candidly About Prostate Cancer* (audiovisual). Winnipeg, Canada: Krahn communications, 1998.

Listserv: http://www.acor.org; http://listserv.acor.org/archives/prostate.html

Male Sling Procedure http://www.brightsurf.com/.../New_male_sling_ procedure_helps_prostate_cancer_survivors_who_suffer_from_urinary_in continence

Michigan Urology Center http://www.med.unich.edu/urology/

Moyad, Mark A. and Pienta, Kenneth J. *The ABCs of Advanced Prostate Cancer.* Chelsea, MI: Sleeping Bear Press, 2000.

My Cancer Advisor http://mycanceradvisor.com/2010/02/01/arnold-palmer-prostate-cancer-survivor/

National Cancer Institute http://www.cissecure.nci.hig.gov/ncipubs/

PSA Rising http://www.psa-rising.com

Pienta, Kenneth J. *Prostate Cancer from A-Z.* Ann Arbor, MI: Ann Arbor Media Group, 2004

Prostate Cancer Education Council 1-800-813-HOPE, 212-302-2400

Prostate Cancer Foundation http://www.prostatecancerfoundation.org

Prostate Cancer Health Education Network http://www.wtop.com/?nid=106&sid=1661222

Prostate Cancer Research Institute http://www.prostate-cancer.org

Prostate Cancer Infolink http://www.comed.com/prostate or http://www.prostatecancerinfolink.net

Prostate Cancer Research and Education Foundation (PC-REF) 619-287-8860, Fax 619-287-8890 http://www.prostatecancer.com

Prostate Cancer Resource Network 1-800-915-1001, 813-848-2494 http://www.pcrn.org

Prostate Conditions Education Council http://prostateconditions.org

Prostate Health http://www.prostatehealth.com

Prostate Net http://www.prostatenet.lorg

Schroeder, Don. *Prostate Cancer: A Journey of Hope.* (audiovisual) Banyan Communications, Inc., 1999.

Sex Following Prostate Cancer http://www.prostatecancerinfolink.ning.com/profiles/blogs/sex-following-prostate-cancer

Urologic Oncology Program at the University of Michigan Comprehensive Cancer Center http://www.mcancer.org

Us TOO International Prostate Cancer Education and Support Network 1-800-80-UsTOO (also several publications) http://www.ustoo.com

ZERO—The Project to End Prostate Cancer http://www.zerocancer.org

Skin Cancer

American Cancer Society http://www.cancer.org/docroot/ped/content/ped_7_1_what_you_need_to_know_about_skin_cancer.asp http://csn.cancer.org/forum/145

Cancer Blog http://www.thecancerblog.com/2006/07/02/miss-maryland-brittany-lietz-skin-cancer-survivor-wins/

M.D. Anderson Cancer Center http://www.mdanderson.org/patient-and-cancer-information/cancer-information/cancer-types/skin-cancer/index.html

Hawaii News Now http://www.hawaiinewsnow.com/Global/story.asp?S=6462805

Journal of Clinical Oncology http://jco.ascopubs.org/cgi/content/abstract/23/16/3733

National Institutes of Health http://www.ncbi.nlm.nih.gov/pubmed/15923570

On Top of Cancer http://www.ontopofcancer.org/skin_cancer_support_
group.php

Skin Cancer Foundation http://www.skincancer.org/

SkinCancerNet http://www.skincarephysicians.com/skincancernet/index.html

Skincancer-Survivor http://www.skincancer-survivor.com/

Testicular Cancer

American Cancer Society http://www.cancer.org/docroot/NWS/content/NWS
_5_1x_College_Scholarships_for_Cancer_Survivors.asp

Everyday Health http://www.everydayhealth.com/testicular-cancer
/management.aspx

FinAid! http://www.finaid.org/scholarships/cancer.phtml

KTVA http://www.ktva.com/cancerconnection/ci_5865872

Lance Armstrong Foundation http://www.livestrong.org
http://www.livestrong.org/Get-Help/Learn-About-Cancer/Survivor-
Interviews/Interviews-with-Men/Jerry-Kelly-is-a-testicular-cancer-survivor

M.D. Anderson Cancer Center http://www.oncolink.org/resources/article.
cfm?c=6&s=29&ss=74&id=927

National Institutes of Health http://www.nlm.nih.gov/medlineplus/ency/
article/001288.htm

Testicular Cancer Resource Center http://tcrc.acor.org/celeb.html

Throat Cancer

American Cancer Society http://csn.cancer.org/node/141995

Blog for a Cure http://www.blogforacure.com/frontend/weblogs/listing.
php?type=Throat+Cancer

CNN http://www.cnn.com/2010/SPORT/03/17/alaska.iditarod/index.html

EmpowHER http://www.empowher.com/condition/throat-cancer

Mayo Clinic http://www.mayoclinic.com/health/oral-and-throat-
cancer/ds00349

M.D. Anderson Cancer Clinic http://www.mdanderson.org/patient-and-
cancer-information/cancer-information/cancer-types/laryngeal-
cancer/index.html

On Top of Cancer http://www.ontopofcancer.org/throat_cancer.php

National Cancer Institute http://www.cancer.gov/cancertopics/types/throat

National Institutes of Health http://www.nlm.nih.gov/medlineplus/ency/
article/001042.htm

University of Iowa, Hardin.MD http://www.lib.uiowa.edu/hardin/md/
throatcancer.html

Thyroid Cancer

American Academy of Otolaryngology http://www.entnet.org

American Cancer Society http://www.cancer.org

Canadian Thyroid Cancer Support Group (Thry'vors) Inc. http://www.thryvors.org

Cancer.gov http://www.cancer.gov

Gilletz, Norene. *The Low Iodine Diet Cookbook: Easy and Delicious Recipes & Tips for Thyroid Cancer Patients.* Your Health Press, 2005

Light of Life Foundation, 1-877-565-632 http://www.lightoflifefoundation.org/

Listserv http://www.acor.org

National Cancer Institute http://www.cancer.gov/cancertopics/wyntk/thyroid

ThyCa: Thyroid Cancer Survivors' Association, 1-877-588-7904 http://www.thyca.org

Thyroid-Cancer.net http://www.thyroid-cancer.net

Thyroid Cancer Survivors' Association http://www.thyca.org

Thyroid Cancer Outreach Network http://www.thyroid.about.com/library/weekly/blthyca-outreach-network.htm

Thyroid Foundation of America and the American Thyroid Association http://www.thyroid.org/patients/brochures/ThyroidCancerFAQ.pdf

Uterine Cancer

CancerLinksUSA http://www.cancerlinksusa.com/endometrium.htm

Centers for Disease Control and Prevention http://www.cdc.gov/cancer/uterine/

Eyes on the Prize http://www.eyesontheprize.org/stories/dx.html

Mayo Clinic http://www.mayoclinic.com/health/endometrial-cancer/DS00306/DSECTION=symptoms

Memorial Sloan-Kettering Cancer Center http://www.mskcc.org/mskcc/html/13173.cfm

National Cancer Institute http://www.cancer.gov/cancertopics/types/endometrial http://planning.cancer.gov/disease/Endometrial-Snapshot.pdf

National Institutes of Health http://www.nlm.nih.gov/medlineplus/uterinecancer.html

On Top of Cancer http://www.ontopofcancer.org/uterine_cancer_support_group.php

OrganizedWisdom Health http://organizedwisdom.com/Uterine_Cancer_Survivors

Uterine Cancer Survivors http://www.mnovarian.org/young_survivors.htm

Ethnic-Focused Websites

African-American Focus:

Black News http://www.blacknews.com/pr/phen301.html

Black Planet http://www.blackplanet.com/groups.group.html?group_id=3270

Post Treatment African Descent Breast Cancer http://www.cme.medscape. com/viewarticle/551302_4

Prostate Health Education Network http://www.cancer.confex.com/cancer/ disparities/recordingredirect.cgi/id/3

Sisters' Breast Cancer Survivors Network http://www.survivorsofbreastcancer.org

Arabic Focus:

Arabic Cancer Information http://www.cancervic.org.au/email-a-page/default. asp?ContainerId=arabic

Breast Cancer Awareness Spreading in Arab World http://www.themuslimhttp://woman.org/entry/spreading-breast-cancer-awareness-in-the-arab-world/

Cancer Backup (UK) http://www.cancerbackup.org.uk/Languages/Arabic

Cancer Council in New South Wales, Australia http://www.cancercouncil.com.au/editorial.asp?pageid=1326

Diagnosing and Treating Breast Cancer—Arabic/English http://www.breastcancercare.org.uk/server/show/nav.681/change Template/PublicationDisplay/publicationId/95

Health Education Resources—Cervical Cancer (Arabic) http://www.healthed. govt.nz/resources/cervicalcancervaccinehpvarabic.aspx

Henry Ford: Breast Cancer Survivors Lax About Mammograms in Arabic Community http://www.henryford.com/body.cfm?id=46332&action =detail&AEProductID=HealthScoutfeed&AEarticleid=14056

Israeli Project Empowers Young Arab Cancer Patients http://www.israel 21c.org/bin/en.jsp?enDispWho=Articles%5El1024&enPage=BlankPage& enDisplay=view

Lebanese Ostomy Association http://www.arabostomy.com

Michigan Cancer Consortium on Arabic Prostate Cancer http://www.michigancancer.org/AboutTheMCC/FeaturedActivity-Arab ProstCaEdBklt.cfm

More Arabic Women Speaking Out About Cancer http://www.abcnews. go.com/GMA/OnCallPlus/story?id=3759570&page=1

Psychosocial Correlates of Pediatric Cancer in the United Arabic Emirates http://www.springerlink.com/index/VJTLNB1HXHG2AMCX.pdf

SBS Radio http://www.radio.sbs.com.au/language.php?news=community youth&language=Arabic

VHL (von Hippel-Lindau) Handbook in Arabic http://www.vhl.org/ newsletter/vhl2005/05bcsurviv.php

Asian and Pacific Islander Focus:

AACPHO http://www.aapcho.org/altruesite/files/aapcho/PDF_Documents/APINCSN%20Organizational%20Membership%20Form.pdf

American Cancer Society, Eastern Division Asian Initiatives http://www.relayforlife.com/docroot/COM/content/div_Eastern/COM_11_2x_Chinese_Unit.asp

Asian Language Materials http://www.acsevents.org/docroot/ASN/ASN_0.asp

Colon Cancer Treatment and Symptoms and Resources https://www.goldbamboo.com/topic-t1195-2resources.html

Giang T. Nguyen Center for Public Health Initiatives (University of Pennsylvania) http://www.med.upenn.edu/apps/faculty/index.php/g20001020/p1866373

Hueina Su973-664-0446 http://www.rxforbalance.com, http://www.intensiveselfcare.com, http://www.youtube.com/watch?v=jO6fn5MYwF8

Hispanic Focus:

Migrant Clinicians Network http://www.migrantclinician.org/mcn/patient-education/cancer/index.html

Israeli/Jewish Focus:

Colllins, Leigh and Courtney, Nathan. *When a Parent Is Seriously Ill: Practical Tips for Helping Parents and Children.* Metairie, LA: Jewish Family Service of Greater New Orleans, 2003.

Interfaith Family, Rabbi Earl A. Grollman http://www.interfaithfamily.com/life_cycle/death_and_mourning/How_to_Talk_to_Your_Kids_about_Death.shtml

Israeli Project Empowers Young Arab Cancer Patients http://www.israel21c.org/bin/en.jsp?enDispWho=Articles%5El1024&enPage=BlankPage&enDisplay=view

Sharsheret http://www.sharsheret.org

Torah http://www.torah.org/features/secondlook/stemcell.html

Native-American Focus:

Community-Driven Native American Cancer Survivors Quality of Life http://www.phac-aspc.gc.ca/ccdpc-cpcmc/bc-cds/projects/app_03-04_e.html

Computer Retrieval of Information on Scientific Projects http://www.crisp.cit.nih.gov/crisp/CRISP_LIB.getdoc?textkey=7487827&p_grant_num=5R25CA 101938-05&p

National Indian Education Association http://www.niea.org/media/broadcasts_detail_html.php?id=280

National Native American Cancer Survivors' Support Network
http://www.natamcancer.org/community.html and www.stormingmedia.
us/71/7153/A715314,html (sponsored by Dept. of Defense)

NCCSA Native American Cancer Research Survivors Network
http://www.canceradvocacy.org/resources/guide/native-american-cancer-
research.html

Native American Cancer Center http://www.informaworld.com/index/
785035289.pdf

WomenStories http://www.womenstories.org/doc.asp.214.html

Gay, Lesbian, Bisexual, Transgender

Hospitals Rated for LGBT Rights http://www.lgbtcancer.com/hospitals-rated-
for-lgbt-rights/

Lesbian, Gay, Bisexual, Transgender Cancer Project http://www.outwith
cancer.com/

LGBT Cancer Survivor and Social Network http://www.lgbtcancer.com/

Lesbian Quarterly http://www.lesbianquarterly.com/2008/10/01/lesbian-
cancer-survivor-support-group

Male Care http://www.malecare.com/gay-prostate-cancer_68.htm

National LGBT Cancer Network http://www.cancer-network.org/

Websites by Geographical Area

Australia

Australian Science and Technology Heritage Centre—Esmond Venner

Cancer Council Australia http://www.cancer.org.au/home.htm

Keogh Guide to Records– Index part C (Cancer studies, etc.)
http://www.austehc.unimelb.edu.au/guides/keog/index_c.htm

Breast Cancer Network http://www.portlincoln.yourguide.com.au/news/local/
news/general/bakersraise-dough-for-breast-cancer/1500404.aspx
http://www.bcna.org.au/index.php?option=com_search&searchword=
raelene

Cancer Council NSW Arabic Translations http://www.cancercouncil.com.
au/editorial.asp?pageid=1326

Cancer Council Victoria(Multi-lingual) http://www.cancervic.org.au/email-a-
page/default.asp?ContainerId

NSW Teachers Federation http://www.nswtf.org.au/events/1185265718_
12213.html

Tackling Cancer Misconceptions in Multicultural Australia http://www.mhcs.
health.nsw.gov.au/mhcs/subpages/polyglot/pdf/poly_37.pdf

Canada

Canadian Breast Cancer Initiative http://www.phac-aspc.gc.ca/ccdpc-cpcmc/
bc-cds/projects/app_03-04_e.html

Canadian Breast Cancer Network http://www.senologia.net/articoli/non
  medici/Bibliografia%20on%20line_siti%2 0per%20le%20pazienti.pdf

Canadian Cancer Advocacy Network http://www.linkinghub.elsevier.com/
  retrieve/pii/S0897189703000089

Canadian Cancer Survivors http://www.expressnews.ualberta.ca/article.cfm?
  id=6574

Canadian Thyroid Cancer Support Group (Thry'vors) Inc.
  http://www.thryvors.org

Canadian Women's Health Network http://www.research.cwhn.ca/en/
  node/14827

Cancer Care Nova Scotia http://www.gov.ns.ca/news/details.asp?id=
  19990615003

Childhood Cancer Foundation, Candlelighters Canada
  http://www.candlelighters.ca

Hamilton, Joan. *When a Parent Is Sick: Helping Parents Explain Serious
  Illness to Children.* Nova Scotia, Canada.Pottersfield Press, 2001.

INFUSION Canada http://www.infusioncanada.org/programs/bursary.html

Kids Cancer Care http://www.kidscancercare.ab.ca/

Krahn, Leona. *Not Alone: Couples Sharing Candidly About Prostate Cancer*
  (audiovisual). Winnipeg, Canada: Krahn communications, 1998.

Lymphovenous-Canada http://www.lymphovenous-canada.ca/
  bclymphedemastudy.htm

Mission Air Transportation Network http://www.cancersurvivors.org/
  Resources/reference2.htm

New Brunswick Breast Cancer Network http://www.abcn.ca/artman2/
  publish/Community_Focus_37/New_Brunswick_Breast_CancerNetwork_
  Creates_a_New www.breastcancernetwork.nb.ca/whats-new.htm

Unconventional Cancer Therapies http://www.bccancer.bc.ca/HPI'/
  UnconventionalTherapies/default.htm.

University of Manitoba—Oral Cancer Self Evaluation
  http://www.umanitoba.ca/outreach/wisdomtooth/exam.htm

China

Children's Cancer Foundation, Hong Kong http://www.ccf.org/hk

Guam

The Edward M. Calvo Cancer Foundation http://www.guamisgood.org

India

India Cancer Society http://www.delhilive.com/events/launch-national-
  childhood-cancer-survivors-network-200902103615

India Childhood Cancer Survivor Network http://www.kidscankonnect.com/

India Online Childhood Cancer Survivor Network
http://www.awarecancer.blogspot.com/

Italy

Associazione Italiana Malati di Cancro, parenti ed amici http://www.aimac.
it/informazioni/dst/visualizza.php?id_articolo=5648 (Italian)

Società Italiana di Patologia e Medicina Orale—Oral Cancer http://www.
sipmo.it/app/prvt/VediFile.d/File92/FAQ%20ca%20iper.pdf (Italian)

Japan

Children's Cancer Association of Japan http://www.ccaj-found.or.jp
http://www.ccaj-found.or.jp/english/

National Cancer Center Research http://www.ncc.go.jp/

SpringerLink http://www.springerlink.com/content/p18541665g760825/

Mexico

ABC Cancer Center
http://www.methodistinternational.org/about/abc_affiliation.shtml

Health-tourism http://www.health-tourism.com/cancer-treatment/mexico/

Instituto Nacional de Cancerologia http://www.incan.edu.mx/

National Cancer Institute http://www.cancer.gov/newscenter/pressreleases/
ArgentinaBrazilMexicoUruguayUS

Netherlands

Greater Amsterdam Cancer Registry http://www.ikcnet.nl/uploaded/FILES/
IKA/kankerregistratie/overleving/3.xls

The Netherlands Cancer Registry http://www.ikcnet.nl/page.php?id=237&
nav_id=97

Netherlands Cancer Institute: Werkgroep Hoofd-Hals Oncologie
http://www.hoofdhalskanker.info/Patient-information.htm

United Kingdom

Abbreviations and Acronyms for Oncology: Medical Terminology for Cancer
http://www.staff.ncl.ac.uk/s.j.cotterill/medtm15a.htm

All Ireland Fatigue Coalition http://wwwtheoncologist.alphamedpress.org/
cgi/content/full/8/suppl_1/1

AlterNet http://www.alternet.org/health/80007

Bioportfolio Limited—Search Screen for Oral Cancer News
http://www.bioportfolio.co.uk/Health_News/Oral_Cancer.shtml

Breast Cancer Care http://www.breastcancercare.org.uk

British Medical Journal http://www.bmj.com

Cancer BACUP http://www.cancerbackup.org.uk

CancerHelp UK http://www.cancerhelp.org.uk

Children's Leukaemia Research Project http://www.clrpireland.com/content/ cat_index_4.php

CLIC Sargent http://www.clicsargent.org.uk/Getinvolved/@1363/London Committee

GazetteLive http://www.gazettelive.co.uk/news/teesside-news/2008/06/10/ cancer-survivor-joe-speaks-out-as-warning-to-other-men-84229-21048561/

Leukemia Research Foundation http://www.lrf.org.uk

Macmillan Cancer Support http://www.macmillan.org.uk

Marie Curie Cancer Care http://www.mariecurie.org.uk

Mouth Cancer Foundation: Initiative of the Restorative Dentistry Oncology Clinic http://www.rdoc.org.uk

National Cancer Dataset http://www.nhsia.nhs.uk/cancer/pages/dataset/ default.asp

Osbourne, Michael, et. al., *The Strang Cancer Prevention Center Cookbook: A Complete Nutrition and Lifestyle Plan to Dramatically Lower Your Cancer Risk*. New York, NY: London, England: McGraw-Hill, 2004.

Restorative Dentistry Oncology Clinic http://www.rdoc.org.uk

The Independent http://www.independent.co.uk/life-style/health-and- families/features/penile-cancer-a-taboo-im-just-glad-to-be-alive- 1942837.html

University of Glasgow Dental School http://www.gla.ac.uk/Acad/Dental/ OralCancer

West of Scotland Cancer Awareness Project http://www.woscap.co.uk/nhsstaff/ default.asp?p=da51

What Do I Tell the Children? A Guide for a Parent with Cancer. http://www.cancerbacup.org.uk

Winston's Wish http://www.winstonswish.org.uk

Acknowledgements

- Jennifer Stewart, in Australia, author of the online *The Write Way*, for sponsoring the writing contest that lead to this book.
- Kendell, Bernard, Chris and Charles—State of Michigan Library, for your patience and helpfulness in finding materials, as well as suggestions for how to market the book.
- Doug Klein, Mason Chamber of Commerce, for your help in locating resources, including Rich Baldwin.
- Rich Baldwin, Buttonwood Press and author of over 20 mystery books and 2 children's books, for your time, ideas, belief and enthusiasm in the book.
- Larry Silsby, Aurelius Township for your guidance in wading through government bureaucracy.
- Ann Rule, True Crime Writer, author of over 20 books, for your encouragement and suggestions (and your being a native Michigander).
- Dr. Lynne Moseley, oral oncologist at Karmanos Cancer Center in Detroit for her time, help and suggestions for the dental concerns section of the book.
- Peggy McNichol, ATS Associates, CPA extraordinaire, for helping set up the financial records to keep us both out of trouble with the IRS, and for recommending Connie Sweet, Connection Graphics.
- Connie Sweet, Connection Graphics, Potterville, Michigan, for her design for Riversmeet Publishing, LLC logo, the jacket design, the website design, and for her belief in this book.
- Sohail Husain, M.D., Yale University, for also opening the doors to the Islamic faith and for introducing Terry to the four remarkable women at the Masjid Mahmood Mosque.
- Ayesha Mangla, Jamila Kahn, Reema Butt and Sabiha Ijaz, new friends at the Masjid Mahmood Mosque in Rochester Hills, MI (their outdoor sign reads "Love for Everyone, Hatred for None") who helped Terry understand some of the intricacies of the Islamic faith. (Any errors are strictly Terry's fault due to either faulty listening or misinterpretation.) They also share the dream of a

universal world of tolerance and peace. As Reema so eloquently wrote in an e-mail, *"Despite our varied backgrounds, we are all connected by a divine thread that embraces humanity at all levels."* Reema, thanks, also, for the connection with Jaspal.

- Amy Bigman, Congregation Shaarey Zedek in East Lansing, MI, for her referral to Sharsheret and a wonderful, laugh-filled conversation in the process.

- Adina Fleischmann, Sharsheret, for her clarification on differences in Jewish observances, as well as her amazing compassion and wonderful sense of humor. (While the website is focused on young Jewish women there is also a wealth of information that applies to other breast cancer survivors.)

- Halima Ismael, for introducing me to Imam Dr. Shahibzada. And to Dr. Sharif Shahibzada, Imam at the Islamic Center of West Michigan and Mosque of Grand Rapids, for his insights into the Islamic faith and for taking so much time to help Terry learn and really understand.

- Sandi Isaacson, Ph.D., ABPdN, long-time friend, the most incredible psychologist for children you will ever want to meet, for providing insights and websites for the Orthodox Jewish Community.

- Jon Priebe, data recovery person extraordinaire. You not only managed to recover every scrap of information in Terry's laptop when it crashed (what a nightmare; it would only do loops and display the "blue screen of death;" it was unknown if the file system was corrupt and a thousand other "oh no's"), but also managed to put it back on her desktop screen, as well as on a disk. May Citadel Defense Technologies and Cide Shields® become household words. You are so much like your Mom (who died from breast cancer)—gracious, kind, gentle, and wanting so much to help others.

- Jaspal Neelam, "Sat sri akal." For perseverance in trying to make phone contact, for sending me a video, "A Saint and A Soldier," and for her insights into the Sikh faith. Your knowledge, your faith, and your belief in the future of humankind are inspirational. We do need to meet one of these days, soon.

- Shazer and Ada Emata, for bringing such enthusiasm to learning about stem cells and for arranging to do a marrow donor drive in the greater Lansing area Filipino community. You and those you helped sign up may one day save a life.

- Tom's high school classmates for their unwavering support and encouragement on a number of levels: Janet, Madeline, Bill and Jeanette, Fran, Ward, Denny and Bridget, Tony and Dick, Joan, Rosemary and Bob, Rosemary and Dick, Roberta, Nick, Mary Ellen and Walter, Jim and Sandi, Bob and Barb, Tom and Carol, Louie and Karen, Joe, Marty and Jim, and Tom and Ruth.

- Family not mentioned in the body of the book: Kaidyn, Kole, and Martin; grandchildren Alex, Tom 5th, Zachary, Jacob, Shawn, Gavin, Bradley, Sam, and Abby; cousins Elizabeth, Walt and Betty; the McNamara clan.

- Extended "family"—Rosie; Darlene and Hank; Mrs. Fair; Tim and Carol; Jim and Char; the Pages in Time family (Pam, Shelley, Kelly, Michele, Sue and Amy); Jim and Pat; Scot; Nancy and Jim; Kathy and Dennis; the Fabiano Candy people (all the Blairs, Jane, Betty); the Van Roekels; Alita, Beto, Ricardito, Lilia, Ricky; Suzanne and Bob; Linda—the best hair stylist!; Bill and Sue; Ray and Janet; Migrant Program Staff.

- San Serif, Inc., to Barb and Susie, for your patience, flexibility and willingness to go through 6 proofs before we had a final product. Your ideas and suggestions were extremely helpful. Thank you!

- Cheryl Corey, MacNaughton & Gunn, Inc., for helping guide a first-time publisher and author through the maze of printing options. Thank you for making the time to take me through your company and to meet the incredible people who actually put the book together.

- Last, but certainly not least, to our editor, Karen Smith. Your abilities to bring out the best in writers, your intuitions about what people would really like to say but have a hard time, your innate sense of the English language, your positive and nurturing side to bring a book and a person to life are immeasureably appreciated. This book wouldn't have been nearly as good as you have made it.

Index